Library of
Davidson College

PSYCHIATRIC ASPECTS
OF NEUROLOGIC DISEASE
VOLUME II

SEMINARS IN PSYCHIATRY

Series Editor
Milton Greenblatt, M.D.
Director, Neuropsychiatric Institute Hospital and Clinics

Professor and Executive Vice Chairman
Department of Psychiatry and Biobehavioral Sciences
University of California, Los Angeles
Los Angeles, California

Other Books in Series:

Psychiatric Aspects of Neurologic Disease, edited by D. Frank Benson, M.D., and Dietrich Blumer, M.D.
Borderline States in Psychiatry, edited by John E. Mack, M.D.
Topics in Psychoendocrinology, edited by Edward J. Sachar, M.D.
Consultation-Liaison Psychiatry, edited by Robert O. Pasnau, M.D.
Drugs in Combination with Other Therapies, edited by Milton Greenblatt, M.D.
Suicidology: Contemporary Developments, edited by Edwin S. Shneidman, Ph.D.
Alcoholism Problems in Women and Children, edited by Milton Greenblatt, M.D., and Marc A. Schuckit, M.D.
Ethological Psychiatry: Psychopathology in the Context of Evolutionary Biology, edited by Michael T. McGuire, M.D., and Lynn A. Fairbanks, Ph.D.
The Family in Mourning: A Guide for Health Professionals, edited by Charles E. Hollingsworth, M.D., and Robert O. Pasnau, M.D.
Clinical Aspects of the Rapist, edited by Richard T. Rada, M.D.
Sex Education for the Professional: A Curriculum Guide, edited by Norman Rosenzweig, M.D., and F. Paul Pearsall, Ph.D.
Psychopharmacology Update: New and Neglected Areas, edited by John M. Davis, M.D., and David Greenblatt, M.D.
Methods of Biobehavioral Research, edited by E. A. Serafetinides, M.D., Ph.D.
Alcohol and Old Age, by Brian L. Mishara, Ph.D., and Robert Kastenbaum, Ph.D.
Psychiatric Research in Practice: Biobehavioral Themes, edited by E. A. Serafetinides, M.D., Ph.D.
Family Therapy and Major Psychopathology, edited by Melvin R. Lansky, M.D.
The Afro-American Family: Assessment, Treatment, and Research Issues, edited by Barbara Ann Bass, M.S.W., Gail Elizabeth Wyatt, Ph.D., and Gloria Johnson Powell, M.D.
Mental Health and Hispanic Americans: Clinical Perspectives, edited by Rosina M. Becerra, Ph.D., Marvin Karno, M.D., and Javier I. Escobar, M.D.
Teaching Psychiatry and Behavioral Science, edited by Joel Yager, M.D.

PSYCHIATRIC ASPECTS OF NEUROLOGIC DISEASE VOLUME II

Edited by
D. Frank Benson, M.D.
Augustus S. Rose Professor of Neurology
Department of Neurology
School of Medicine
University of California, Los Angeles

Dietrich Blumer, M.D.
Clinical Professor of Psychiatry
University of Michigan School of Medicine
Chairman, Department of Psychiatry
Henry Ford Hospital
Detroit, Michigan

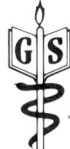

GRUNE & STRATTON
A Subsidiary of Harcourt Brace Jovanovich, Publishers
New York   London
Paris   San Diego   San Francisco   São Paulo
Sydney   Tokyo   Toronto

Library of Congress Cataloging in Publication Data
Main entry under title:

Psychiatric aspects of neurologic disease, volume 2.

    (Seminars in psychiatry)
    Includes bibliographies and index.
    1. Mental illness. 2. Mental illness—Etiology.
3. Nervous system—Diseases—Complications and sequelae.
4. Psychological manifestation of general diseases.
5. Neuropsychiatry. I. Benson, D. Frank (David Frank),
1928-   . II. Blumer, Dietrich. III. Series: Seminars
in psychiatry (Grune & Stratton) [DNLM: 1. Mental
disorders—Complications. 2. Nervous system diseases—
Complications. WL 100 P976 1975]
RC454.4.P75   616.8   82-1024
ISBN 0-8089-1477-4   AACR2

© *1982 by Grune & Stratton, Inc.*
All rights reserved. No part of this publication
may be reproduced or transmitted in any form or
by any means, electronic or mechanical, including
photocopy, recording, or any information storage
and retrieval system, without permission in
writing from the publisher.

Grune & Stratton, Inc.
111 Fifth Avenue
New York, New York 10003

Distributed in the United Kingdom by
Academic Press Inc. (London) Ltd.
24/28 Oval Road, London NW 1

Library of Congress Catalog Number 82-1024
International Standard Book Number 0-8089-1477-4

Printed in the United States of America

Contents

Foreword *Milton Greenblatt*		vii
Contributors		ix
Preface		xi
1	Acute Confusional State *Richard L. Strub*	1
2	Psychiatric Manifestations of Epilepsy *Dietrich Blumer and D. Frank Benson*	25
3	Episodic Dyscontrol *Kenneth C. Rickler*	49
4	The Interictal Psychoses of Epilepsy *Michael R. Trimble*	75
5	Cortical Dementias *Jeffrey L. Cummings*	93
6	The Treatable Dementias *D. Frank Benson*	123
7	Alcoholic Dementia *John Cutting*	149
8	Pseudodementia and the Recognition of Organicity *Charles E. Wells*	167
9	Chronic Pain as a Psychobiologic Phenomenon: The Pain-Prone Disorder *Dietrich Blumer*	179
10	Tardive Dyskinesia *Christopher G. Goetz and Harold L. Klawans*	195
11	Traumatic Brain Injury *Michael P. Alexander*	219
12	Amnesia: A Clinical Appoach to Memory *D. Frank Benson and Dietrich Blumer*	251
13	Psychiatric Aspects of Multiple Sclerosis *Michael R. Trimble and Igor Grant*	279

| 14 | Neuropsychiatric Aspects of Stuttering
David B. Rosenfield | 301 |

Index 315

Foreword

In the first Seminars in Psychiatry volume on *Psychiatric Aspects of Neurologic Disease* (1975), we learned that neurologic diseases account for *at least 30 percent* of first admissions to mental hospitals and that many of these disorders are treatable. Drs. Benson and Blumer, emphasized in particular depression and the pseudodementias, personality changes associated with frontal and temporal lobe lesions, the mental concomitants of organic brain syndrome, and the behavioral aberrations related to the epilepsies.

The reception of the first book in the Seminars in Psychiatry Series indicated that psychiatrists and neurologists were eager to know more about this fascinating borderland.

Since 1975, the borders between psychiatry and neurology, psychiatry and medicine, and pediatrics, obstetrics, and gynecology have been vigorously explored. Many young physicians-in-training see a rewarding and expanding future in this field, and many psychiatrists as well as other professionals anticipate that this new interest will help lessen the distance between psychiatry and the field of medicine which originally gave it life.

Behavioral medicine, neurobehavioral clinics, and consultation-liaison psychiatry provide the media through which that distance is currently being closed. The original excitement of psychoanalysis and psychodynamics led psychiatry to stray from the core of medicine; similar excitement is now being felt in neurobehavioral science and practice, and the need for closer ties is leading the prodigals back to medicine in increasing numbers.

The growth of this trend called for a second volume of *Psychiatric Aspects of Neurologic Disease,* and fortunately for all of us, Drs. Benson and Blumer were willing to do the job. Seven years richer in clinical and research experience and now even more highly esteemed by their colleagues and students for their manifold contributions, the editors have produced a second volume that treats a totally new set of subjects as well as updates knowledge related to previous themes. We do not know of an area that demands higher priority for continuing education than the practical diagnosis and treatment of borderland states.

Milton Greenblatt, M.D.

Contributors

Michael P. Alexander, M.D.
Chief, Aphasia/Neurobehavioral Unit
Boston Veterans Administration Medical Center
Boston, Massachusetts

D. Frank Benson, M.D.
Augustus S. Rose Professor of Neurology
Department of Neurology
School of Medicine
University of California, Los Angeles
Los Angeles, California

Dietrich Blumer, M.D.
Clinical Professor of Psychiatry
University of Michigan School of Medicine
Chairman, Department of Psychiatry
Henry Ford Hospital
Detroit, Michigan

Jeffrey L. Cummings, M.D.
Director, Neurobehavior Unit
Brentwood Veterans Administration Medical Center
Assistant Professor of Neurology in Residence
School of Medicine
University of California, Los Angeles
Los Angeles, California

John Cutting, M.D., M.R.C.P., M.R.C.Psych.
Senior Lecturer, Kings College Hospital
Medical School and Institute of Psychiatry
London, England

Christopher G. Goetz, M.D.
Assistant Professor
Rush Medical College
Department of Neurological Sciences
Rush-Presbyterian St. Luke's Medical Center
Chicago, Illinois

Igor Grant, M.D., F.R.C.P.(C)
Associate Professor
Department of Psychiatry
School of Medicine
University of California, San Diego
Chief, Mental Health Clinic
Psychiatry Service
Veterans Administration Medical Center
San Diego, California

Harold L. Klawans, M.D.
Professor, Rush Medical College
Department of Neurological Sciences
Rush-Presbyterian St. Luke's Medical Center
Chicago, Illinois

Kenneth C. Rickler, M.D.
Staff Neurologist, Forensic Division
St. Elizabeth's Hospital
Director, Neurobehavioral Service
Psychiatric Institute
Washington, D.C.

David B. Rosenfield, M.D.
Assistant Professor
Department of Neurology
Director, Stuttering Center
Baylor College of Medicine
Houston, Texas

Richard L. Strub, M.D.
Professor
Department of Neurology
Louisiana State University Medical Center
New Orleans, Louisiana

Michael R. Trimble, M.R.C.P., F.R.C.Psych.
Consultant Physician, Psychological Medicine
Senior Lecturer, Behavioral Neurology
The National Hospital for Nervous Diseases
London, England

Charles E. Wells, M.D.
Professor, of Psychiatry and Neurology
Vice-Chairman, Department of Psychiatry
Vanderbilt University School of Medicine
Nashville, Tennessee

Preface

When the first volume of *Psychiatric Aspects of Neurologic Disease* was published in 1975, very few physicians were aware of or stressed the importance of the disorders in the borderland between psychiatry and neurology. In the past few years there has been a considerable increase in both interest and activity in this area. In fact, this borderland area ranks among the most rapidly expanding areas of research in both neurology and psychiatry.

Currently at least three terms are regularly used to designate activities in the borderland between neurology and psychiatry. For many years, neuropsychiatry was the term used by physicians who practiced in both disciplines and regularly handled patients with the disorders affecting both areas. To the levels of their day, these physicians were competent in both fields and, because of their combined background, much of their interest was reserved for patients who had psychiatric problems based on brain abnormality, particularly the complications of neurosyphilis. With increasing specialization in both fields, this double expertise has all but disappeared. In recent years, a new subspecialty has arisen within psychiatry that focuses on a psychiatric approach to disorders caused by brain abnormality; some individuals practicing in this part of the biologic–psychiatric arena use the term *neuropsychiatry*. Their emphasis is on the psychiatric problems complicating or confused with organic mental disorders. Even better established is a new subspecialty of neurology that deals with the behavioral problems caused by brain damage—a rapidly growing field called the *neurology of behavior.* Here the emphasis is clearly placed on the neurologic, not the psychiatric, aspects of the patient with organic problems. Each of these terms clearly reflects the original orientation of the subspecialist representing either psychiatry or neurology. To avoid this unimodal emphasis, the more neutral term *neurobehavior* has been suggested with the intention that it will indicate both the psychiatric and the neurologic abnormalities consequent to cerebral malfunction. Neurobehavior is used in this volume to indicate the field covering the borderland between neurology and psychiatry; more honestly, though, it is intended that neurobehavior be seen as a bridging discipline that not only requires knowledge from both fields and an appreciation of both neurologic and psychiatric approaches to behavioral problems but also investigates and manages behavioral disorders that are not currently recognized by either field.

One important facet of this neurobehavioral approach reflects an ongoing alteration in the concepts underlying psychiatric disease. Of all the specialized medical disciplines, psychiatry encompasses the most complex and poorly understood of human disorders and has a history of wide-swinging alterations in basic approaches. One source of ongoing change within the field of psychiatry has been identified by the English psychiatrist Richard Hunter[8] who states: "In every generation, a number of disorders that were considered psychogenic are discovered to have a biologic origin and are no longer to be considered purely psychiatric disorders." In recent years, a sizeable number of disorders have fulfilled this description. Probably the most important are the current demonstrations of significant biologic abnormality in the classic psychotic disorders of schizophrenia, mania, and depression. In addition, a number of syndromes with accepted psychodynamic explanations have been suggested to have, at least in some degree, organic causations. Among these are such entities as anosognosia,[6] autism,[17] multiple personality,[11] confabulation,[10] the Capgras syndrome,[1] possession states,[11] Tourette's syndrome,[5] and hysteria.[13] Increased understanding of such syndromes has implicated brain abnormality as a factor of consequence.

At first glance it would appear that Richard Hunter's dictum would indicate a dwindling incidence of "psychogenic" psychiatric problems, reciprocal to the increase in behavioral problems with a medical, biologic, or neurologic basis. This is not true. Concurrent with the increased realization of the biologic abnormality present in many "psychiatric" disorders is the improved recognition of the importance of social and environmental factors, both present and past, in the behavioral response of an individual patient. This point has been outlined by another English psychiatrist, David Taylor,[15] who separated the problems caused by medical disorders into three major aspects—disease, illness, and predicament. First, there is the specific biologic abnormality, usually called disease, that can produce a specific clinical syndrome. For many medical and surgical problems, the disease is not only the focal problem but the entire problem and can be managed at this level alone. Dr. Taylor emphasized, however, that a given disease process is likely to produce somewhat different clinical problems, based on the individual's background and situation. To understand this aspect the entire response of the individual must be considered, and the disorders noted on this level can be considered an illness—the product of the specific disease and its effect on a given individual. As a third aspect, Dr. Taylor noted that the disease process itself might be minor while the problems secondary to the patient's situational state were serious; this orients the medical disorder far more toward the individual situation than to the disease process—a situation Taylor termed predicament. For total patient understanding, physicians should be aware of all three aspects— the actual disease process, the personal reaction to the disease, and the consequences of the patient's life situation as related to the disease process. More than in most areas of medicine, the patient with neurobehavioral problems demands attention to all three facets.

While the preceding concept may seem rather obvious, the full, three-sided approach is rarely carried out in the practice of medicine today. Physicians with a strong medical model orientation tend to deal at the level of disease rather than that of the individual patient. On the other hand, physicians with a strong psychodynamic orientation often restrict their interest to the individual's situational status and almost ignore the presence of a disease process. Neither approach is entirely successful; they are a schism that is excellently exemplified in the current practices of neurology and psychiatry. Most modern neurologic training, clinical expertise, and technical competence is oriented toward a neuroscience approach. This is particularly notable in the more peripheral aspects of neurology where a quantitative approach is enhanced by a strong gadget influence. Neurologists tend to ignore the fact that the neurologic disease processes they have outlined in their patients are involving an individual. Nonetheless, it is obvious that a disease process such as multiple sclerosis or even a peripheral neuropathy may be far more devastating to one personality than to another. On the other hand, for many years most American psychiatrists have been strongly oriented toward the social and environmental aspects of an individual's illness, often expressing little interest in the presence of a disease process. Only in recent years has a biologic approach to psychiatric problems regained prominence to supplement the continuing interest in dynamic factors. To date, unfortunately, far too little bridging between the two approaches has been accomplished. Patients are treated "individually" but too often either the patient or the disease process is treated, not both. Patients whose medical problems place them in the borderland between neurology and psychiatry are particularly susceptible to incomplete management. There is a strong tendency for specialists in each field to be overly sensitive to the problems germane to the other. Thus, the neurologist may consider a given patient with neurobehavioral problems to be a candidate for psychiatric management, while the psychiatrist believes the same patient has organic brain syndrome, a neurologic problem. Far too many patients fall into this chasm between neurology and psychiatry and, currently, receive inadequate care.

The need to change this situation is obvious. Improvement would demand re-education of both neurologists and psychiatrists, not a decrease in or de-emphasis of their current practice methods; it would require an enlargement of the scope within which they currently see a patient so that all three of the aspects suggested by Dr. Taylor—the disease itself, the overall illness, and the predicament of the patient within the illness situation—can be handled comfortably.

The scope of problems to be handled in the borderland between psychiatry and neurology is large, and with increased understanding of these problems, the incidence of the disease processes to be handled is increasing. One significant boost in the number of neurobehavioral patients stems from the increased longevity of the population with a subsequent increase in the mental diseases of the elderly, particularly depression and dementia. Not only has dementia become one of the prime public health problems facing the civilized world, but it is inexorably increasing in frequency.[12] Almost 5 percent of all individuals over age 65 are said to have an incapacitating dementia, and an additional 10 percent have a milder but still disabling degree of mental deterioration.[16] This is a large population, and when the high frequency of serious affective disease that occurs in the elderly is added, the combined problem reaches tremendous proportions. While depression and dementia are usually separated, and current treatments for the two disorders are quite dissimilar, both appear to reflect biologic abnormalities of the brain, and both disorders, particularly in the elderly, appear to fall within the borderland.

Another massively large group of patients who fall into the borderland are those with schizophrenia. At one time, individuals with this diagnosis occupied a high proportion of all hospital beds in the United States, and they still represent a sizeable proportion of the diseased population. While schizophrenia is still considered to have many psychogenic features, a biologic approach to the disease has become standard in recent years, and the management of both the disease itself and the many neurologic complications of its treatment fall within the realm of neurobehavior.

There are many other borderland disease processes; in fact, most behavioral disorders are not well portrayed as purely psychodynamic or purely neuroscientific problems. For instance, patients with multiple sclerosis, head trauma, aphasia, amnesia, alexia, agnosia, frontal and temporal types of personality disorder, and chronic pain, to name only a few disorders, will have varying combinations of neurologic and psychiatric problems; they demand a combined treatment approach if optimum results are to be obtained. Similarly, the biologic management of most psychotic disorders is fully accepted, and medical alterations of neuroses and personality disorders are being attempted.

This volume attempts to highlight only a few of these problems. As with the first volume of *Psychiatric Aspects of Neurologic Disease*,[2] this presentation is directed primarily at individuals in clinical practice who are faced with managing patients with borderland problems. The presentations, in general, are practical and clinical with comparatively little emphasis given to detailing either the psychodynamic or the neuroscientific basis. As in the first volume, this is not a complete text of neurobehavioral problems and makes no attempt to cover all topics in the field. The topics that are covered were selected by the editors, at least to some degree, because information on the topic has only recently been highlighted. In this respect, *Psychiatric Aspects of Neurologic Disease, Volume II,* is not an updated edition, but rather a totally new volume. Many of the topics included in this volume were not in the previous volume and vice versa. Similarly, except for the two editors, all of the authors in Volume II are different from those who wrote for Volume I.

While neither this nor the original volume of *Psychiatric Aspects of Neurologic Disease* attempts to cover the field of neurobehavior, a number of more complete approaches have appeared between the publication of these two volumes. Most notably, W. A. Lishman published an exhaustive and excellent review of the field, *Organic Psychiatry,* in 1978.[9] Just recently, three smaller but more up-to-date volumes appeared, all published in 1981. These are *Organic Brain Syndromes* by Strub and Black,[14] *Organic Mental Disorders* by Freemon,[7] and *Neuropsychiatry* by Trimble.[16] The first two are by neurologists, the last by a psychiatrist, and the contents are influenced to some extent by the orientation of the authors. Each is comparatively concise and reasonably complete, and all three are delightfully readable. Two of the authors, Strub and Trimble, are contributors to this volume and reflect the esteem the editors hold for their competency. One additional publication covering part of the field of neurobehavior deserves mention; this is a chapter entitled "Psychiatric Conditions Associated with Focal Lesions of the Central Nervous System" in Volume 4 of *The American Handbook of Neurology, Edition 2,*[3] which offers a broad picture of the behavioral disorders consequent to focal brain abnormality.

As in Volume I, there are some deliberate omissions. One of these is the absence of emphasis on childhood problems. Except for some areas of overlap, particularly the behavioral complications of epilepsy and stuttering, this volume deals only with the neurobehavioral disturbances of adults. This is because the field of childhood behavioral problems is so vast and so different that it demands a separate approach.

Another omission is detailed discussion of neuropsychology. Though this is a healthy, blooming, vibrant, investigative discipline dealing with many of the borderland problems, a number of good books on neuropsychology have been published in the past few years. In addition there are a number of journals devoted exclusively to this approach, and there are several national societies that hold regular meetings featuring reports on neuropsychological investigations of neurobehavioral problems. Much of the current output centers on research so that the literature contains many controversial opinions, decreasing the value of much current neuropsychological material. In this volume, neuropsychological results have been used only as they are considered useful for the practicing clinician.

In a somewhat similar manner, almost no attention has been given to the many important breakthroughs in the basic sciences. A number of remarkable discoveries and crucial biologic hypotheses concerning many of the disease processes under discussion have surfaced in the past decade. Since these are both controversial and already well reported, basic neuroscience data is presented here only when the information supports clinical discussion.

The field of genetics in psychiatric and neurobehavioral disorders has again been omitted, as have discussions of the biochemical and enzymatic approaches to the classic psychoses. Important work is appearing in both fields but, in general, is well reported and is included in this volume only when pertinent to a clinical problem.

Finally, little emphasis has been given to the many new technical diagnostic aids. Tremendous strides have been made in both diagnostic and laboratory approaches to brain-behavioral problems in the past few years. The most obvious and heavily used is the x-ray computerized tomogram which has revolutionized the diagnostic approach to many cerebral diseases. In addition, new laboratory studies offer information concerning significant enzymes, neurotransmitters, endocrine responses, and electrophysiologic changes. There has been no attempt to cover this vast field in the present volume, and both the procedures and their results have been alluded to only as they support the clinical approach.

One significant difference between Volumes I and II of *Psychiatric Aspects of Neurologic Disease* will be noted by the careful observer: a great deal more stress has been given to treatment in the second volume. In most chapters, the authors have provided up-to-date summaries on therapy for the various neurobehavioral disorders discussed. In addition, the editors have attempted to augment this with personal suggestions for treatment in the commentaries following the chapters. Neurobehavioral disorders have changed from diagnostic curiosities to remediable conditions, and the recognition and employment of appropriate treatments have become a reality. Considerable emphasis has been given to freeing neurobehavioral disorders from the long-standing stigma of being untreatable organic brain disorders. With appropriate diagnosis, many of the causes of neurobehavioral symptomatology have become amenable to therapy.

In summary, *Psychiatric Aspects of Neurologic Disease, Volume II,* presents useful information for the physician who is seeing increasing numbers of patients with behavioral abnormality secondary to disturbance of the central nervous system. We hope this volume, along with the first volume, can help bridge the two disciplines of neurology and psychiatry and, at least to some degree, help the many individuals suffering from disorders that fall between the two organized specialty groups.

To initiate this volume, we have again selected a problem that is both common and important but one that has always proved difficult to handle and discuss—the acute confusional state. Volume I contained a discussion of this problem,[4] but the importance of the confusional state in the practice of medicine is so great that re-emphasis is clearly indicated. Actually, we believe that the two chapters on the acute confusional state published in these two volumes are mutually supportive. The chapter by Manfred Bleuler in Volume I was oriented toward historic and classic clinicopathologic correlations, while the chapter in this volume by Richard L. Strub provides a more pragmatic approach, emphasizing both diagnosis and treatment. Increased recognition and better management of the confusional state are essential. Not only are such problems increasingly frequent in medical practice, but, almost without exception, the confusional state represents a treatable disease process. While the diagnosis may be difficult and the treatment tricky, the prognosis in appropriately recognized and treated cases is often excellent. The approach that Dr. Strub offers in Chapter 1 is eminently practical and presents a good overview of the far-ranging problems that present to the clinician.

REFERENCES

1. Alexander MP, Stuss DT, Benson DF: Capgras syndrome: A reduplicative phenomenon. Neurology 29:334–339, 1979
2. Benson DF, Blumer D: Psychiatric Aspects of Neurologic Disease. New York, Grune & Stratton, 1975
3. Benson DF, Geschwind N: Psychiatric conditions associated with focal lesions of the central nervous system, in Arieti S, Reiser MF (eds): American Handbook of Psychiatry, vol 4. New York, Basic Books, 1975, pp 208–243
4. Bleuler M: Acute concomitants of physical diseases, in Benson DF, Blumer D (eds): Psychiatric Aspects of Neurologic Disease. New York, Grune & Stratton, 1975, pp 37–61
5. Butler IJ, Koslow SH, Seifert WE Jr et al: Biogenic amine metabolism in Tourette syndrome. Ann Neurol 6:37–39, 1979

6. Cutting J: A study of anosognosia. J Neuro Neurosurg Psychiatry 41:548–555, 1978
7. Freemon FR: Organic Mental Disease. New York, SP Medical Books, 1981
8. Hunter R, Macalpine I: Psychiatry for the Poor. London, Dawson & Sons, Ltd, 1974
9. Lishman WA: Organic Psychiatry. Oxford, Blackwell, 1978
10. Mercer B, Wepner W, Gardner H, Benson DF: A study of confabulation. Arch Neurol 34:429–433, 1977
11. Mesulam MM: Dissociative states with abnormal temporal lobe EEG. Arch Neurol 38:176–181, 1981
12. Plum F: Dementia: An approaching epidemic. Nature 279:372–373, 1979
13. Slater E: Diagnosis of hysteria. Br Med J 1:1395–1399, 1965
14. Strub R, Black W: Organic Brain Syndrome. Philadelphia, Davis, 1981
15. Taylor D: The components of sickness: Diseases, illnesses and predicaments. Lancet 2:1008–1010, 1979
16. Trimble M: Neuropsychiatry. New York, Wiley, 1981
17. Wing L: The syndrome of early childhood autism. Br J Hosp Med 4:381–391, 1970

PSYCHIATRIC ASPECTS
OF NEUROLOGIC DISEASE
VOLUME II

Richard L. Strub, M.D.

1
Acute Confusional State

The acute confusional state ranks as one of the most common organic mental syndromes encountered in clinical medicine. This form of acute insanity is familiar to all physicians; the surgeon confronts it when his postoperative patient begins yelling incoherently at night and tries to climb over the side-rails of the bed; the internist and general physician deal with it when the renal failure patient is found wandering down the hall in a hospital gown mumbling that "they" are trying to poison him with the intravenous solution; and the psychiatrist recognizes it in the tremulous, hallucinating ravings of the recently abstinent alcoholic. Though somewhat different clinically, all of these patients are displaying acute confusional behavior. Most simply defined, an acute confusional state is a rapidly developing, yet fluctuating, behavior change that is characterized by altered arousal; inattention; incoherent speech, thought and action; global impairment of memory and intellectual processes; perceptual disturbances, including illusions and hallucinations; and marked emotional lability.

The above clinical picture represents the brain's behavioral response to a widespread disruption of cerebral metabolism. The cause may be the toxic effects of a medication, the result of anoxia, uremia, or other metabolic disturbance, the withdrawal from the chronic use of a depressant substance such as alcohol or barbiturate or, as is often the case, a combination of factors. Since the acute confusional state is most often caused by a physiologic disturbance and not structural brain disease, it is usually reversible if recognized and promptly treated. The confusional state is but one stage in the continuum of altered levels of consciousness and, if the medical problems producing the patient's condition go undiagnosed, the level of consciousness will worsen and progress inexorably to stupor, coma, and finally death. The physician, therefore, should view the confusional state with the same sense of urgency as the more dramatic states of stupor and coma.

Controversy has developed concerning the terminology best suited to denote this clinical state. The internist most often uses the terms metabolic or toxic encephalopathy; the neurologist prefers the term used in this chapter—acute confusional state. The psychiatrist has used various terms—acute brain syndrome with psychosis, toxic psychosis, but has recently returned to the classic term delirium.[1,26] It has been observed for centuries that patients with metabolic disturbances of the brain may present in either a quiet lethargic state or in an agitated hyperactive state.[22] The psychiatrist labels all such patients as delirious and classifies them secondarily as either hypoactive or hyperactive. Neurologists, on the other hand, use the term acute confusional state for all such patients, and reserve the label delirium for agitated, hyperactive patients. If future research reveals that the two forms of the syndrome represent different physiologic responses and require separate approaches for diagnosis and treatment, it will then be necessary to divide the syndrome into subcategories. Until such time, however, it is best to consider all forms of the syndrome under a single label. This chapter will use the term acute confusional state; hyperactive and hypoactive variants are noted in the clinical discussion.

CLINICAL MANIFESTATIONS

The acute confusional state, a purely behavioral syndrome, is diagnosed by the recognition of its particular behavioral features. Since the metabolic abnormality underlying the syndrome affects many different neurons throughout the central nervous system, the clinical picture is of a global impairment involving both cortical and subcortical functions. The syndrome is called acute brain failure or acute cerebral insufficiency by some, denoting a similarity to the concept of organ failure used in general medicine.[14] The broad symptom complex is due to the generalized nature of the brain involvement. This generalized nature, more than any one symptom, identifies this behavioral syndrome.

The most reliable feature in distinguishing the acute confusional state from other acute organic or functional behavioral syndromes is probably a clouding of consciousness. Although the term by itself is somewhat vague, it does describe the mental state of the confused patient. More specifically, clouding of consciousness refers both to a dulling of intellectual processes and to an alteration in alertness. This combined impairment of arousal and cognition reduces the patient's awareness of the environment and prevents effective operation within it. There is failure to elaborate impressions and mental processes loosen in their correspondence to reality. The patient appears bewildered or perplexed, almost as though in a waking dream.

One of the most characteristic aspects of the patient's clouded mental state is an incoherence in the train of thought. This incoherence gives rise to incoherent discourse, muddled reasoning, and disorganized behavior. Most often it is this loss of orderly and efficient thinking with its attendant disordered behavior that leads an observer to describe the patient as being confused.

The incoherence of thought and action is the product of disturbances in three basic processes. First, arousal is altered. In the quiet confusional patient, the ascending activating system of the brain stem is sufficiently suppressed so that the higher cortical centers are not adequately stimulated; in the agitated patient, overactive arousal makes efficient thinking impossible. The second disturbance is a general reduction of all higher intellectual functions. The entire cortex is affected and full mental status testing will reveal defects in memory, abstract reasoning, calculating, writing, and many other specific functions.[13] The third disordered process is attention. The confusional patient shows a markedly reduced capacity for sustained attention and concentration. He is distractable, constantly shifting attention from the examiner to extraneous stimuli in the environment, and when selective attention is lost all competing stimuli seem to carry equal value in attracting his attention. This erratic shifting of attention is obvious and it is easy to appreciate how this pervasive problem is responsible for much of the general disorganization exhibited. Physiologically, attention is a complex function that, most simplistically, reflects the controlling influence of the cortex and limbic systems in focusing the arousal energy of the ascending activating system.[33] In the confusional state, the higher controls are compromised and sustained selective attention becomes impossible.

Concomitant with the inattention and incoherence of thought, the patient often experiences a wide range of perceptual disturbances, many of which are characteristic of the confusional state. The first and most common is a tendency to misinterpret environmental stimuli; e.g., calling the intravenous stand a flagpole or thinking that a fold in the bed clothes is a garden hose. These experiences are simple illusions and may also occur with auditory or tactile stimuli. One curious misperception, seen almost exclusively in organic patients, is the propensity to identify the unfamiliar as familiar. The confusional patient may welcome the physician as an old friend or long lost relative. The scientific basis of this type of disordered perception is unknown but, in a psychologic sense, it seems logical that the confusional patient would attempt to reconstruct the environment in search of a familiar order in the midst of the chaos of his mind.

An even more dramatic perceptual disturbance are the vivid hallucinations so frequently reported, particularly in the agitated or delirious form of confusion. The hallucinations are most often visual, but auditory, tactile, and mixed types can also be found.[15,37,50] The content of the hallucination is often an animal, person, snake, or some variety of bug. The hallucination may be frightening or threatening. In delirium tremens, for example, giant spiders or snakes are commonly seen or felt crawling on the skin; the parade of pink pachyderms, however, is more a cartoon characterization than a reality. The hallucination is often nonthreatening, e.g. the appearance of a beloved pet or other creature can be a source of comfort or amusement to the patient. Patients may be embarrassed about their hallucinations and reluctant to report them for fear of having their own suspicions of insanity confirmed by the physician; it is important, therefore, to inquire specificaly about hallucinations and reassure the patient that they may occur in sickness without indicating insanity.

Hallucinations, a positive symptom in the Jacksonian sense, are the result of abnormal reactivation and distortion of stored sensory images. The comparison of this state of vivid visual experience to that of normal dreaming is often made.[24] It is easy to see why the confusional state would be considered similar to a dream state; the incoherence of events coupled with the vivid, often frightening, visual hallucinations is all too reminiscent of a nightmare. Exactly how the visual images are thrust into consciousness in both the dream and the confusional state is unknown. In the agitated confusional patient, arousal from the brain stem ascending activating system is high and the cortical attention facilitating or inhibiting systems are weakened; it is possible that the hallucination represents a release phenomenon where diffuse activation stimulates higher centers in a random and uncontrolled fashion.[48] Although such explanations remain speculative, the study of sleep and dreaming may shed light on the disordered mechanisms present in the confusional patient.

Emotional and personality changes are also exhibited by the confusional patient. This is not too surprising since the entire brain, including the limbic system, is affected by the basic disorder. A wide variety of abnormalities can be observed: anxiety, fear, depression, paranoia and even frank delusions. The delusions, however, are usually fragmented or associated with a particular piece of apparatus in the room and are rarely systematized in the manner common to schizophrenia. In some patients, the only emotional change is limited to an accentuation of premorbid personality traits. In mild cases where insight is largely intact, much of the anxiety and fear appears self-generated as the patient consciously grapples with the frightening disintegration he perceives occurring in his own mind. When the condition is severe, the florid emotional changes seem more primitive and distinct from the more self-reflective reactions of more alert patients.

In association with the cognitive and emotional changes described above, the confusional patient experiences a substantial disruption of normal sleep pattern and circadian rhythm. They are characteristically awake at night and lethargic during the day. The sleep that they do manage to obtain is fragmented and nonrestorative. Rapid eye movement (REM) and slow wave sleep stages are all but absent. In the confusional state due to withdrawal from alcohol, REM activity may be increased in a rebound nature and may even be present in the awake state. The association of the REM state with dreaming suggests that the hallucinatory events of delirium tremens may be dream content erupting into the conscious state. Such a patient cannot separate dream from reality and perceives all events as real. The sleep disturbances are not only a part of the confusional state but, by virtue of the relative sleep deprivation they engender, serve to perpetuate confusional behavior.

Alterations in psychomotor activity are seen as well. Some patients become hypoactive (quiet) while others are hyperactive (active), as noted by Gowers.[19] In the quiet state patients sleep restlessly, often rearranging themselves and the bed coverings. When active, they may shout, pull at intravenous and other tubing, and flail about. Although patients may display only one level of activity during their illness, swings between the extremes are often noted. In general, the restlessness and heightened activity level become exaggerated at night. Those patients exhibiting marked hyperactivity (e.g., florid delirium tremens) often show an outpouring of autonomic activity: pupils dilate, pulse and blood pressure rise, diaphoresis is profuse, mucous membranes are dry, and vomiting or diarrhea may be present.[37] Myoclonic jerking may be observed and generalized seizures are not uncommon.

The clinical picture is not the only diagnostic element typical of this condition. The clinical course itself is as characteristic of the confusional state as are the behavioral changes. At times, this may be the most helpful factor in establishing the diagnosis. As the name implies, the acute confusional state evolves rapidly, usually over several days. The onset is rarely sudden unless it has been caused by a vascular accident, blow to the head, or epileptic seizure. The initial signs of sleeplessness, irritability, and subtle changes in thought processing or emotion may go unnoticed or be present only at night. As the condition progresses, the nocturnal exacerbations persist and confusional behavior is observed intermittently during the daylight hours. Lucid intervals occur and examination during a clear period may fail to reveal any behavioral aberration. This tendency to fluctuate, almost as much as any other single aspect, is an identifying characteristic of the acute confusional state.

To summarize, the diagnosis of a confusional state rests upon the recognition of specific clinical features plus an appreciation of the clinical course. The physician must watch carefully for evidence of altered consciousness, incoherence, inattention, and misperceptions, etc. and also obtain a history of both these symptoms and their fluctuations. Once familiar with the syndrome, the physician should have little difficulty recognizing the acute confusional state.

DIFFERENTIAL DIAGNOSIS

Several disease entities can present with rapidly progressive disorganized behavior that may resemble a confusional state. Some are functional psychiatric illnesses while others are different organic brain syndromes. By being familiar with the clinical picture of these conditions, the examiner should have little difficulty differentiating between them and the confusional state.

Dementia

The disease most frequently misinterpreted as a confusional state on initial examination is probably dementia. If there is a history documenting a gradual deterioration of intellectual and social adaptive abilities over many months or years it is not difficult to recognize dementia. If, however, the history is insufficient and the examination reveals an inattentive, incoherent, and suspicious individual, the diagnosis is far from obvious. One major differentiating point is the level of arousal and its fluctuation. The demented individual is relatively alert and remains so throughout the day; the confusional patient is not. Both patients may show disorientation and agitation at night so this feature will not assist in differentiation. Active hallucinations are not characteristic of dementia. Complicating the diagnostic differentiation is the propensity for the demented patient to develop a superimposed confusional state with illnesses that would not affect a normal individual. These mixed problems are difficult to evaluate and the decision as to which mental abnormality is to be attributed to each condition may be impossible.

Aphasia

Another organic condition that can be perplexing initially is an acute aphasia presenting without hemiparesis. Lesions in the dominant temporal or parietal lobes often produce marked language disturbances, easily mistaken for the incoherent verbal output of the confusional patient. The verbal output of both is fluent and disorganized. The aphasic patient, however, produces many abnormal words called paraphasias—

plenkal for pencil, red grass for green grass, or durlup for necktie are some examples.[3,18] The confusional patient may slur words and have difficulty finding the correct word, but paraphasia is infrequent.[13] The fluent aphasic may produce sentences that are virtually devoid of meaning or content. For example, an aphasic man describing how to change a tire may say, "you know, you take the the thing and over there, and well you know over by the one that is wrong, oh I don't know. . . ."

A second important feature seen in aphasia is the frequent occurrence of a comprehension deficit, particularly if the lesion is in the parietal-temporal junction area. The aphasic will fail to point to objects on request and will answer questions inappropriately. The confusional patient, though inattentive, will perform more adequately. Emotional reactions such as anxiety and paranoia can be seen in both conditions,[4] but an altered level of consciousness strongly suggests a confusional state. A combination of aphasia and confusion may be present during the first few days after an acute vascular accident or if the aphasia is caused by a tumor producing increased intracranial pressure. The clinical findings may be quite complex in these cases but the aphasia will often stand out against the confusional behavior, indicating that two behavioral syndromes are present.

Psychiatric Disorders

Schizophrenia

In addition to the organic conditions discussed above, several psychiatric disorders may simulate organic confusion. Schizophrenia is one. As with dementia, an adequate history will usually establish the diagnosis. An adequate history, however, is not always obtainable and the diagnosis must be made on clinical signs alone. The age of the patient is of some help since schizophrenia is more common in the young and confusional state in the elderly; however, the occurrence of acute adjustment reactions in older individuals and the prodigious misuse of drugs by the young dilute the usefulness of age as a differential feature. Both disorders cause inattention, anxiety, and disorientation, but only the confusional patient shows the fluctuations in level of consciousness.[43,44] The confusional patient may be suspicious and have some fragmented delusions but not the systematized, bizarre, and fantastic delusions characteristic of the schizophrenic. Perceptual disturbances differ also. Whereas the confusional patient misidentifies strangers as old friends, the schizophrenic may find that once familiar individuals have lost all meaning and are unrecognizable.[16] Hallucinations differ as well; visual and tactile hallucinations predominate in the acute confusional state and auditory hallucinations predominate in schizophrenia.

Mania

A second functional syndrome to be considered is acute mania. At the height of mania, patients may display disorientation, incoherent thought, hallucinations, and psychomotor agitation. Because of the clinical similarity with the confusional state, the term delirious mania has often been applied to these patients.[6,12,24] Obviously, a history of gradually increasing loquaciousness, hyperactivity, racing thoughts, and hypersexuality strongly favors a diagnosis of mania. On occasion, however, mania can build so rapidly that the history will not clearly make the diagnosis. As with other functional syndromes, fluctuations in level of consciousness are not characteristic of mania and cognitive abilities, though often dificult to test, will be more impaired in the confusional patient.

Depression

Psychotic depression can superficially mimic the quiet confusional state, just as mania simulates agitated confusion, but the classic mood disturbance of depression is just not seen in confusion. Similarly, the clouding of consciousness of the confusional state is not present in depression.

A few other functional psychiatric conditions can occasionally cause a problem in differentiation; the highly anxious neurotic, the agitated hysteric, and the malingerer may present with agitated disorganized behavior; but again, the specific features of fluctuating clouding of consciousness, visual hallucinations, and incoherent thought and action are not seen.

ETIOLOGY

Once a clinical diagnosis of an acute confusional state has been made, a number of factors must be considered to determine the etiology or etiologies. In some cases, a single obvious cause such as drug reaction exists, but more frequently a complex mosaic of predisposing factors and precipitating events is responsible. In the complex case, individual contributing factors (e.g., fever) may not be sufficiently abnormal to disrupt overall brain metabolism; but in conjunction with other elements, such as an elevated BUN, low sodium, sedation and/or several sleepless nights, the cumulative effect is enough to cause decompensation. Each factor may affect different neuronal functions or different populations of neurons, but the combined effect produces a remarkably consistent clinical picture regardless of etiology.

In establishing the cause or causes of a confusional state, the physician must consider all possible factors, including precipitating events and predisposing tendencies. Certain individuals are more vulnerable to the effects of metabolic disturbances and therefore are more prone to develop a confusional state. Among predisposing factors for this vulnerability are advanced age, dementia or senility, preexisting brain damage, a history of prior alcohol or drug abuse, and, of course, a previous history of an acute confusional reaction. In addition to constitutional predispositions, there are also nonorganic contributing factors. The most important is sleep deprivation. A healthy young adult can endure many days of sustained sleep deprivation before significant mental symptoms appear,[31,42,49] but in the elderly, especially the ill or mildly senile, even a single night of sleep loss can have a devastating effect. Another well-known factor is the disorientating effect of being in an unfamiliar environment (such as a hospital). This is magnified in patients with poor memory and other cognitive deficits who may become grossly disoriented and agitated after only a few hours in a strange, darkened room.[10] The psychologic stress engendered by physical illness can be a separate, nonorganic factor. This may be a major factor before emergency surgery where the threat to life may be great. In contrast, there does not seem to be any particular premorbid personality type or psychiatric illness that predisposes a patient to develop a confusional state.

Specific Conditions

In addition to the factors above, many specific conditions can produce a confusional state.[26,32] Though too numerous to list here, they can be separated into several main categories.

Prescription and Nonprescription Drugs

The first is prescription medications. In some patients, an idiosyncratic reaction can occur to a single drug although the confusional state is more often precipitated by the combined effects of several medications. Psychotropics, barbiturates, anticholinergics, digitalis, propanolol, and cimetidine are some of the current problem medications. As usual, it is the elderly that are the most sensitive to medication problems.

Nonprescription toxic substances are also common offenders. Alcohol is the leading cause, but a staggering variety of drugs and noxious substances are being abused and all can cause acute confusional behavior. When a young person is brought into the hospital behaving abnormally, the first consideration is a drug-induced toxic state. Withdrawal, as well as the acute intoxication, of drugs and alcohol is another common problem. This diagnosis must always be entertained when young or middle-aged adults begin to develop confusional behavior several days after admission to the hospital.

Metabolic Disturbances

The second major category is specific metabolic disturbances; these can be acute as is seen in anoxia, hypoglycemia, or electrolyte abnormalities or chronic as in endocrine disturbances or vitamin deficiency. Major organ failures, such as renal or cardiac failure, can also produce metabolic disturbances.

Infection

A third category is infection. Febrile delirium is the archetype confusional state and is still seen commonly in children. Specific infections of the central nervous system such as meningitis or encephalitis are particularly likely to present with confusional behavior.

Structural Lesions of the Brain

A fourth etiologic category is structural lesions of the brain. There are several mechanisms by which focal lesions lead to confusional behavior. With mass lesions, confusion appears to be related to diffuse increased intracranial pressure. With acute cerebral thrombosis, the mechanism is uncertain, although it may be secondary to shifts in blood flow, vascular spasm, or neuronal shock in adjacent tissues. Of considerable theoretical interest are reports of specifically localized lesions that can cause a prolonged confusional state. Lesions in the right frontal lobe, the right mid-parietal lobe,[28] the limbic system of the medial temporal and occipital lobes,[25,27] and the medial frontal cortex, including the cingulate gyrus,[2] have all been reported. Why a localized lesion should produce a clinical picture of confusional behavior is uncertain; destruction of limbic structures might be expected to cause some behavior change, but why this should take the form of a confusional state is speculative. The cases in which mid-frontal and mid-parietal damage were demonstrated in the right hemisphere are explicable if one accepts that these areas of cortex are critical for controlling selective attention.[28] A patient with a severe defect in attentional mechanisms is unable to sustain coherent thought and action and is obviously confusional on examination. Proof that the right cortical centers are dominant for selective attention remains weak at best, however.

Neurologic Diseases

There are other neurologic diseases that can present with confusional behavior—subarachnoid hemorrhage, head trauma, and epilepsy being the most common. The postictal period following a generalized tonic-clonic (grand mal) seizure is a classic confusional state and a similar state follows many complex-partial seizures. Absence (petit mal) and complex-partial (temporal lobe) status epilepticus can be continuous for days and produce all the features of an acute confusional state.

Surgery

The final major medical setting often associated with a confusional state is surgery. It is not the operation itself but the unique set of circumstances found during the surgery and in the postoperative recovery period that are responsible for the behavior change. Postoperative confusional behavior usually begins 3–5 days after the surgery but can be present immediately after the effects of the anesthesia have worn off. The confusional behavior seen immediately after surgery usually indicates hypoxia or an acute anticholinergic syndrome.[20] Acetylcholine is a major neurotransmitter in the central nervous system, particularly in the temporal lobe limbic structures, and the anticholinergic effect of either preoperative atrophine or other anticholinergic drugs given prior to surgery (e.g., tricyclic antidepressants, anti-Parkinson drugs, phenothiazines, or such over-the-counter drugs as Excedrin-PM [Bristol-Myers], Sleep-EZ [Whitehall], and Sominex [J. B. Williams]) may precipitate postoperative confusion.

The more common postoperative confusional state begins several days after surgery and is usually due to multiple factors including sleep loss, pain, medications, sensory deprivation, metabolic abnormality, atelectasis with reduced ventilation, fever, the effects of blood loss, plus the predisposing factors discussed earlier. Some additional factors may increase the vulnerability of the surgical patient: (1) The urgency of the surgery. Patients undergoing emergency surgery are more likely to become confused after surgery than those who have undergone elective surgery.[29] (2) The number of different medications the patient is taking before surgery; more than five drugs will increase the incidence of confusion. (3) The seriousness of the preoperative illness. (4) The number of postoperative complications or physical changes such as hemorrhage, anemia, and elevated BUN, etc. (5) A decreased vision or hearing. (6) A history of previous postoperative confusion. (7) Preoperative confusional behavior. This factor is invariably associated with postoperative confusion.

Although postoperative confusional behavior can occur after any surgical procedure, a very high incidence has been reported after cardiac surgery, especially following valve replacement.[38,39,41] The incidence of microembolism, though greatly decreased with special filters in the pump-oxygenator, is still a problem,[8,23] and recent evidence has demonstrated that decreases in cardiac output during the procedure also have a high correlation with the appearance of postoperative confusion.[21]

EVALUATION

The clinical evaluation of the confusional state has three distinct goals: first, to make a specific behavioral diagnosis; second, to establish that the patient has an organic confusional state and not an organic or functional condition that can mimic it; and third, to determine the etiology.

The initial steps in a clinical assessment include a careful medical history, best taken from those caring for the patient, and a mental status examination. The latter must be guided toward eliciting or observing the clinical features of confusional behavior described earlier. Once it is determined that the patient is confusional, extensive cognitive testing becomes unnecessary.

Next, a complete physical and neurologic examination must be performed to seek the etiology. The same urgency and thoroughness used in examining a stuporous or comatose patient is indicated. Signs of systemic illness and specific organ disease should be sought. The presence of tremor or asterixis should be noted since these are reliable signs of metabolic encephalopathy. The possibility of increased intracranial pressure or focal cerebral lesions must also be considered.

The diagnosis of a confusional state is primarily clinical and no specific laboratory test can establish the diagnosis. The electroencephalogram (EEG) may be helpful in verifying the diagnostic impression, for in the quiet confusional state, the EEG usually demonstrates diffuse, irregular theta frequency slowing, often with superimposed bifrontal delta bursts. A slow EEG, therefore, is helpful in differentiating the confusional patient from a patient with a functional psychiatric illness, the latter usually demonstrating a normal recording. A problem arises with the agitated hyperactive patient, especially those with withdrawal syndromes. In these patients, not only is the record ridden with artifact, but the background activity is usually fast and therefore nonspecific.[14,30,34]

A second test that can be helpful on occasion is the intravenous amytal test.[46] The test is performed by infusing 50–75 mg amobarbital per minute with waits of about 1 minute per 2 minutes of infusion. When nystagmus or slurred speech occurs, the patient's mental status should be re-evaluated. Patients whose disorientation is secondary to a functional psychiatric illness may calm down and demonstrate a marked improvement.[45] Most confusional patients will worsen and become obtunded. Unfortunately, the patient with withdrawal delirium, the patients most difficult to differentiate from functional psychosis, may improve with the barbiturate.

The remaining laboratory examinations focus on the identification of the underlying medical cause or causes of the condition. Discussion of these tests is voluminous and is covered in standard medical texts.

One aspect of evaluation that has not been mentioned is the quantification of the confusional behavior. A qualitative appreciation of the behavioral symptoms is all that is necessary to make the diagnosis, but a quantitative measure of the degree of confusion is useful in following the course of the confusional patient. Since behavior change is the sole parameter available to judge success or failure of medical management, it is important to determine changes in the clinical status. One problem is the tendency for dramatic fluctuations in symptomatology. For monitoring, either frequent assessments or some estimate of the percentage of time the patient displays abnormal behavior must be made. Items on any clinical scale must be weighted to reflect their relative pathologic significance. For example, mild disorientation for the date of the month is not as significant as the appearance of visual hallucinations.[36] The information included in the rating should come from several sources, including nurses, attendants, doctors, and the patient himself. To rely only on the patient's reports is not satisfactory, for confusional patients have inefficient memories, tend to confabulate, and often frankly deny the presence of illness.[47]

A sample assessment form is presented in Table 1-1. The point score on the right reflects the general pathologic significance of each item. Using this assessment scheme, evaluation of the patient should not require more than 2 minutes and can be repeated hourly with the results recorded on a simple graph. Longitudinal evaluations can be very important for comprehensive management.

MANAGEMENT

The management plan for a patient in an acute confusional state should include two distinct avenues of treatment—the specific treatment of the underlying medical problems and control of the abnormal behavior. Since medical management is better described in the appropriate medical texts, discussion here will center around the control of the confusional behavior itself.

Environmental Manipulations

In dealing with an acute confusional state, environmental manipulations are as important as the use of pharmacologic agents. First, the physician must stabilize the patient's environment. Reassuring relatives and

Table 1-1
Assessment For Confusional Behavior

1.	Level of arousal		
	Day: Mild lethargy	1 point	
	Significant lethargy	2 points	
	Night: Asleep	0 point	
	Awake	1 point	
	Agitated	2 points	_____
2.	Disorientation		
	Time	1 point	
	Place	2 points	
	Person	3 points	_____
3.	Inattention		
	Mild	1 point	
	Moderate	2 points	
	Severe	3 points	_____
4.	Incoherence in conversation		
	Mild	2 points	
	Moderate	3 points	
	Marked	4 points	_____
5.	Misperceptions		
	Misidentifies individuals	3 points	
	Illusions	4 points	
	Hallucinations	5 points	_____
6.	Behavior change		
	Restlessness	1 point	
	Agitation	3 points	
	Paranoia	4 points	_____
7.	Inappropriate behavior		
	Mild, such as walking out in open gown asking to go home	3 points	
	Significant agitated behavior with yelling and attempting to pull out catheters, climb over bed rails, etc.	5 points	_____
		Total	_____

nursing personnel that the patient's chaotic behavior is a temporary medical problem and not the sudden appearance of irreversible insanity or senility, is of inestimable value. Once calmed, the family's assistance can be enlisted in caring for the patient. It is important that the patient have an attendant at all times if possible, but particularly at night. Family members make ideal attendants as they are familiar to the patient and are usually more attentive to the patient's needs. This is obviously impossible in intensive care units, but increased visitation can sometimes be arranged even under these circumstances. The attendant has several important functions: One function is to prevent the patient from hurting himself or disrupting his intravenous apparatus, etc., but equally as important is the attendant's ability to calm the patient and make him more comfortable. The attendant should orient the patient frequently and inform him of his medical progress.[9] Frequent, short, uncomplicated social discussions are beneficial. Such discussions should focus on topics of known interest to the patient as this will relax him and help in organizing his thoughts. When the patient becomes agitated, gentle conversation and physical attention such as washing the face or arms with a warm cloth will often control the agitation and obviate the need for medication or physical restraint. Restraints should be a last resort as they usually increase agitation. If they must be used, they should be removed as soon as possible.

In addition to the presence of a sympathetic attendant, several other changes should be made in the patient's physical environment. When medically stable, the patient should be moved to a private room. Lights should be kept at a reasonable level during the day and dimmed at night. A totally darkened room removes the previous visual cues required for orientation. A clock and calendar should be in evidence, and a radio or television played at a reasonable level may be helpful. A familiar atmosphere can be fostered by having the family bring in pictures or objects from home. Such familiarity is conducive to calming the patient and helping him orient his thoughts.

Insuring Adequate Sleep

With the environment stabilized, the next major step is to insure adequate sleep. Sleep is disrupted in the confusional patient and sleeplessness alone can perpetuate confusional behavior, even after the metabolic defect has been corrected. Adequate night sleep is critical and best achieved with use of a soporific or tranquilizer at the hour of sleep. Chloral hydrate, 500–1000 mg, is usually sufficient and may be repeated in an hour if necessary. Flurazepam, paraldehyde, or tranquilization with either major or minor tranquilizers may also be effective. Barbiturates should be avoided, particularly in the elderly, for they depress respiration and produce paradoxical excitement on occasion. Sleep, when it does come, may be very sound and last 12-18 hours. An EEG, at this time, often demonstrates a high percentage of slow-wave sleep and REM activity. The restorative value of sleep is often startling, and its value in the overall management plan cannot be overstressed.

Tranquilization

The final element in the management of the confusional patient is the tranquilization of the agitation and hyperactivity that may arise during the course of the illness. Although any tranquilizer may be effective, some appear safer and more efficacious than others. Haloperidol is currently the best choice; it does not have the hepatotoxicity or hypotensive potential of the phenothiazines or the propensity for paradoxical excitation of the barbiturates. Although benzodiazepines may be used, they are less effective and at times can cause increased agitation. If a medication is unsuccessful it is best to switch to a completely different class of drug (e.g., from haloperidol to benzodiazepine).

Dosage and route of administration deserve comment. Dosage must be titrated and initial doses should be small and frequent, particularly in the elderly. Dose and route of administration vary with the severity of agitation. In severely agitated patients, it is most efficacious to sedate rapidly using parenteral haloperidol (0.5-2.0 mg/hour in older patients and 5 mg/hour or more in young adults). When agitation is controlled, the controlling dose should be given every 6 hours and gradually tapered as the patient's conditions warrants. Intramuscular injection is not as reliable in achieving adequate blood levels as intravenous administration, but the drug is not officially approved for intravenous use.[17] In mild agitation and after severe excitement has been controlled, oral medication can be used; administration in the morning and at bedtime are often all that are required. A double dose can sometimes be given at night in place of a sedative. Medication is usually restricted to agitated patients and not given to quiet lethargic confusional patients. Further lowering of the level of consciousness in these individuals is not in their best interest and may compromise recovery.

Two varieties of acute confusional state require additional specialized treatment: one is delirium tremens, the other the anticholinergic syndrome occasionally seen following use of atropine or similar drugs. In delirium tremens, the therapeutic regimen should include vitamin therapy (particularly thiamine), fluid replacement, and magnesium administration in conjunction with medications for sedation.[40] For sedation, the benzodiazepines have been the most successful. Dosages of 400 mg chlordiazepoxide or 100 mg diazepam daily may be necessary. Intravenous administration can be used and is often advisable during the acute phase.

In the anticholinergic syndrome some success has been achieved by blocking the cholinesterase enzyme with physostigmine. One or two milligrams can be given intravenously every 30 minutes until agitation is controlled. Physostigmine must be used with caution as many conditions such as asthma, coronary or peripheral vascular disease, glaucoma, peptic ulcer, and bowel or bladder dysfunction may be adversely affected by the autonomic action of physostigmine.[20]

Extended Recovery

In general, the acute confusional state is not difficult to manage and, when successfully treated, should not result in any neurologic or behavioral sequela. The patient will frequently be amnesic, or at least partially so, for the period of greatest confusion, and should be reassured that this is normal. In cases where the confusional behavior has been chronic, as in myxedema or Cushing's syndrome, permanent residual deficits may occur. The rate at which the confusional behavior clears varies. For example, correction of serum electrolytes is only the initial step in reestablishing normal neuronal function. Membranes must stabilize, intracellular milieu must return to normal, and neurotransmitters and synapses must be normalized. These processes may require days or even weeks to correct fully after the immediate crisis is resolved. The physician must be prepared to deal with ongoing behavioral abnormalities after initial treatment has been instituted. The precise pathophysiology of this extended recovery is far from known, but there is evidence supporting a continuing metabolic abnormality. One recent study showed a prolonged acidosis in the spinal fluid of patients with delirium tremens whose confusional behavior continued after serum acid-base balance was normal.[11]

In some patients, a prolonged, apparently unremitting confusional state may reflect a previously unsuspected dementia. Patients with early dementia may be well compensated until they develop a physical illness and become confusional. Their behavior then provokes close scrutiny and a premorbid dementia is uncovered. It is wise to wait several weeks before reaching this conclusion, however, since some patients, particularly the elderly, may require a longer time to recover from an acute confusional state.

PREVENTION

A physician who understands the phenomenology, etiology, and management of the acute confusional state can do much to prevent its appearance and/or minimize its degree when present. One effective preventive measure is to identify the vulnerable patient and then observe carefully for confusional behavior during any systemic illness, when using a new medication, or when the patient undergoes surgery. As already stressed, it is the elderly, the senile, the brain damaged, and those patients with histories of alcohol or drug abuse that are the most vulnerable. Medications must be carefully monitored in these patients because they often forget to take them or inadvertently take too much. Minor illnesses also demand careful medical attention. It is also wise to alert families to the possible development of confusion, so that medical attention is sought early in the course.

The effect of sleep loss must be appreciated. Learning to ask about and recognizing the importance of a restles night in infirm elderly patients allows the physician to take the appropriate steps and head off the full-blown delirium that may lay two nights ahead. With the first signs of confusion, the family should be brought in to stay with the patient and nighttime sedation started to insure adequate sleep.

In the surgical setting, several steps may minimize the degree of a postoperative confusion. If time permits, as with elective surgery, the surgeon should take a few extra minutes to discuss the operation, the postoperative care (including the routine of the recovery area), the expected discomfort, and other pertinent information. Such a discussion permits the patient to express his anxieties and thereby reduces them in the postoperative period.[35] Family members should be encouraged to discuss the impending surgery with the patient rather than studiously avoiding or underplaying the subject. Medications should be reduced to an absolute minimum and the patient's medical condition stabilized as well as possible. After surgery, attendants should routinely check for signs of confusion and report them promptly to the surgeon. Many of the environmental manipulations utilized to manage a confusional state can then be employed: family involvement, familiar objects in the room, adequate sleep, adequate lighting, clocks, calendars, and the like. Regardless of the precautions, many patients will become confusional after surgery. If, however, the surgeons, nurses, and family are alert and prepared to act, the postoperative confusional state will be a less awesome problem.

CONCLUSION

This discussion of the acute confusional state has been largely clinical by necessity; there is very little known about its basic pathophysiology. What is recognized is that the whole brain, when subjected to an abnormal metabolic product, a noxious substance, or the release from such a substance, responds by producing a behavior that is disordered in many respects. Arousal is compromised, attention is hopeless, sleep is disturbed, cognition is disorderly, and emotions are unruly. The clinical picture varies from somnolent incoherent muttering to raving paranoid hallucinosis. Literally thousands of agents or metabolic disturbances can cause the condition yet there is no correspondence of etiologic agent to clinical features.[5,7] Although withdrawal states are often characterized by agitation and hyperactivity, the specificity ends there. Is it that our acumen in analyzing the clinical phenomena of the confusional condition is so dull that we miss subtle differences, or is it that the entire neuronal pool is affected equally by all causal agents? The latter seems unlikely as we now realize that the confusional states caused by atropine, lysergic acid, and amphetamines produce disturbances in different neurotransmitter systems; and in a similar vein, anoxia surely has a different effect on nerve cells than a blow to the head, an elevated BUN, or a low serum sodium, although this still remains conjecture. Attempts to study the physiology of the brain in confusional patients using such gross instruments as the electroencephalogram have done little more than verify that there is, in fact, a neurophysiologic disturbance. Spinal fluid examination has done no better. To say that the field needs more study is an all too tired redundancy. It seems more prudent to conclude by stressing that the acute confusional state, by whatever name one may choose to call it, is an important clinical entity that, with proper attention from the treating physician, can be recognized and successfully managed despite so few clues to its true nature.

REFERENCES

1. American Psychiatric Association: Diagnostic and Statistical Manual of Mental Disorders (DSM III). Washington, American Psychiatric Association, 1980
2. Amyes EW, Nielsen JM: Clinicopathologic study of vascular lesions of the anterior cingulate region. Bull Los Angeles Neurol Soc 20:112–130, 1955
3. Benson DF: Fluency in aphasia: Correlation with radioactive scan localization. Cortex 3:373–394, 1967
4. Benson DF: Psychiatric aspects of aphasia. Br J Psychiatry 123:555–566, 1973
5. Bleuler M: Acute mental concomitants of physical diseases, in Benson DF, Blumer D (eds): Psychiatric Aspects of Neurologic Disease. New York, Grune & Stratton, 1975
6. Bond TC: Recognition of acute delirious mania. Arch Gen Psychiatry 37:553–554, 1980
7. Bonhoeffer K: Die psychosen im gefolge von akuten infektionen. Allegemeinerkrankungen und innern Erkrankungen, in Aschaffenburg G (ed): Handbuch der Psychiatrie. Leipzigund Wien, Deutke, 1912

8. Brennan RW, Patterson RH, Kessler J: Cerebral blood flow and metabolism during cardiopulmonary bypass: Evidence of microembolic encephalopathy. Neurology 21:665-672, 1971
9. Budd S, Brown W: Effect of a reorientation technique on postcardiotomy delirium. Nurs Res 23:341-348, 1974
10. Cameron ED: Studies in senile nocturnal delirium. Psychiat Avert 15:47-53, 1941
11. Carlen PL, Kapur B, Huszar LA, et al: Prolonged cerebralspinal fluid acidosis in recently abstinent chronic alcoholics. Neurology 30:956-962, 1980
12. Carlson GA, Goodwin FK: The stages of mania. Arch Gen Psychiatry 28:221-228, 1973
13. Chédru F, Geschwind N: Disorders of higher cortical functions in acute confusional states. Cortex 8:395-411, 1972
14. Engel AL, Romano J: Delirium, a syndrome of cerebral insufficiency. J Chronic Dis 9:260-277, 1959
15. Farber IJ: Acute brain syndrome. Dis Nerv Syst 20:296-299, 1959
16. Freedman BJ: The subjective experience of perceptual and cognitive disturbances in schizophrenia: A review of autobiographical accounts. Arch Gen Psychiatry 30:333-340, 1974
17. Fruensgaard K: Parenteral treatment of acute psychotic patients with agitation: A review. Curr Med Res Opin 5:593-600, 1978
18. Geschwind N: Current concepts: Aphasia. N Engl J Med 284:654-655, 1971
19. Gowers WR: A Manual of Diseases of the Nervous System. Philadelphia, Blakiston, 1888, pp 536-538
20. Granacher RP, Baldessarini RJ: Physostigmine: Its use in acute anticholinergic syndrome with antidepressant and antiparkinson drugs. Arch Gen Psychiatry 32:375-380, 1975
21. Heller SS, Kornfeld DS, Frank KA, Hoar PF: Postcardiotomy delirium and cardiac output. Am J Psychiatry 136:337-339, 1979
22. Henker FD: Acute brain syndromes. J Clin Psychol 40:117-120, 1979
23. Hill JD, Osborn JJ, Swank RL, et al: Experience using a new dacron wool filter during extracorporeal circulation. Arch Surg 101:649-652, 1970
24. Hirsch W: A study of delirium. NY State J Med 70:109-115, 1899
25. Horenstein S, Chamberlain W, Conomy J: Infarction of the fusiform and calcarine regions: Agitated delirium and hemianopia. Trans Am Neurol Assoc 92:85-89, 1967
26. Lipowski ZJ: Delirium: Acute brain failure in man. Springfield, Illinois, Thomas, 1980
27. Medina JL, Rubino FA, Ross A: Agitated delirium caused by infarction of the hippocampal formation and lingual gyri: A case report. Neurology 24:1181-1183, 1974
28. Mesulam MM, Waxman SG, Geschwind N, Sabin TD: Acute confusional states with right middle cerebral artery infarctions. J Neurol Neurosurg Psychiatry 39:84-89, 1976
29. Morse RM, Litin EM: Postoperative delirium: A study of etiologic factors. AM J Psychiatry 126:388-395, 1969
30. Obrecht R, Okhomina FOA, Scott DF: Value of EEG in acute confusional states. J Neurol Neurosurg Psychiatry 42:75-77, 1979

31. Pasnau RO, Naitoh P, Stier S, Kollar EJ: The psychological effects of 205 hours of sleep deprivation. Arch Gen Psychiatry 18:496-505, 1968
32. Plum F, Posner JB: The Diagnosis of Stupor and Coma. Philadelphia, Davis, 1980, p 177-304
33. Pribram KH, McGuiness D: Arousal, activation, and effort in the control of attention. Psychol Rev 82:116-149, 1975
34. Pro JD, Wells CE: The use of the electroencephalogram in the diagnosis of delirium. Dis Nerv Syst 38:804-808, 1977
35. Reading AE: The short term effects of psychological preparation for surgery. Soc Sci Med 13A:641-656, 1979
36. Sadler PD: Nursing assessment of postcardiotomy delirium. Heart Lung 8:745-750, 1979
37. Salum I: Delirium tremens and certain other acute sequels of alcohol abuse. Acta Psychiatr Scand (Suppl) 235:1-145, 1972
38. Steinhart MJ: Treatment of delirium: A reappraisal. Int J. Psychiatry Med 9:191-197, 1978-1979
39. Summers WK: Psychiatric sequelae to cardiotomy. J Cardiovas Surg 20:471-476, 1979
40. Thompson WL: Management of alcohol withdrawal syndromes. Arch Intern Med 138:278-283, 1978
41. Tufo HM, Ostfeld AM, Shekelle R: Central nervous system dysfunction following open-heart surgery. JAMA 211:1333-1340, 1970
42. Tyler DB: Psychological changes during experimental sleep deprivation. Dis Nerv Syst 16:293-299, 1955
43. Vaillant GE: Prospective prediction of schizophrenic remission. Arch Gen Psychiatry 11:509-518, 1964
44. vanPraag HM: About the impossible concept of schizophrenia. Compr Psychiatry 17:481-497, 1976
45. Ward NG, Rowlett DB, Burke P: Sodium amylobarbitone in the differential diagnosis of confusion. Am J Psychiatry 135:75-78, 1978
46. Weinstein EA, Kahn RL, Sugarmon LA, Malitz S: Serial administration of the "amytal test" for brain disease. Arch Neurol Psychiat 71:217-226, 1954
47. Weinstein EA, Kahn RL: Denial of Illness: Symbolic and Physiologic Aspects. Springfield, Illinois, C. C. Thomas, 1955
48. West LJ: A Clinical and theoretical overview of hallucinatory phenomena, in Siegel RK, West LJ (eds): Hallucinations. New York, Wiley, 1975
49. West LJ, Janszen HH, Lester BK, Cornelisoon FS Jr: The psychosis of sleep deprivation. Ann NY Acad Sci 96:66-70, 1962
50. Wolff HG, Curran D: Nature of delirium and allied states. Arch Neurol Psychiat 33: 1175-1215, 1935

Commentary

Dr. Strub has given proper emphasis to a clinical truism that is periodically rediscovered, namely that clinically identical states of acute confusion can arise from totally different etiologic agents that appear to involve different parts of the central nervous system. The remarkable similarity of the clinical state suggests a common pathophysiology, and certain features described by Dr. Strub point to specific neuroanatomic areas that are the apparent sites of malfunction. Most specifically, the altered arousal apparent in many (but not all) patients in the acute confusional state suggests malfunction of the reticular activating system indicating disturbance as low as the level of the mesencephalon.[3] Another commonly noted feature of the confusional state, inattention, is not so easily localized but, to some degree at least, suggests involvement of the posterior, inferior, medial frontal region, often called the septal area.[1] While not frequent, cases of structural pathology involving these two areas have been reported which provide some correlation with behavioral abnormality. Most cases of acute confusion seen by the clinician are not based on structural disorder, however; rather, the cause is metabolic, toxic, mechanical, or infectious and appears to affect broad areas of the brain. Nonetheless, the consistency of the clinical picture suggests that the crucial pathophysiology centers in these basal areas, producing widespread symptoms by altering the modulating and/or activating functions of these anatomic centers. While the pathophysiologic picture remains unclear, the pragmatic clinical management approach offered by Dr. Strub is of real value.

Among the many difficult and controversial disorders that fall in the borderland between psychiatry and neurology, the behavioral abnormalities seen in individuals with epilepsy have long been a problem. Psychiatric complications of epilepsy have been recognized for well over a century,[4] but they continue to challenge clinicians. In the past few years, a great deal has been written in attempts to discuss these disorders. Not only are there neurobehavioral disorders that appear to be specific for epileptic patients but these must be differentiated from other behavioral disorders occurring in these same patients such as lesion-caused behavioral alterations and psychogenic response abnormalities. The following chapter (Chapter 2) is designed to provide a base against which the symptomatology of individuals with possible epileptic behavioral complications can be evaluated. The division of epilepsy-related psychiatric symptomatology into distinct stages such as ictal, postictal and interictal has been emphasized. While overlap between the stages is common, in fact almost mandatory—particularly between the ictal and postictal and to some degree between the interictal and psychogenic—the ability to recognize the completely different psychiatric symptomatology occurring in the separate stages can aid in the total evaluation of a seizure-related psychiatric problem.

Considerable controversy has surrounded this topic for the past decade, especially concerning the question of whether a specific, pathognomonic interictal personality disturbance occurs in complex partial epilepsy. At times this controversy became heated; proponents adamantly demanded that the personality defect of epilepsy is one of the most specific of all psychiatric syndromes[2] while opponents insisted that the psychiatric abnormalities associated with chronic epilepsy were nonspecific.[5] The heat of this discussion has abated somewhat in recent years with a compromise opinion that certain behavior patterns are suggestive of an interictal epileptic state but that many epileptics do not show these features. This controversy will receive little attention in the following chapter; instead, emphasis has been given to describing the many psychiatric disturbances that are known to appear in various stages of epilepsy.

The following chapters will spotlight a number of complicated disorders related to epilepsy that are particularly vexing for the psychiatrist. While far from being an exhaustive discussion, it is hoped that these three chapters will help prepare the clinician to recognize and manage the psychiatric problems that can occur as complications of epilepsy.

REFERENCES

1. Benson DF, Geschwind N: Psychiatric conditions associated with focal lesions of the central nervous system, in Arieti S, Reiser MF (eds): American Handbook of Psychiatry, vol 4. New York, Basic Books, 1975, pp 208–243
2. Geschwind N: Behavioural changes in temporal lobe epilepsy. Psychol Med 9:217–219, 1979
3. Magoun HW: The Waking Brain. Springfield, Illinois, Thomas, 1963
4. Samt P: Epileptische Irreseinformen. Arch Psychiat 6:110–216, 1876
5. Stevens JR: Interictal clinical manifestations of complex partial seizures, in Perry JK, Daly DD (eds): Advances in Neurology, vol 11. New York, Raven, 1975

Dietrich Blumer, M.D.
D. Frank Benson, M.D.

2
Psychiatric Manifestations of Epilepsy

Whether the admittedly frequent psychiatric complications of epilepsy result directly from seizure disorder has long been a topic of controversy. Many epileptologists doubt that the psychiatric manifestations of epilepsy are specific, and they note that seizure disorders tend to be stigmatizing and frequently require toxic doses of medication. Many psychiatrists and neurologists, however, propose that some specific psychiatric disturbances are directly related to some epileptic disorders.

Through the centuries, behavioral disturbances have always been associated with epilepsy. Temkin, in his classic historic study of epilepsy "The Falling Disease"[50] actually chronicles the history of insanity and its treatment. Some ancients considered epilepsy to be a manifestation of religious significance and it has been called "the sacred disease." More often, however, the epileptic was thought to be influenced by evil spirits. As psychiatric care became more organized, epileptics were treated as insane. The great asylums of Europe always included sizeable numbers of epileptics and epileptic units can still be found in most of the psychiatric hospitals of Europe. Through the first half of the present century epilepsy was considered, along with schizophrenia and manic-depressive illness, one of the three major psychiatric disorders, and care of the epileptic patient was taught by psychiatrists in the medical schools of most countries.

In the late 19th and early 20th Century, drugs first provided some control of the seizures. The original drugs did not alter the psychiatric manifestations and, in fact, often appeared to increase the problem.

Drugs such as bromides and barbiturates, while controlling seizure activity, often proved toxic or produced a worsening of psychiatric disorders among epileptics. The epileptic remained an individual set aside because of psychiatric problems. Progress in the diagnosis of epilepsy with the development of the electroencephalogram (EEG) and the introduction of modern anticonvulsants, particularly phenytoin, which permitted good seizure control without serious behavioral side effects for a sizeable number of epileptics, allowed many epileptics to lead a comparatively normal life. Different types of seizure disorder were recognized, and "the epilepsies" became part of the neurologic specialty. A well organized social action to erase the stigma of epilepsy arose which eventually led to an outright denial of any psychiatric disturbance specifically associated with epilepsy. Most practicing epileptologists have no primary interest in psychiatry and support this view. They are correct in that many individuals with seizures can be well controlled medically and remain free of psychiatric disorder. Based on careful studies,[24,38,42] Rodin has pointed out that it is not the seizure itself but the presence or absence of intellectual limitations, of organic and other psychiatric changes, as well as of individual motivation, that represent the crucial factors in the disability of patients with epilepsy. Many patients with seizure disorders do have psychiatric problems and the nature of this relationship needs to be clarified.

Different forms of epilepsy tend to have different effects on the mind of the afflicted—or they have none at all. Infantile epileptic encephalopathy (West syndrome) and, to a lesser degree, childhood epileptic encephalopathy (Lennox-Gastaut syndrome) tend to be associated with intellectual deterioration. On the other hand, the common or primary generalized seizure disorders such as petit mal (absence attacks or grand mal (with seizures mainly within the awakening period), are uncomplicated by cerebral damage, tend to respond to anticonvulsants, and typically are not associated with significant mental changes.[28,37,40] Among the partial seizure disorders, cortical motor and sensory seizure disorders tend to be free of significant mental impairment. The complex partial seizures (CPS) originating from the limbic temporal lobe area, on the other hand, tend to be associated with psychiatric changes that vary from mild peculiarities of personality and behavior to severe and disabling mental changes, including psychosis.

All studies agree that a sizeable number of individuals with CPS have behavioral problems.[1,15,16,17] The same behavioral problems, however, were often found in control groups of generalized seizure patients.[22,36,46,47] One major problem with using "generalized seizure patients" as a control group is the difficulty in excluding temporal lobe involvement. Many seizure disorders that, on the surface, appear generalized will carry subtle signs that suggest focal involvement (history of brain damage, focal neurologic or neuroradiologic findings, focal component to the seizure, or to the EEG); while classed as generalized seizure disorders, either primary or secondary temporal involvement would carry a risk of psychiatric complications of the type attributed to CPS.

Another problem in these studies of the psychiatric complications of CPS concerns methodology. For instance, appreciation of the sexual changes associated with CPS requires specific inquiry of the patient and/or spouse. This is a simple matter, and the finding of global hyposexuality has been widely confirmed.[16,26,52] The viscosity/circumstantiality of many CPS patients is difficult to overlook if one listens to the patient. It is not an overwhelming finding in many patients, however, and can be hidden by a hurried, pressing interview. In addition, viscosity remains difficult to quantify. Similarly, the deepening of emotionality[20] cannot be appreciated unless the interviewer sensitively inquires of the patient and/or family members.

The surprising lack of definition of the emotional changes in the otherwise excellent British textbook descriptions of the psychiatric aspects of seizure disorders[33,34] is, in our opinion, methodological. In the United States, on the other hand, these psychiatric traits were not even identified for a long time and are still not widely recognized. This is due, in part, to an ignoring of European literature on the topic and partly related to a lack of competent psychiatric inquiry into the problems of seizure patients. The inventory devised by Bear[3] addresses the traits in question but experience with this particular instrument remains limited. Most well-standardized inventories used by psychologists for general psychiatric investigation (e.g., MMPI, Eysenck) have proved useless for documentation of the mental changes of CPS.

If one looks for characteristic mental changes associated with epilepsy, it cannot be a surprise that complex partial epilepsy—with its chronic excessive and irregular neuronal discharges involving the center of the limbic system—is singled out. Since the first half of the 19th century, the *ammonshorn sclerosis* has been recognized as an important pathologic finding among institutionalized persons with epilepsy.[18] In the early 1950s, Gastaut and his co-workers described specific behavioral changes among temporal lobe epileptics that were absent among generalized seizure patients and could be viewed as traits of a partial inverse Klüver-Bucy syndrome (Table 2-1).[13,15,16,17] These same traits, with the exception of global

Table 2-1
Syndrome of Temporal Hyperconnection

Hypometamorphosis	Viscosity
	Circumstantiality
	Hypergraphia
	Verbosity
Hyperemotionality	Increased emotional depth
	Irritability, anger, rage
	Emotional lability, mood swings
	Goodnatured, helpful attitude
	Sense of justice
	Religious (philosophical) interests
Hyposexuality	Decrease of sexual interest and arousal

This Table represents a partial elaboration of the behavior syndrome described by Gastaut[17]. The syndrome of temporal hyperconnection in epilepsy represents a partial inverse Klüver-Bucy syndrome. The excessive tendency to attend immediately to each new stimulus perceived (hypermetamorphosis) stands in contrast to the excessive tendency to adhere to each thought, feeling, and activity (hypometamorphosis or viscosity); tameness and lack of fear are in contrast to irritability, deepened emotionality, and excessive sexual arousal to decreased erotic and genitopelvic arousal and response.

The sometimes very sticky adherence to each particular ongoing activity, feeling, or thought *and* the deepened emotionality combine in the manifestation of heavy, prolonged (at times very ponderous) verbosity and hypergraphia.

hyposexuality, were well known to psychiatrists dealing with institutionalized seizure populations.[30] Rodin has recently shown that a more severe mental impairment is characteristic of those temporal lobe epilepsy patients who also have generalized seizures.[41] Such generalized seizures document the facilitation of spread from the focal discharge, and this factor may well play a role in the degree of expression of the mental changes. On the other hand, the personality and mental changes characteristic of CPS appear to be pronounced in the presence of bi-temporal foci, even in the absence of generalized seizures.

Personality and behavioral changes, while common among CPS patients, tend to emerge only some years after onset of the seizure disorder. The more severe psychotic disorders are far less common and, on the average, occur some 14 years after onset of epilepsy.[45] The mental effects of either focal or diffuse brain damage associated with a seizure disorder (i.e., frontal lobe damage) must be assessed separately. Similarly, the toxic or idiosyncratic effects of anticonvulsant medication on mental functions in a given individual have to be carefully distinguished from the specific mental changes of chronic seizure activity. Of greater practical and theoretical significance than the direct effect of the anticonvulsant drugs on the mental state is their indirect effect via modification of the seizure disorder.

CLASSIFICATION OF EPILEPTIC, PSYCHIC, AND BEHAVIORAL MANIFESTATIONS

The various stages in the seizure episode are of paramount importance for understanding of the psychic and the behavioral manifestations of seizures. Failure to separate the psychiatric symptomatology of the various stages is a prime source of confusion to the nonepileptologist attempting to understand the behavior of an epileptic. While there are a number of ways to classify these manifestations, for this chapter the following seizure stage categorizations will be described:

1. Prodromal manifestations
2. Ictal manifestations
    Primictal
    Amnesic
3. Postictal manifestations
4. Interictal manifestations
5. Epileptic Psychoses
    Ictal
    Postictal
    Interictal
6. Psychological response to the seizure disorder

Prodromal Manifestations

Some epileptic patients report a distinct alteration that precedes the onset of the seizure. While epileptic patients rarely complain of a prodrome spontaneously, close questioning often reveals unpleasant mental changes in a period preceding onset of the seizure. For some this prodromal feeling can last several days but for most it lasts hours or minutes. The alterations are subjective and usually vague, most often reported as feelings of moodiness, apprehension, or being "up-tight." Some describe decreased ability to concentrate, a feeling of fuzzy or clouded thinking. Increased difficulties in interpersonal relationships and everyday activities are noted; they become testy and bitchy, have disagreements with family and friends, and are unhappy with everything. An observant parent or spouse may be aware of the alterations and their implications, but the disagreeable behavior is more often interpreted as a sign of bad temper. For some patients and the next of kin, the prodromal feeling is sufficiently unpleasant that the onset of the seizure is welcomed.

Ictal Manifestations

Significant behavioral abnormalities occur with some seizures. In fact, the original name for one type of seizure—psychomotor epilepsy—implies psychic as well as motor disturbance. Several general characteristics of the ictal phase of CPS are pertinent. Most important, the seizure events, while highly variable, tend to be stereotyped for the individual patient. Few CPS patients experience identical seizure events, but for any individual the very same events tend to occur at each seizure. The stereotype of the nature and sequence of ictal events in a given patient serves to differentiate CPS from psychogenic events. A second point is the brevity of the CPS. Most are measured in seconds, to a maximum of 60–90 seconds, Only in cases of partial complex seizure status do ongoing ictal behavioral disturbances occur over a more prolonged period. Another important characteristic is that the episodes are a passive experience; the patient feels he is an observer, dissociated from the actual occurrences. This is unlike schizophrenic hallucinations which are firmly believed to be actual occurrences. A fourth significant point is that the ictal manifestations are unrelated to the environment except for rare seizures triggered by specific stimuli (e.g., musicogenic or sexual seizures). Typically, there is a sudden arrest of ongoing activities and a strange psychic experience and/or behavior ensues. Resumption of interaction with the environment, often initially in a confused status, occurs in the postictal phase. Another point is that while the type of CPS is often labeled by the reported dominant manifestation (e.g., epigastric, uncinate, visual hallucination, etc.), careful exploration often detects a remarkable wealth of experiences, recurrent with each ictus.[28] The dream-like quality of the epileptic aura encompasses many sensations (forced thinking, visual hallucinations, olfactory-gustatory sensations, etc.), all reported as distinct but undescribable experiences, like an ever fleeting dream.

Finally, a CPS typically consists of an initial, remembered portion, the aura or primictal event, and an amnestic portion. The aura is not a warning but is the initial phase of the actual seizure; it may serve to warn of impending loss of consciousness or generalized seizure. The observable part of the CPS is, almost invariably, not recalled by the patient. Although many patients never experience an aura, the complete recording of seizure events requires that the subjective report of the patient be added to objective accounts of observers. The amnestic period persists beyond the seizure discharge and into the postictal phase; indeed, it may last beyond the confusional portion. Thus, "automatic behavior," the carrying out of routine activities for which there is no recall (cf. Jackson's Dr. Z[49]), may be seen.

The general rules concerning CPS noted above are actually of more value for recognizing seizure disorders than the listing of subjective and objective seizure events that follows.

Primictal (Aura) Seizure Events

In this phase of the seizure, which corresponds to the electrographic onset, the patient is aware of what is happening. Seizures may begin without a primictal stage, but more than half of CPS begin with an aura. It is beyond the scope of this chapter to list all varieties of aura; the most common, particularly those with psychiatric connotations, will be mentioned.

Hallucinations, illusions, and other misperceptions. Misperceptions are common manifestations of CPS and may be mistaken as signs of schizophrenia or of a delirious state. The hallucinations may be visual and may consist of complex scenes appearing with each attack in a recurrent stereotyped fashion. They may be auditory, e.g., the patient may hear his own name called or some specific yet undefinable melody. A breath of wind (the original aura) or the sensation of someone brushing past may be experienced. Sudden dizziness or a feeling of motion may be accompanied by a supple turning of the head or body. Illusions such as seeing objects or persons enlarged (macropsia), smaller (micropsia), removed at a distance (peleopsia), or closer up (poropsia) may occur.

Highly characteristic is the paroxysmal occurrence of olfactory-gustatory hallucinations—the patient may experience repeated fleeting sensations of the same distinct yet undescribable odor or taste. The most common aura, a peculiar epigastric sensation is similarly unmistakable; it is described by patients, although never precisely, as a rising upwards followed by loss of consciousness. The latter two types of digestive or crude sensations[27] are particularly likely to be associated with the experience of a dreamy state.

Altered awareness and mood—the dreamy state. The aura or primictal experience of the dreamy state was well described by H. Jackson over 100 years ago.[27] It consists of a peculiar, fleeting change of perception, thinking, and mood—the sudden, strange familiarity with something unfamiliar (*déjà-vu*) and opposite experience (*jamais-vu*) are well known examples. *Déjà vu* is a common phenomenon among healthy individuals, but both the intensity of the experience and the admixture of other seizure events distinguish the ictal phenomenon. Peculiar hallucinations, illusions, and body sensations occur and are reported as dream-like experiences upon regaining normal awareness.

The mood change of the dreamy state is always described as having a sudden onset and being out of context with the situation. It is frequently reported as a peculiar apprehension or sadness. Experiences of elation and anger occur more rarely. The fear many patients experience at the onset of each seizure is not the rational fear of the impending loss of consciousness or convulsion but rather a direct psychic effect of the seizure discharge.

Amnesic Seizure Behavior

About one third of patients with CPS do not experience an aura and thus are amnesic for the entire seizure. Some may remain unaware that they suffered a lapse or realize that a seizure took place only because of an aftermath (e.g., headache, sore mouth). The majority experience an amnesic state following the aura and will know that a seizure took place, although many may be unaware of the period of lost consciousness. The observable events of the CPS, as a rule, are not recalled by the patients and are now listed in our sketch of the amnesic part of the CPS. The very first observation of a CPS is arrest of ongoing activity including speech.

Visceral automatisms. Almost pathognomonic for CPS are the observations of brief oral automatisms such as lip smacking, licking, chewing, and swallowing. Tongue, lip, or cheek bites may occur with such CPS, not just with generalized attacks. There may be choking or even vomiting. In a few patients, accelerated, slowed, or arrested respiratory movements may be noted, and cyanosis of the lips or entire face can be observed.

Motor alterations. A blank stare is often noted, caused by a widening of the interpalpebral fissures. A supple turning of eyes, head, or trunk may take place. Repetitive motion such as scratching, rubbing, stamping, or kicking occur and, like the events of the ictal phase in general, are not related to the environment. Clonic movements are not characteristic for CPS, but tonic changes occur fairly often; these are observed as grimacing, spasms of the upper extremities, or even as generalized tonic innervation. On the other hand, the attacks may be associated with a loss of muscle tone and falling.

Speech utterances. Various dysphasic manifestations can be observed, usually with discharge in the dominant temporal lobe, while stereotyped utterances (such as: "I am getting sick," or "help, help, help") tend to occur with foci in the nondominant temporal lobe. Laughter or merely a smile may be observed in the course of a CPS.

Autonomic manifestations. Psychic, sensory, and motor phenomena of the CPS are almost always associated with some or a rich variety of autonomic changes. Pupillary dilatation (or constriction), pallor (or flushing) of the face, salivation, sweating, tachycardia, hypertension, gastrointestinal motility changes, and incontinence of urine and rarely of feces can all be observed as parts of a CPS, with the individual patient displaying his own characteristic pattern with each attack.

Postictal Behavioral Manifestations

In the postictal state, a wide variety of abnormal behavioral activities can occur that may be subtle or may be misinterpreted as psychotic, hysteric, or otherwise deviant behavior. If the aura is not followed by loss of consciousness, there may be no postictal phase whatsoever. If loss of consciousness occurs with the CPS, then a postictal phase follows. The postictal phase is usually more prolonged than the preceding phase, lasting perhaps 2-10 minutes and rarely as long as 1 hour. While the ictal phase, whose duration is measured in seconds rather than minutes, may easily go unnoticed, the unusual behavior of the postictal phase cannot escape attention. The striking psychomotor automatisms described as characteristic for psychomotor seizures are often postictal manifestations.

Janz has emphasized that there tends to be a clear clinical difference between ictal and postictal events.[28] The stereotyped sequence of events of the seizure proper is passively experienced by the patient, who is not relating to his surroundings. In the postictal phase, the patient carries out more appropriate activities and gradually becomes better able to relate to his surroundings. The passive stare of the ictal phase ceases as the eyes begin to scan in the postictal phase. Electographic evidence from telemetry and depth electrode studies, however, suggest that seizure discharges may extend into what is traditionally judged to be the postictal phase. A clear border is often difficult to draw between the two phases.

Simple, relatively stereotyped, and repetitive acts are characteristic for the early portion of the postictal phase. More complex activities may follow (such as disrobing, shining shoes, unpacking, packing away, and singing). The third portion of the postictal phase is clearly aimed at reorientation and, during this stage, the interaction with the surroundings becomes appropriate. There are striking instances when a patient can carry out, for perhaps 10 minutes, entirely appropriate routine activities, following a perhaps imperceptible ictal phase and yet without recollecting what has been done (cf. Jackson's Dr. Z[27]). Such wondrous "automatisms" simply indicate that the postictal amnesia outlasted the confusional phase.

Older people, in whom the capacity to remember may be weakened, appear particularly vulnerable to protracted postictal amnesia. The more severe the seizure discharge, the more marked the memory lapse—it is plausible that with bi-temporal involvement this lapse will be more protracted. A series of seizures occurring at short intervals may produce a very prolonged amnesia, covering entire days.

Typically, there is an initial retrograde amnesia following a CPS. This amnesia shrinks fairly promptly as the patient regains orientation and begins to recall what happened before the attack—except for a variably brief, permanent retrograde memory gap. The postictal period of amnesia does not disappear, as memorizing did not take place during that phase.

Complex Postictal Behavior and its Differential Diagnosis

Postictal automatisms. Postictal automatisms include activities performed in an amnestic state, and differentiating between this epileptic postictal state and the psychogenic dissociative reaction can be difficult. One long-standing rule of thumb concerns a difference in duration. Most postictal automatisms are of short duration, usually measured in minutes, while most psychogenic dissociative reactions last considerably longer—a period of approximately 1 hour has been suggested as a dividing line. This is obviously not an absolute distinction. More important may be the question of motive: Psychogenic dissociative reactions can be understood within the patient's personal environment, while postictal automatisms are either harmless, routine activities or consist of senseless deviant behavior. Decisive for the diagnosis is the presence or absence of a relationship to a documentable seizure typical for the individual.

Temporal lobe status. In differentiating an epileptic state from a dissociative reaction, one needs to consider the possibility of an ongoing ictal state. Temporal lobe status,[11] a series of CPS without recovery from the postictal state before the next seizure takes place, can lead to a prolonged state of incoherent and peculiar activities. This entity is rare but should be kept in mind if one encounters an epileptic patient with sudden onset of unresponsiveness, incoherent behavior, and confusion that is interspersed with repetitive and stereotyped manifestations of CPS (e.g., oral automatisms or verbal utterances).

Continuous aura. A milder form of temporal lobe status in which consciousness and recollection are not lost is the phenomenon of a continuous aura;[44] this is probably less rare than the more severe temporal lobe seizure status. In both conditions, EEG recordings clarify the diagnosis, and treatment with increased doses of anticonvulsants is indicated.

Poriomania. A related disorder has been termed poriomania.[19,35] This is a state in which an epileptic patient can wander for hours, days, or even weeks while sufficiently abiding by society's rules so that his activities are not recognized as related to a seizure disorder. The patient "suddenly awakens" in a strange place, having lost hours or days, without any notion of how he had traveled or what he had done. Although the similarity of this state to a psychogenic dissociative reaction is remarkable, the actions in poriomania lack psychologic motivation and an epileptic basis can be established. Poriomania is rare, much less frequent than dissociative reactions. Gastaut was able to document the presence of consecutive, independent bi-temporal discharges separated by 5- to 10-minute intervals at a time of appropriate responses for which there was no recollection in a woman who, at an earlier date, had experienced an amnestic fugue of 30 days duration.[14,19]

Postictal Violence—Ictal and Interictal Explosive Behavior

One of the most frequently discussed aspects of epilepsy is its association with violent, explosive behavior. Anger is not a common primictal emotion, and only rare cases have been documented of patients who display an aggressive and threatening attitude at the time of their seizure. As a rule—and point of legal importance—there is no interaction with the surroundings at the time of the seizure, and *ictal violent behavior,* to the best of current knowledge, cannot be attributed a role in destructive acts against property or persons.

It is generally accepted that *violence with amnesia* may occur in the *postictal* phase. If a patient is forcibly restrained while in a confused state following a seizure, he may attempt to fight his way out and someone may be injured. It is advisable not to restrain a patient at all in the postictal phase or, if necessary, to hold him back very gently should he move towards an area of risk. Postictal violence is infrequent and rarely appears to be a forensic issue.[23,29] Amnesia, the lack of any motive for the act, and the relationship to a seizure typical for the individual must all be established for such cases.[51] Alleging that a seizure is the cause of an act of violence appears to be less popular in court proceedings nowadays.

Interictal explosive behavior and irritability are common phenomena in seizure patients with temporal lobe involvement. Although this type of episodic behavior is generally not of legal significance and is usually relatively harmless, it can produce hardship within the family. It is usually precipitated, although often by rather minor irritants, is not associated with amnesia, and is followed by remorse on the part of the patient. This behavior is further described in the following section on interictal phenomena.

Postictal Sexual Arousal—Sexual Seizures

An occasional patient with CPS will confide that he experiences sexual arousal for a short interval, perhaps 10–15 minutes after a seizure. Intercourse is consummated if the spouse is available, there is no amnesia for the event, and there is nothing unusual about the happening except that it is triggered by the passage of a CPS. This *postictal sexual arousal* seems to be peculiar for some patients with CPS who are moderately hyposexual during the interictal period.[8]

Seizures with components of sexual arousal, such as an aura of orgasmic feeling or the pelvic motions of intercourse with vaginal discharge, have been documented in the literature. *Ictal sexual arousal* is associated with other subjective or objective seizure events and tends to be triggered by sexual stimuli and arousal. This latter phenomenon probably explains why intercourse can trigger a generalized seizure in the rare patient.[7]

Global hyposexuality of the interictal phase is a common phenomenon in contrast to the ictal and postictal sexual arousal.

Interictal Behavior Manifestations

The buildup of excessive neuronal activity to a CPS paroxysm and its aftermath is associated with the enormous and often confusing variety of mental and behavioral features we have tried to describe. Between clinical seizure periods, the epileptogenic focus responsible for the CPS is not dormant. An EEG usually reveals some signs of persistent subclinical seizure activity localized to the general area of the medial aspects of one or both of the temporal lobes. We assume that this chronic excessive neuronal activity in the centers of the limbic system is responsible for the important psychiatric changes that can be documented in patients with CPS and among seizure patients with secondary temporal lobe involvement. Once this process has been established for a couple of years[5,9,13,16] and is of at least moderate severity, a hyperconnection syndrome[2] of varying degrees can develop. This syndrome is the opposite of the typical major behavioral changes of the Klüver-Bucy syndrome that have been described as a temporal disconnection syndrome (Table 2-1). The changes observed with CPS of some severity and duration are then specific and related to the basic neural changes. Some of these behavioral alterations may be rather subtle and require both a careful inquiry from the patient and the next-of-kin and an understanding of what areas need to be explored. More severe changes of a psychotic degree may appear after an average of perhaps 15 years after onset of the epilepsy and become manifest in a much smaller percentage of the patients with CPS.

While the mental and behavioral changes surrounding the seizure tend to come to the attention of neurologists, the interictal changes, if marked, are often directed to the attention of psychiatrists. The more subtle interictal personality and behavioral changes of patients with CPS tend to be overlooked upon routine neurologic examination and it may merely be noted that such patients are *peculiar*. In view of the highly focused training and interest of the modern neurologist who cares for these patients, it cannot be a surprise that the interictal personality and behavioral changes of CPS have been so widely ignored even though they represent one of the most characteristic syndromes of clinical psychiatry.[5,20]

In an attempt to investigate interictal emotional and behavioral changes, David Bear reviewed the world literature on CPS, noting specifically all reports of psychiatric changes and, from these, produced a list of 18 separate behavioral abnormalities associated with seizures.[3] A special inventory concerning these changes was constructed and given to patients with well-documented temporal lobe seizure foci; their relatives were also asked to complete an identical inventory concerning the patient.[4] Abnormal responses to the items tended to be significantly more frequent among the patients with CPS than in two matched control groups. It was also noted that patients with right temporal lobe foci had a tendency to deny negative behavior (e.g., outbursts of anger), a point that was made clear when the patients' inventories were compared to those completed by their relatives. On the other hand, the self-report of patients with left temporal lobe foci corresponded closely to the description given by their relatives. The right temporal lobe seizure patients thus tended to improve ("polish") the description of their behavioral activities while the left temporal lobe patients tended to be bluntly honest in their responses ("tarnishers").

The interictal behavioral and personality changes detailed by Bear as 18 separate traits can be lumped together and described under three major categories: the sexual changes; the viscosity (or circumstantiality); and the deepened emotionality. These three categories correspond to the three major traits of the Temporal Hyperconnection Syndrome (Partial Inverse Klüver-Bucy Syndrome) listed in Table 2-1. The sexual changes are the most easily understood and least controversial and will be described before the more complex traits listed as hypometamorphosis (viscosity-circumstantiality) and deepened (or hyper-) emotionality.

Hyposexuality.

Perhaps a majority of patients with temporal lobe epilepsy develop a global hyposexuality characterized by lack of interest in sexual matters and rare genital arousal.[7,9,16] This hyposexuality is a primary phenomenon if onset of CPS occurred before or at the time of sexual maturation, and is secondary if onset of CPS occurs later. The trait is more easily ascertained if it develops in the male since sexual arousal can be normally absent in many females if they do not have a mate. The early onset hyposexual patient is not bothered by the lack of interest and arousal, but for patients with a late onset of seizures, the ensuing hyposexuality may be a troubling matter. On rare occasions, CPS patients may develop a deviation of their sexual interest, such as homosexual trends, fetishism, or transvestism, usually with decreased frequency of genital arousal.[9]

It is incorrect to blame anticonvulsant medication for the hyposexuality. Rather, with sufficient control of the seizure activity by medication, a revival of sexual interest and genital arousal may occur. The same phenomenon can be observed, sometimes dramatically, weeks or even months after successful unilateral temporal lobectomy. The postictal sexual arousal described earlier, which is noted in some patients who are moderately hyposexual between seizures, is probably best understood as a release phenomenon which occurs after clearing of the inhibitory seizure discharges.

Hyposexuality is not a social problem and often escapes medical attention. However, this trait leads to further social isolation of many persons with epilepsy (particularly those of the male sex) who do not feel compelled to seek sexual companionship and tend to remain single.

Hypometamorphosis (Viscosity-Circumstantiality)

Hypometamorphosis, the opposite trend to the hypermetamorphosis of the Klüver-Bucy syndrome, denotes a decreased trend to change over to something new. To some, viscosity (adhesiveness or stickiness) denotes this trend in the behavioral sphere, while circumstantiality refers to the verbal manifestation of the same trait. Viscosity was formerly considered by many to be the core trait of the so-called epileptic personality but it is, rather, a characteristic trait of CPS or of temporal lobe involvement in patients with apparent generalized seizure disorder.

Patients who are viscous proceed laboriously and emphatically in their activities and speech and are bent on clarifying every detail. Their stream of conversation is not only excessive but appears incoherent, branching away from the direct line of thought—yet, if given sufficient time, they will stubbornly get back to and complete the original thought. Their talk is overinclusive, includes excessive background detailing, precise times, and other nonessentials. Thus, a simple question may prompt a lengthy and circuitous discussion before the answer is finally given. They tend to be verbose and have a marked difficulty terminating a conversation; as a result, they are often shunned. Most busy physicians find this behavior totally unacceptable and routinely interrupt during an apparently meaningless circumlocution, and therefore misinterpret the patient's verbal output as confused or even psychotic. Some more knowledgeable clinicians contend that they can recognize the temporal lobe epileptic by his intense and prolonged handshake.

As a corollary of the described verbosity, *hypergraphia* has been noted as a not infrequent occurrence in the interictal period of patients with CPS.[53] Some patients with CPS keep voluminous notes (filling a spiral notebook every 7 to 10 days) and detailed logs of their health, including time of seizures, timing and exact dosage of medications, and time of bowel movements, etc. They may even write books or articles on the experiences of an epileptic. They may write many long and detailed letters to Congressmen, ministers, their physicians, and important figures in the news, etc. Most of these letters are never mailed but most clinicians and newsworthy individuals have received such letters. Some patients are more literary and will write novels or nonfiction works covering ponderous subjects. Many attempt to write poetry, and detailed diaries are frequently kept. The tendency toward circumstantiality, overinclusiveness, and overdetailing in verbal output is matched by the same quality in the written output. Many CPS patients with marked verbal circumstantiality do not write at all, however, possibly reflecting a lower educational level.

We know of no drug that improves viscosity, and even successful surgical removal of an epileptogenic focus, with full control of seizures and normalization of the EEG, does not seem to appreciably lessen this trait.[52] In some patients, however, viscosity can be overcome, at least to a degree, by gentle insistence and by educating the patient to a more expedient form of verbal exchange. Of therapeutic importance is the fact that intelligent patients can be confronted with their communication problems, once a good rapport is present, and learn to be more to the point and therefore more socially acceptable.[6] It is possible that patients with epileptogenic foci that primarily involve the left temporal lobe tend to be more self-critical and therefore more willing to accept criticism from others while patients with right temporal foci tend to deny their difficulties[4] and are less open towards confrontation with problem traits such as viscosity.

Deepened Emotionality

The detail-bound and long-winded manner of speech of many temporal lobe epileptics tends to be heavily laden with emotional emphasis and often assumes a ponderous characteristic. The increased depth of emotionality, in fact, appears to contribute to the viscosity in that every detail tends to become overly important.

We consider the core feature of this deepened emotionality to be the hyperethical attitude commonly found among temporal lobe epileptics. Issues of right or wrong are central to them at all times; nothing can be taken too lightly, and sobriety prevails. The patients tend to fluctuate between a highly good-natured, helpful, often hyperreligious attitude and briefer episodes of heightened anger, moodiness, or explosiveness in the form of intense verbalized anger and threatened physical violence. These negative phases are soon followed by return of the good-natured attitude with much remorse—or, in other patients, with denial of their own negative behavior.[48] Some patients maintain a good-natured attitude throughout and others display explosive behavior only very rarely; however, many patients tend to fluctuate markedly between the opposite poles. One cannot understand temporal lobe epilepsy patients unless one understands this basic conflict. The writings of Dostoevsky, the most famous temporal lobe epilepsy sufferer, consistently reflect this polarity between good and evil, crime and punishment, the saint and the murderer. The contrast strikes some observers as hypocritical, as Freud has noted.[12] In our opinion, both poles of the personality are genuine and the good-natured side usually tends to be prevalent. It is due to their angry outbursts, however, that these patients lose friends, become at times intolerable to their families, and may be admitted to a psychiatric unit.[32,43]

In young patients with CPS, one may find a rapid cycling of mood with shifts from lows to highs within hours, a peculiarity of mood which is poorly documented in the literature. The younger the patient, the more pronounced the episodes of anger tend to be. In older patients with CPS, depression often becomes a predominant problem; suicide occurs significantly more often among patients with CPS, and this is perhaps most frequent when the seizures have become well controlled.[28] Hermann and Stevens have correctly pointed out how often depression is overlooked and suggest that depression and anxiety may be the most prevalent psychiatric changes among patients with CPS.[26] We consider both types of changes to be phenomena of the hyperemotionality of the patient with CPS. A heightened sensitivity, to the point of paranoid ideation, may appear in some patients with CPS and must be added to this group of symptoms.

In children in particular, a reduction of anticonvulsants allowing more seizures may be necessary at times to reduce their irritability. Carbamazepine may have an emotionally calming effect, and in some patients it can reduce an undesirable irritability to tolerable levels. The additional use of neuroleptics may be necessary, perhaps only at times of heightened irritability.

Episodic mood changes in epilepsy patients have been well-described since Kraepelin.[30] They consist of dysphoric episodes lasting for hours or days,[6] characterized by a fairly distinct onset of a brooding, tense, and irritable demeanor. A marked sensitivity that may reach paranoid proportions may be noted. The episodes may terminate with a clinical seizure, often followed by exemplary (and remorseful) behavior. The episodes of mood change often become more prevalent when the incidence of seizures has abated.

The episodic mood changes may merely represent accentuations of the characteristic "two-faced" personality of patients with CPS. On the other hand, they are akin to, and may be precursors of, the more severe disturbances that are labeled *intermittent psychoses*.

Epileptic Psychoses

Psychotic complications of seizure disorders will be handled in detail in Chapter 4 and will be mentioned only briefly here. The classification of psychoses associated with epilepsy dates back to Landolt and is still useful (Table 2-2). A psychosis following a flurry of seizures was a common occurrence in the past. This *postictal psychosis* was characterized by a brief lucid interval of 12–24 hours between a series of seizures and the onset of a delirious state that could last for days or as long as a couple of weeks. Since more effective anticonvulsants have become available, the postictal psychosis has become rare. Treatment is that of a delirious state and may often require antipsychotic medication.[6]

In modern times, the much more common psychosis associated with epilepsy is the *schizophrenia-like psychosis*.[45] This psychosis is characterized by a clear state of consciousness and occurs interictally; it sometimes terminates with a seizure and often, perhaps in a third of the cases, occurs at times when seizures have been controlled (*alternating psychosis*).[6,10,25,28] These psychoses usually commence after many years (average of 14) of epilepsy, usually with temporal lobe involvement, and may show any of the symptoms of schizophrenia except that the basic personality is not schizoid. Thus, the emotional state is not flat but tends to be rather intense, and the rapport that the patient can establish remains surprisingly intact. The schizophrenia-like psychosis develops in individuals who have a greater or lesser degree of the interictal personality and mood changes of the temporal lobe epileptic. The course may be intermittent or chronic, but without the deterioration that can be observed in schizophrenics.

Treatment of the schizophrenia-like state may consist of carbamazepine and/or antipsychotic drugs. If the psychosis is alternating in type, e.g., occurring upon the introduction of a more effective anticonvulsant, then the particular drug should be discontinued; other anticonvulsant drugs may have to be reduced. On occasion, after a careful assessment of all the factors involved, the anticonvulsant medication may be stopped to allow for recurrence of seizures and remission of the psychosis. Rarely, one or a few treatments with electroconvulsive therapy (ECT) may

Table 2-2
Psychoses in Epilepsy

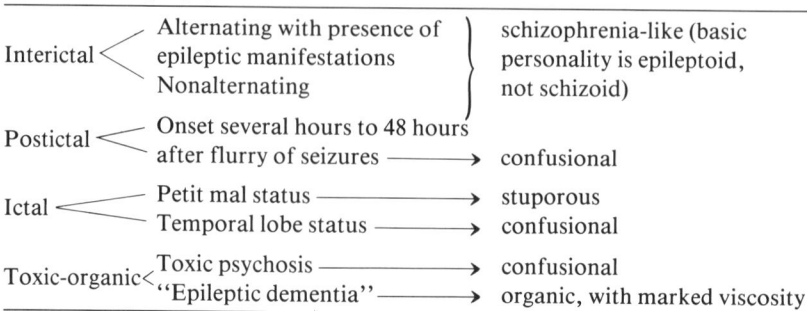

To Landolt's original classification[31] we have added the temporal lobe status, a diagnosis which is rarely made. Postictal psychoses (postepileptic twilight states) were common as long as effective anticonvulsants were not available. The interictal psychoses have become better known with the era of modern anticonvulsants and may be either spontaneous or iatrogenic (occurring when sizure control is achieved by medication).

---

be employed in order to resolve the psychosis with artificially induced seizures.

Toxic psychosis or an epileptic dementia can occur. The former is transient, while the latter consists of a progressive deterioration of intellectual capacity in epileptics who suffer from frequent, severe, poorly controlled seizures and consume large doses of anticonvulsant medication. There is usually evidence of structural brain damage, either congenital, developmental or acquired, plus a history of many major seizures and prolonged periods of hypoxia. This combination alone can produce dementia but it includes the additional complication of a polypharmacy of strong anticonvulsant medications, often at or above toxic levels in a valiant attempt to control the multiple seizures. Fortunately, modern surgical and pharmaceutical treatments have greatly decreased the number of patients that suffer epileptic dementia.

The stuporous state of a *petit-mal status* (spike-wave stupor), which sometimes lasts for hours, has been listed among the psychoses associated with epilepsy[31] but is a rather distinct entity. More difficult to differentiate is *temporal lobe status*.[28] This entity has been discussed above. Both conditions are characterized by distinct EEG abnormalities and characteristic mental pictures.

Pseudoseizures ("Hysteroepilepsy")

Hysterical seizures are a frequent occurrence among individuals with epileptic seizures. CPS only rarely occurs on a hysterical basis, thus hysterical episodes most often need to be differentiated from generalized tonic-clonic seizures. Rodin has discussed the differential diagnosis of genuine and hysterical seizures, emphasizing the clinical importance of the ocular changes at the time of the attack.[39] Even in patients with clearly hysterical attacks, one must suspect the presence of some form of a genuine seizure disorder. We have frequently found a history of rape or sexual abuse among women with severe hysterical seizures, and this may be a significant finding.

Treatment of the hysterical attacks is that of benign neglect with focus on the emotional and interpersonal difficulties. Not infrequently, the situation demands that treatment take place in a psychiatric unit. If anticonvulsants are increased on the basis of an incorrect diagnosis, a toxic state may result with slowing of the EEG and increased primitive-hysterical manifestations.[37] The EEG often cannot be validly reassessed for a month following withdrawal from anticonvulsants as barbiturate withdrawal is associated with abnormal findings. Patients with concomitant genuine seizure disorder need to be continued on appropriate doses of anticonvulsants.

The differential diagnosis of hysteroepilepsy includes postictal automatism, poriomania based on seizure activity in the temporal lobes, and dissociative reaction (discussed above).

Psychologic Response to the Seizure Disorder

Any chronic illness is bound to have a significant impact on the patient, and the effect of the seizure disorder on a given patient may be profound. An individual, constantly aware that he may suddenly awaken on the sidewalk or in an office or shop, surrounded by concerned and excited onlookers, lives in a state of constant apprehension. The prospect of episodes of odd and embarrassing comportment may be difficult to bear, particularly during the early phase of the disease. We know of patients with CPS who made serious suicide attempts at the time when their previously unnoticed seizures had become a public embarrassment. Patients adjust, and most learn to deal with their handicap in a realistic and commendable manner. This adjustment, however, is bound to be difficult; many patients with epilepsy have been treated as if they were "different" since their school days, and many find their employment opportunities restricted.

Paradoxically, the arrest of seizures in individuals with chronic temporal lobe seizure disorders brings about a period of risk in some patients at a much later stage in their life. As discussed above, there is an increased risk for psychosis with better seizure control. The incidence of suicide is also heightened at this time,[28] a fact that may be ascribed partly to the change of suddenly having to live *without* a recognized handicap and partly to the deepening of a depressed state secondary to the absence of convulsions (i.e., the loss of ECT effect).

It is not only the seizures but also the mental changes specifically found in patients with CPS that often lead to social isolation. These patients are fundamentally friendly, emotional, and highly ethical people, but their emotional intensity and overemphatic and overconscientious manner of conversing may not be easily tolerated by others. Also, because of their recurrent irritable moods they may be shunned or choose to avoid social contact themselves. They may feel more intensely about religious matters than the other parishioners (or even the pastor) or they may choose to keep their thoughts about God and the universe to themselves. The reduced sexual interest favors another type of isolation which causes patients to avoid intimate contact with the opposite sex. In psychosis, the isolation becomes most manifest, even though the patient may maintain a remarkable ability to reach out for contact with a friendly human being.

Individuals with the traits characteristic for epilepsy with temporal lobe involvement need to have their unique difficulties understood, particularly on the part of family members and members of the helping professions. They often require more friendly patience than is commonly afforded. Efforts at re-education for viscosity may have to be undertaken. Obviously, the maintenance of family ties and the development of job opportunities are of considerable importance for the well-being of these patients.

CONCLUSION

It has been almost customary to begin a discussion of the psychiatric complications of epilepsies with a prolonged list of the various mental and behavioral deviations previously noted among epileptics, as if to ridicule any effort at establishing a meaningful correlation of these traits.

The high incidence of such complications among relatively chronic epileptics has been well-established, even by critical investigators.[22,46,47] The findings demand careful analysis; simplifications such as blaming the complications on "chronic illness" or simply on the stigma associated with epilepsy are ill-advised. It is possible to relate specific changes among patients with temporal lobe seizure involvement to the *temporal hyperconnection syndrome,* and careful clinical study documents rather unique findings. The deepened emotional response characteristic for this syndrome can best explain why, in addition to the highly characteristic changes described, we find among these patients an accentuation of the entire range of human eccentricities such as sensitivity, selfishness, paranoid trends, phobias, hypomania, hypochondriasis, with depression and anxiety foremost. The psychiatric manifestations of epilepsy are multiple and complex, and only careful analysis will lead to demonstration of remediable problems. This must become a major goal for epilepsy management in the future.

REFERENCES

1. Alstrom CH: A study of epilepsy in its chemical, social and genetic aspects. Acta Psychiatr Scand [Supple]63:1–284, 1950
2. Bear D: Temporal lobe epilepsy: A syndrome of sensory-limbic hyperconnection. Cortex 15:357–384, 1979
3. Bear DM: The temporal lobes: An approach to the study of organic behavioral changes, in Gazzaniga M (ed): Handbook of Behavioral Neurobiology—Neuropsychology. New York, Plenum, 1979
4. Bear DM, Fedio P: Quantitative analysis of interictal behavior in temporal lobe epilepsy. Arch Neurol 34:454–467, 1977
5. Blumer D: Temporal lobe epilepsy and its psychiatric significance, in Benson DF, Blumer D (eds): Psychiatric Aspects of Neurologic Disease. New York, Grune & Stratton, 1975
6. Blumer D: Treatment of patients with seizure disorders referred because of psychiatric complications. McLean Hosp J (Special Issue), pp 53–73, 1977
7. Blumer D, Walker AE: The neural basis of sexual behavior, in Benson DF and Blumer D (eds): Psychiatric Aspects of Neurologic Disease. New York, Grune & Stratton, 1975
8. Blumer D: Hypersexual episodes in temporal lobe epilepsy. Am J Psychiatry 126:1099–1106, 1970
9. Blumer D, Walker AE: Sexual behavior in temporal lobe epilepsy. Arch Neurol 16:37–43, 1967
10. Bruens JH: Psychoses in epilepsy, in Magnus O, De Haas AML (eds): The Epilepsies. Handbook of Clinical Neurology, vol 15. Amsterdam, North-Holland, 1974, pp 593–610
11. Engel J Jr, Ludwig BI, Fetell M: Prolonged partial complex status epilepticus: EEG and behavioral complications. Neurology 28:863–869, 1978
12. Freud S: Dostoevsky and parricide (1928). Strachey E (ed), Standard Edition vol 21. London, Hogarth, 1965
13. Gastaut H, Morin G, Lesèvre N: Etude du comportement des épileptiques psychomoteurs dans l'intervalle de leurs crises: les troubles de l'activité globale et de la sociabilite. Ann Med Psychol 113:1–27, 1955
14. Gastaut H, Roger J, Roger A: Sur la signification de certaines fugues épileptiques. A propos d'une observation électroclinique d'étal de mal temporal. Rev Neurol (Paris) 94:298–301, 1956

15. Gastaut H, Roger J, Lesèvre N: Différenciation psychologique des épileptiques en fonction des formes électrocliniques de leur maladie. Rev de Psychol Appl 3:237–249, 1953
16. Gastaut H, Collomb H: Etude de comportement sexual chez les epileptiques psychomoteurs. Annales Medico-Psychologiques 112:657–696, 1954
17. Gastaut H: Interprétation des symptômes de l'épilepsie "psychomotrice" en fonction des données de la physiologie rhinencéphalique. Presse Med 62:1535–1537, 1954
18. Gastaut H: Etat actuel des connaissances sur l'anatomie pathologique des épilepsies. Acta Neurol Et Psychiat Belg 56:5–20, 1956
19. Gastaut H, Vigoureux M: Electro-clinical correlations in 500 cases of psychomotor seizures, in Baldwin M, Bailey P (eds): Temporal Lobe Epilepsy. Springfield, Illinois, Thomas, 1958
20. Geschwind N: Behavioral changes in temporal lobe epilepsy. Psychol Med 9:217–219, 1979
21. Gibbs FA: Ictal and nonictal psychiatric disorders in temporal lobe epilepsy. J Nerv Ment Dis 113:522–528, 1951
22. Guerrant J, Anderson WN, Fischer A, et al: Personality in Epilepsy. Springfield, Illinois, Thomas, 1962
23. Gunn J: Epileptics in Prison. London, Academic Press, 1977
24. Hakkarainen H: Rehabilitation of patients with epilepsy. Acta Univ Oul, D5, Neurol, 1, 1973
25. Helmchen H: Reversible psychic disorders in epileptic patients, in Birkmayer W (ed): Epileptic Seizures—Behavior—Pain. Bern-Stuttgart-Vienna, Huber, 1976, pp 175–186
26. Hermann BP, Stevens JR: Interictal behavioral correlates of the epilepsies, in Hermann BP (ed): A Multidisciplinary Handbook of Epilepsy. Springfield, Illinois, Thomas, 1980, pp 272–307
27. Jackson JH: On a particular variety of epilepsy ("intellectual aura"): One case with symptoms of organic brain disease, in Taylor J (ed): Selected Writings of John Hughlings Jackson, vol 1. London, Staples, 1958, pp 399–405
28. Janz D: Die Epilepsien. Stuttgart, G. Thieme, 1969
29. Knox SJ: Epileptic automatism and violence. Med Sci Law 8:96–104, 1968
30. Kraepelin E: Psychiatrie. Leipzig, Verlag von Johann Ambrosius Barth, 1909
31. Landolt H: Die Temporallappenepilepsie und ihre Psychopathologie. Bibl Psychiat Neurol (Basel) 112:451, 454, 459, 462, 1960
32. Liddel DW: Observations on epileptic automatism in a mental hospital population. J Ment Sci 99:732–748, 1953
33. Lishman AW: Organic Psychiatry. Oxford, Blackwell, 1978
34. Mayer-Gross W, Slater E, Roth M: Clinical Psychiatry, ed. 3. London, Baillière, Tindall and Cassell, 1969
35. Mayeux R, Benson DF, Alexander M, et al: Poriomania. Neurology 29:1616–1619, 1979
36. Mignone RJ, Donnelly EF, Sadowsky P: Psychomotor and non-psychomotor epileptics. Epilepsia 11:345–359, 1970
37. Niedermeyer E: The Generalized Epilepsies. Springfield, Illinois, C. C. Thomas, 1972

38. Rodin E: The Prognosis of Patients with Epilepsy. Springfield, Illinois, Thomas, 1968
39. Rodin E: Psychosocial management of patients with complex partial seizures. Adv Neurol 11:383-414, 1975
40. Rodin E: Psychiatric disorders associated with epilepsy. Psychiatr Clin North Am 1(1):101-115, 1978
41. Rodin EA, Katz M, Lennox D: Difference between patients with temporal lobe seizures and those with other forms of epileptic attacks. Epilepsia 17:313-320, 1976
42. Rodin E, Rennick P, Dennerll R, et al: Vocational and educational problems of epileptic patients. Epilepsia 13:149-160, 1972
43. Roger A, Dongier M: Corrélations électrocliniques chez 50 épileptiques internés. Rev Neurol (Paris) 83:593-596, 1950
44. Scott JS, Masland RL: Occurrence of "continuous symptoms" in epileptic patients. Neurology 3:297-301, 1953
45. Slater E, Beard AW, Glithero J: The schizophrenia-like psychoses of epilepsy. Br J Psychiatry 109:95-150, 1963
46. Small JG, Small IF, Hayden MP: Further psychiatric investigations of patients with temporal and nontemporal lobe epilepsy. Am J Psychiatry 123:303-310, 1966
47. Stevens JR: Psychiatric implications of psychomotor epilepsy. Arch Gen Psychiatry 14:461-471, 1966
48. Szondi L: Schicksalanalytische Therapie. Bern, Huber, 1963
49. Taylor DC, Marsh SM: Hughlings Jackson's Dr. Z: The paradigm of temporal lobe epilepsy revealed. J Neuro Neurosurg Psychiatry 43:758-767, 1980
50. Temkin O: The Falling Sickness, 2nd Ed. Baltimore: Johns Hopkins, 1971
51. Walker AE: Murder or epilepsy. J Nerv Ment Dis 133:430-437, 1961
52. Walker AE: Blumer D: Long-term behavior effects of temporal lobectomy for temporal lobe epilepsy. McLean Hosp J (Special Issue), pp 85-103, 1977
53. Waxman SG, Geschwind N: Hypergraphia in temporal lobe epilepsy. Neurology 24:629-636, 1974

Commentary

From the preceding chapter it is easy to see that there are incidents and symptoms present in the epileptic patient that are correctly termed psychiatric disturbances. In most instances, the seizure is prominent and the psychiatric symptomatology is recognized as seizure related. If the seizure itself is not recognized, however, and this does happen, a diagnosis of a primary psychiatric disorder may be suggested. Even more troublesome are the more chronic problems seen in some epileptics—the psychoses and personality changes that are not temporally related to a seizure discharge. The controversy concerning the exact relationship of these entities to the original seizure problem can only be settled by careful study of the chronic psychiatric problems seen in epileptics. Recognition of the psychiatric aspects of epilepsy is an important part of epilepsy management.

The psychiatric manifestations of the seizure, including the prodrome, are often controlled by appropriate epilepsy therapy, and the future for improvement at this level of management seems bright. The same cannot be said for the more chronic psychiatric disturbances suggested in this chapter. There has been almost no recognition of these disturbances until recently and, even now, many clinicians doubt that these are epilepsy-related problems. Thus, most such patients are treated (unsuccessfully) as primary psychiatric problems. A first step would be a broader recognition and sharper distinction of these disorders—this will be discussed further in Chapter 4. With recognition, improved management can be anticipated. The history of epilepsy therapy has been extremely happy thus far in the 20th Century, and it seems possible that management of the serious, long-term psychiatric manifestations seen in some epileptics can also be improved.

Among the most difficult problems arising from the question of epilepsy and behavioral disturbance concerns the patient with aggressive behavior, particularly when it is paroxysmal and explosive. In the past two decades, interest in violent behavior has increased, along with an apparent increase in the actual incidence of violence. Theories and explanations abound, varying from basic science-derived postulations based on neuroanatomy and psychopharmacology to complex social interaction theories embracing ethology, psychoanalysis, and similar diverse disciplines. Despite this apparent surge of interest, the basic problems remain unanswered. The aggressive, difficult patient is routinely dumped on the psychiatrist or neurologist with almost no help offered but the occasional advice of the referring source. While the theoreticians have consistently criticized the way violent patients are handled, their own theories have proved woefully inadequate and often downright wrong in actual practice. The violent patient remains a threat and a challenge and ranks among the most difficult borderland patients faced by the practitioners of neurology and psychiatry.

Since seizure disorder does play an important part in the differential diagnosis of episodic violence, and because seizure and violent behavior are linked in a number of these patients, the review of episodic dyscontrol has been placed with the discussions of the behavioral concomitants of epilepsy. In this chapter, Dr. Rickler has extracted a great deal of the pertinent background material concerning episodic violent behavior from the current literature and, in addition, has presented suggestions, both diagnostic and therapeutic, from his own considerable clinical experience.

Kenneth C. Rickler, M.D.

3
Episodic Dyscontrol

States of episodic explosive behavior provide an important challenge to investigators in behavioral neuroscience. While most investigators agree that social, cultural, economic, and personality factors are important in the production of violent behavior, there is a resurgence of interest in the neurobiologic substrate of violence. As Elliott notes, wide ranging etiologic formulations may miss or minimize the significant contribution of organic brain dysfunction in the production of such behaviors.[21]

The management of individuals prone to violent behavior is replete with difficulties at multiple levels. Such patients are often unpopular among clinicians; their behavior is characterized by unpredictable interpersonal aggression as well as the destruction of property. Simply put, many clinicians wish to avoid the risks and responsibilities involved in the care of these patients.

Dedication aside, clinicians are beset by significant problems at the basic level of definition. The nosology of violent behavior is complicated by imprecise usage of such commonplace terms as violence and aggression.[45] Attempts at exploring causal issues is further compromised by a more basic semantic confusion involving neurobiologic and psychosocial terminologies.

Formal research on violent behavior suffers from a number of methodologic difficulties. Serious legal and ethical issues are raised by study design to compound the problems of definition and the quantification of behavior. Ethologic concerns are raised: violence occurs in real-life settings, and the introduction of a laboratory environment seriously alters the naturalistic perspective, particularly as the behaviors are intermittent.

The net result is a body of knowledge that is often anecdotally and inferentially derived. Application of research findings to clinical problems is also subject to moral and legal restraints. Related forensic issues involving criminal responsibility, treatment of the violent offender, and the prediction of dangerous behavior represent an area of controversy.

DEFINITION

During the past decade, a number of characterizations of episodic violent behavior have emerged in the literature. In their book, *Violence And The Brain,* Ervin and Mark[27] describe four characteristic symptoms of the dyscontrol syndrome: (1) a history of physical assault, especially wife and child beating; (2) pathologic intoxication; (3) impulsive sexual behavior; and (4) serious automobile accidents and multiple traffic violations. Monroe, another major contributor to this field, defined episodic dyscontrol as "an abrupt, single act or short series of acts with a common intention carried through to completion with at least a partial release of tension or gratification of a specific need. As a subclass of the episodic behavior disorders, it also has the characteristic of a maladaptive, precipitous interruption in the life-style or the life-flow of the individual."[65] Monroe describes episodic dyscontrol as part of a larger paradigm of episodic behavioral reactions involving dysinhibition of action and further subdivides episodic dyscontrol in a hierarchic fashion.[65] The American Psychiatric Association's DSM-III Manual[18] characterizes the dyscontrol syndrome, "intermittent explosive disorder," in the following way.

1. There must be at least three discrete paroxysmal episodes of significant loss of control or aggressive impulses resulting in serious assault or destruction of property.
2. The magnitude of the behavior during an episode is grossly out of proportion to any psychosocial stressors which may have played a role in eliciting the episodes of lack of control.
3. Following each episode there is genuine regret or self-reproach at the consequences of the action and the inability to control the aggressive impulse.
4. Between the episodes, there are no signs of generalized impulsivity or aggressiveness.
5. The syndrome does not meet the criteria for schizophrenia, antisocial personality disorder, or conduct disorder.

Episodic Dyscontrol

A category for a single such act is also included under "isolated explosive disorder." The differential diagnosis of these categories includes antisocial personality disorder, paranoid or catatonic schizophrenia, dissociative disorder, and underlying organic conditions including brain tumors or epilepsy.

Maletzky[60] notes that patients with episodic dyscontrol are basically characterized by "uncontrollable storms of aggression," and this appears as a common theme in the three definitions/characterizations above. Attempts to refine the definition yield a number of questions. Can an individual who is generally impulsive still have episodic dyscontrol? At what point is a personality style or disorder separated from considerations of the organic substrate of behavior? Monroe's definition, as well as that of the APA Task Force, involves time modifiers as to the length of the act or acts of concern. How long can a dyscontrolled act persist before it represents something other than episodic dyscontrol? Monroe's definition is based in part upon subjective reports involving tension relief or specific-need gratification. Ervin and Mark's definition is based in part upon a controversial symptom, that of pathologic intoxication.[37] Must one be remorseful after the violent act? To what extent are these factors essential to a definition of episodic dyscontrol?

Rather than being critical, these questions illustrate the difficulties in characterizing the diverse phenomenologic manifestations related, at least in part, to brain dysfunction. The penchant for tight classifications has exceeded current capability. The disorder appears to be a spectrum of behavior and should be termed episodic dyscontrol syndromes, rather than suggest a single entity. The exploration of explosive behavior will be more productive if the concepts involved are recognized to be evolving rather than final truths. From such a perspective, a spectrum of behaviors involving variability in the underlying pathophysiology may be derived. Whether defined along the intuitive lines of Maletzky, the specific criteria of Ervin and Mark and DSM-III, or the complex hierarchic paradigm of Monroe, the chief value of episodic dyscontrol as a concept is its ability to stimulate thinking about aspects of the brain-behavior relationship.

An important clarification of terminology must be made as there is a tendency in the literature to use the terms impulsive and aggressive interchangeably, or at least to link them in describing behavior. Rotenberg and Mordechai clearly demonstrated that aggressiveness and impulsivity need not coexist.[82] Similarly, Elliott noted that aggressive acts committed by psychopaths often have the planned, deliberate quality characteristic of predatory animals.[22] Both Monroe and DSM-III suggest that the aggressive acts in episodic dyscontrol tend to occur spontaneously in a dramatic and paroxysmal fashion.

PHENOMENOLOGY

In his description of an act as a unit, Monroe characterizes the complex interactions that intervene between a stimulus and a response in human behavior.[65] The process of central integration plays a key role in Monroe's description and involves reciprocal interactions between memory, affect, and anticipation, which result in reflection. The further application of a comparative analysis of an ongoing situation, with values derived from previous experience and learning (conscience), completes the process Monroe calls the reflective delay. Episodic dyscontrol characteristically occurs without warning in a sudden, paroxysmal fashion without a period of contemplation, and patients are often startled by the suddenness of their own behavior. There is little reflective delay, and statements such as "something came over me" or "I don't know, I just did it" are frequently heard from such patients. The dyscontrolled acts show little in the way of planning or intention and precipitously interrupt ongoing activities in a poorly coordinated fashion. Characteristic acts include assaultive behavior, destruction of property, and self-injury.

The above description corresponds to Monroe's category of primary dyscontrol in which a short circuit between stimulus and response is suggested.[65] He also conceptualized a higher level of dyscontrol, secondary dyscontrol, with excessive reflection and complicated, coordinated activities which are variably timed in occurrence (choice delay). Although Monroe suggests activation of the same substrate involved in primary dyscontrol, the complex interplay of psychodynamic and neurophysiologic factors in secondary dyscontrol produces confusion at both the phenomenologic and etiologic levels.

Several case histories will help to illustrate the various types of behavior under discussion.

CASE 1

A 27-year-old man was struck in the head and was briefly unconscious but had no focal neurologic abnormalities on examination shortly after the incident. An electroencephalogram (EEG) revealed transient slowing in the theta range in the left posterior temporal region. A CT scan was reportedly normal.

Prior to the incident the patient was described as even-tempered, pleasant, and without any noticeable behavioral or personality disturbances. He had a high school education and functioned effectively in his job as a semi-skilled worker and as head of a household. His wife described him as affectionate, not particularly moody, and not prone to violent behavior. During the 6 months following the accident, the patient complained of intermittent occipital headaches and experienced episodes characterized by his wife as "rage attacks." He described the onset of sudden irritability which rapidly escalated into the violent destruction of property in the room about him, at times involving an amazing degree of strength. His wife indicated that the family had learned to recognize the somewhat glazed look in his eye at the outset and would immediately leave the room. The episodes were usually brief, lasting less than 5 minutes, and terminated in a state of fatigue at times followed by a short period of sleep. No typical tonic-clonic movements or automatic behavior occurred independently or in association with these destructive episodes. Following each of the incidents, for which he claimed total amnesia, the patient was quite concerned and remorseful regarding his behavior.

Several EEGs with sleep activation and nasopharyngeal leads were within normal limits. A regimen of diphenylhydantoin and carbamazepine completely eliminated the episodes. Diphenylhydantoin was discontinued in a gradual fashion but was reinstituted after the occurrence of another destructive episode. The patient is currently working and free of rage episodes.

CASE 2

This patient is a 25-year-old married man with three children. His birth and developmental milestones were reportedly normal. At age 2, he was struck in the head with a bat and briefly stunned but without obvious sequelae. At age 23, a significant change in his personality and behavior was noted by his wife. He complained of headaches, was irritable, and occasionally exploded in a rage with only minimal or trivial precipitants. Destruction of property occurred, including holes punched in walls and furniture broken plus poorly coordinated assaults on family members and some neighbors. The patient's wife described him as unresponsive during these brief episodes (lasting only several minutes); sometimes he was nauseated and exhausted afterwards. He reported a patchy loss of recall for these episodes, but could describe his anger escalating beyond his control. At the outset, small amounts of alcohol increased his irritability and, on occasion, precipitated a violent episode. His wife reported variability in his moods; at times he was pleasant and even jovial, at other times irritable, a state in which a violent episode was more likely to occur. The patient appeared concerned about these outbursts which had placed significant stress upon the family unit.

Neurologic examination was within normal limits. Neuropsychologic testing suggested a problem in auditory information processing, and EEGs on several occasions revealed transient slowing in the left temporal lobe. A CT scan demonstrated mild central atrophy. The patient was treated with neuroleptic and anticonvulsant therapy without benefit.

The above cases manifest behavior that is considered typical of episodic dyscontrol. The next case emphasizes the possible role of developmental factors in the production of dyscontrolled behavior.

CASE 3

This patient, a 16-year-old ambidextrous black man, had a long history of violent outbursts. Birth and early developmental milestones were reported as normal except for temper tantrums which were not of unusual frequency. In school, multimodal learning disabilities as well as deficits in attention and concentration were described but no hyperactivity was noted. IQ testing in fourth grade was reportedly average.

He subsequently engaged in assaultive behavior with peers and authority figures. The outbursts would usually build up over 15 minutes during which time he would try to verbally de-escalate himself. The transition to overt anger was rapid and accompanied by strong feelings. At times he experienced *deja-vu* in association with escalating anger. Objective reports described a mean and glazed look but no automatic behavior. The outbursts were of variable duration, from a few minutes to somewhat longer. The patient often perceived his aggressive outbursts as justified, particularly with his father, whom he described as provocative. He also noted that he generally felt irritable and had a chip on his shoulder. In addition to physical assault, there were episodes which involved the destruction of property, including smashing of walls and objects around him in a random fashion. Following the outbursts, the patient noted a definite release of tension.

Review of neurologic history was unremarkable except for a recent mild head injury without apparent residual. Mental examination revealed some religious preoccupation but no clear-cut paranoid ideation. Deficits in attention for verbal material and impairment of recent memory were noted, and mild difficulties with calculations and constructional tasks were evident. Neurologic examination was normal except for mild generalized impairment on fine motor coordination. Psychologic testing appeared consistent with a mild degree of organic dysfunction. A sleep-activated EEG was normal. At the present time, he remains in an in-patient psychiatric unit.

The next two cases show behavior that is consistent with episodic dyscontrol but include factors that complicate etiologic considerations. In Case 4 there is an apparent coexistent personality disorder and in Case 5, mild mental retardation associated with structural brain disease. The behaviors under consideration, however, are typical of episodic dyscontrol; it is cases like these that raise difficult questions about narrow-based exclusionary definitions.

CASE 4

This 35-year-old right-handed man fell at work and sustained a brief loss of consciousness. Several months later he had a generalized seizure. Neurologic examination was within normal limits as was a CT scan, but an EEG demonstrated a right fronto-temporal spike wave focus. Occasional Grand Mal seizures as well as infrequent *absence*-type episodes were reported subsequently.

The patient was relatively easy-going before the accident. He had had a long-standing interest in judo and had been involved in both competition and teaching.

He admitted to several fights before the accident, but denied any excessive propensity for violence. Increasing irritability with easily elicited violent behavior, including assault on his wife, destruction of property within the home, and assault on several members of the community was reported over a 6-month period following the accident, and a pattern of intermittent, explosive violence has continued for the past several years. There did not appear to be any clear relationship between seizure activity and violent outbursts and there was no aura to his explosive behavior. He noted an awareness of his actions but described himself as losing control in response to frustration. Overall, he was concerned about his violent tendencies but expressed little remorse for his behavior, describing himself as feeling helpless. He also expressed depressed feelings and indicated that since losing his job and developing a seizure disorder he felt worthless.

The patient was treated with carbamazepine and other anticonvulsants, occasionally in combination with minor tranquilizers or neuroleptic agents. Carbamazepine appeared to reduce his level of irritability but was discontinued following recurrent leukopenia. Obsessive narcissistic concerns related to loss of employment were frequently voiced: The patient demonstrated tremendous resistance to psychotherapy, however; and in fact expressed little willingness to work at changing his violent behavior.

CASE 5

This patient was a 28-year-old right-handed woman with a history of mild mental retardation. Birth and early developmental history were not available, but the patient successfully attended special education classes and completed high school. At age 11, she had several Grand Mal seizures and was treated with diphenylhydantoin. At age 13, intermittent aggressive outbursts, mostly directed toward her mother, began. Although termed seizures, the violent outbursts were not associated with loss of contact and did not terminate in any loss of consciousness. No absences or automatisms were described. During these episodes she acted infantile, reminiscent of a tantrum. She described herself as unable to control herself in these episodes despite a desire to do so. Trivial events precipitated aggressive outbursts; in addition to assaulting her mother, marked destruction of property within the house occurred. At times, aggressive outbursts resulted in self-injury. An increased frequency of aggressive behavior was noted premenstrually.

Examination revealed evidence of mood lability and a mild degree of receptive dysphasia with paraphasic substitutions. Mild right-sided sensory-motor findings were evident. CT scan demonstrated a left parietal-occipital porencephalic cyst with dilatation of the left occipital horn. EEG demonstrated generalized anterior slowing, anterior temporal and left mid-temporal sharp wave activity, and left temporal slowing. Psychologic testing demonstrated a full-scale IQ of 71 without significant verbal-performance spread. A marked deficit in short-term memory was also apparent. Attempts to control her behavior with anticonvulsants, low doses of neuroleptics, oxazepam, and acetazolamide were relatively ineffective. Improvement in her behavior while in a highly structured residential hospital environment has been reported.

ASSOCIATED CLINICAL FINDINGS

Discussion of clinical findings in patients with episodic dyscontrol cannot be separated from etiologic concerns. As would be expected, assessment of underlying conditions reveals a variety of neurologic illnesses. Bach-Y-Rita et al.[6] and Elliot[21,24] reported that a significant percentage of patients with explosive, violent behavior had antecedent histories of minimal brain dysfunction (MBD), unconsciousness (most often from head injury), and seizures. A number of patients in Elliot's series had multiple diagnoses including MBD and seizures or seizures associated with head injuries. Three quarters of the patients with seizures were diagnosed as having partial complex epilepsy. Elliot also reported a significant percentage of patients with a variety of neurologic disorders, including 12 patients with brain tumors.[24] Bach-Y-Rita et al. reported a significant percentage of patients with a childhood history of enuresis, fire setting, or cruelty directed towards animals.[6] This triad is thought to have some limited predictive significance.[29,42] Lewis has also described a triad including symptoms of psychomotor epilepsy and paranoid ideation in aggressive delinquents.[49]

No tabulation of abnormalities on neurologic examination is available, and the variety of possible etiologies associated with episodic dyscontrol renders generalization difficult. The neurologic examination is often negative or shows mild abnormalities. Problems with motor performance, attention, concentration, recent memory, and constructional tasks may be noted.[46] Varying degrees of dyslexia may be present as well as subtle signs of cortical sensory dysfunction. Monroe noted positive correlations between episodic dyscontrol and a variety of congenital stigmata, hyperacusis, photophobia, apraxia, and asymmetries in motor strengths.[66] However, these findings as well as the others mentioned above are nonspecific.

LABORATORY FINDINGS

Most investigators utilize the EEG in the assessment of patients with episodic dyscontrol. Again, variability reflects the diverse etiologies. Bach-Y-Rita et al. noted EEG abnormalities in 37 of 79 patients studied.[6] Twenty patients showed spiking in the temporal region, and the remainder had asymmetries or rhythm changes. Thirteen of the 123 patients in their sample were found to have undiagnosed temporal lobe epilepsy. Riley and Niedermeyer only found EEG abnormalities in 6.6% of patients with rage disorders.[80] However, Elliot noted significant EEG abnormalities in more than 60 percent of his cases and cautioned against confident acceptance of negative EEG findings.[24] Monroe also emphasized the high false-negative rate of a single EEG and reported abnormalities in 58 percent of 93 aggressive criminals who had two tracings.[66]

Pneumoencephalography may reveal deformity of one or both temporal horns[26] and episodic violent behavior has occasionally been linked with communicating hydrocephalus.[14] Elliot noted asymmetries of the middle fossa with basal views of the skull and also reported abnormalities in 42 percent of 148 cases who had CT scans performed.[24]

DEMOGRAPHIC DATA

The frequency of episodic dyscontrol is unknown. As noted above, significant problems exist in defining episodic dyscontrol, and the inclusion of this disorder into other major etiologic headings such as head injury and epilepsy accounts, in part, for the lack of accurate figures. In addition, the social implications of the disorder may inhibit the patient or his family in reporting the behavior. Also, poor recognition of the syndrome of episodic violent behavior by mental health and medical professionals undoubtedly contributes to the lack of statistics. The experience of a number of investigators and clinics, however, suggest that the syndrome is not rare.[6,21,27]

In the populations studied so far, the frequency of episodic violence has been higher in men than in women.[6,21,24] Monroe notes that adult women with dyscontrol are more likely to be hospitalized.[65] Marked variability with socioeconomic status has also been noted: Elliot's group[24] was comprised mainly of middle and upper-class patients, but other studies have reflected lower socioeconomic status.[6]

MECHANISMS UNDERLYING EPISODIC DYSCONTROL

Biologic Factors

The neurobiologic assessment of episodic violent behavior has included studies of genetic factors, neuroendocrine relationships, and neurotransmitter substances, but the major focus has been the neurophysiologic investigation of the limbic system. This complex neuroanatomic structure has been identified as a substrate associated with violent behavior.[27,32,69,73] Although a detailed discussion of limbic anaotomy and physiology[43,54,55,73] is clearly beyond the scope of this chapter, it can be stated, generally, that limbic circuitry is interposed, literally and conceptually, between the so-called higher and lower centers which involve the frontal lobe and the diencephalic core, respectively.

Animal experiments have demonstrated that limbic mechanisms play a significant role in the modulation of aggressive behavior.[8,27,32] Extension of these results to humans is difficult. The interactions between frontal lobe mechanisms, memory, and affective systems in man far exceeds the complexity of animal models. Nauta conceives human anticipation of the future as a function of the reciprocal relationship between the frontal lobes and the limbic system.[66]

How can the role of the limbic system in episodic aggressive behavior be demonstrated? One approach would be to look for evidence of the syndromes in patients with limbic system dysfunction. Autopsy material provides one source. Malamud reported aggressive behavior in a number of patients with tumors involving the limbic system,[59] and Elliot has noted dyscontrolled behavior in a number of patients with tumors involving the cingulate gyrus, subfrontal, or subtemporal structures.[25] It is important to stress, however, that not all lesions or tumors of the limbic system necessarily result in dyscontrolled behavior.

EEG Findings

Electroencephalography provides a noninvasive technique for assessing the role of the limbic system, but a number of methodologic problems are of concern. The limbic system is relatively inaccessible to surface recordings and requires nasopharyngeal or sphenoidal lead techniques to increase the yield. Multiple records are necessary. A variety of activation techniques involving hyperventilation, photic stimulation, sleep activation, or the artificial induction of sleep with hypnotics are used routinely. The EEG findings in episodic dyscontrol populations comprised of a high proportion of patients with known or suspected epilepsy often yields a high frequency of abnormalities. Thus, Meltzky reported EEG abnormalities in 14 out of 28 patients studied.[60] Monroe reports that false-positives as well as false-negatives complicate interpretation of the use of alpha chloralose.[66] He contends, however, that its use raises the percentage of abnormal tracings to almost 90 percent. Both focal and generalized patterns occur with alpha chloralose activation, and Monroe believes a correlation exists between the type of pattern and the individual's behavior.

EEG studies have been performed with depth electrodes implanted in the limbic system but the results have been variable and controversial. Spontaneous discharges have been reported in limbic structures during episodes of rage.[27] Discrete anatomic localization involving reciprocal relationships between medial and lateral amygdala complexes in patients with episodic rage have been described by Smith[86] and Mark et al.[61] St. Hillaire et al. also reported several recent cases demonstrating subcortical epileptiform discharges during apparent attack behavior.[88]

Limbic Stimulation and Epilepsy

A number of authors have reported the production of aggressive responses and/or feelings of rage by limbic stimulation.[27,86,61] Halgren et al., however, stimulated 36 patients a total of 3,500 times and produced only several angry responses.[34] Gloor also reported an inability to produce anger or rage with the stimulation of electrodes implanted in the limbic system.[30] Differences in methodologies involving electrode placement, the amount and duration of current, as well as certain subtle, and perhaps unrecognized, contextual cues may account for these differences. The presence of a varied spectrum of possible anatomic and/or physiologic insults in the limbic system before stimulation may also contribute to the variability noted.

The converse, looking for episodic dyscontrol in patients with known limbic dysfunction, can be applied to the search for the substrate(s) of episodic violent behavior. Some, but not all, patients with tumors of the limbic system have disordered impulse control. Aggressive behavior has been reported in patients with partial complex seizures, but the incidence has varied widely (4.8–36 percent).[21] Some of the variability depends on the composition of the patient population. Differences in interview techniques will affect the amount of aggressive behavior recognized in epileptics.

The relationship of aggressive behavior to partial complex epilepsy has been the subject of much controversy.[9,44,45,57,74,81,84,91] Ictal or peri-ictal aggression is rare and is most often characterized by uncoordinated, nonsequential behavior. Interictal aggressive behavior provides the greatest problem. Attempts to demonstrate a clear-cut, cause-and-effect relationship are easily frustrated because epilepsy and aggressive behavior may result from a common dysfunction.[91] Patients with epilepsy often suffer head injuries from which limbic dysfunction may arise. The question of whether violence can be the sole manifestation of a seizure disorder remains unresolved and the controversy involves both semantic and forensic issues.[41,74,75,91]

Psychosurgical Experience

Psychosurgical experience has provided some indirect evidence of the involvement of limbic structures in the production of episodic aggressive behavior. Most surgery for aggressive behavior has involved placement of small stereotactic lesions in the amygdala complex bilaterally. Narabayashi and Uno produced bilateral 2–4 mm lesions between the medial and lateral amygdala complex.[70] Other surgical techniques including bilateral posterior hypothalomotomy,[83] ventromedial orbital undercutting,[36] and temporal lobectomy[28,94] have also been reported to reduce aggressive behavior. The studies cited above are notable for their attempts at follow-up, a problem which often complicates the interpretation of psychosurgical results. No single technique has emerged with a consistently high level of long-term efficacy.

The placement of the effective lesion(s) within the limbic system or its connections may not necessarily prove that limbic dysfunction is the cause of explosive behavior. Goddard's discussion of kindling suggests that chronically altered limbic physiology may result in increased interictal aggressive behavior.[31] The data appears species specific and is presently confined to animal models. Positron emission tomography (PET) is another new technique which may afford a better understanding of the functional state of subcortical structures during and between explosive outbursts. Correlations with CT scanning and surface and depth telemetry recordings are likely to result in better characterization of the role played by subcortical structures in aggressive behavior.

Neuroendocrine Relationships

The role of neuroendocrine relationships in violent behavior bears consideration, particularly the relationship of testosterone levels to aggressive behavior in men.[10,20,56,62,63,85] Results have been inconsistent, however. Recently Ehlers et al. studied the relationship between plasma-testosterone levels and assaultive behavior in adult women.[19] Aggressive women clustered around the high-normal level, whereas a nonaggressive control group clustered in the low-normal range. Dalton studied women with perimenstrual irritability and violent behavior and noted low or absent premenstrual progesterone levels.[16,17]

Neurotransmitter Function

Studies of neurotransmitter function in aggressive animal behavior suggested the involvement of a number of neurotransmitter systems but have not produced conclusive results.[77] More recently, studies of human CSF metabolites of serotonin and norepinephrine demonstrated an inverse correlation of aggressive behavior with the former and a direct correlation with the latter.[12] This observation may have implications for pharmocologic treatment.

Genetic Factors

A number of studies have focused on genetic factors in the production of aggressive behavior.[32,38,72] The data on men with XYY syndrome have undergone considerable scrutiny and a number of artifacts of selection are felt to contribute to previously noted correlations.[32,95] Although a family history of violent behavior is not uncommon in XYY males, a clear-cut dissection between genetic factors and environmental influences has not been possible. Continued genetic studies appear to be indicated, particularly on a variety of aggressive individuals outside the criminal justice system.

Psychosocial Factors

The discussion has focused upon organic factors in the production of intermittent explosive behavior, but the importance of early experiences also deserves consideration. Ervin and Mark stressed the importance of early childhood emotional deprivation, social maladjustment in the family, increased aggressiveness among parents, siblings, or significant other adults in the family, and chronic alcoholism in the production of violent behavior.[27] Monroe's model involved the concepts of faulty "equipment" and faulty "learning."[65] While faulty equipment was stressed as the major etiologic factor in primary dyscontrol, faulty learning may secondarily track susceptible individuals into antisocial patterns of behavior.

The constant interaction between the neurologic substrate and the environment make an accurate dissection of neurophysiologic, psychologic, and social factors almost impossible. The psychodynamics of explosive behavior have been discussed by a number of authors. Monroe has sought correlations between the neurophysiologic and psychologic levels.[65] Madden has reviewed a number of theories and emphasized the importance of frustrated childhood dependency needs in the later production of aggressive behavior.[58] Lion has described helplessness as a core dynamic in the violent patient and also mentioned inadequate sublimation and unresolved oedipal conflicts as contributory mechanisms.[50] Adler has discussed impulsive behavior from the multiple perspectives of ego psychology.[1] Elliot[21] and Ervin and Mark[27] have noted the role of significant others in eliciting dyscontrolled behavior. While such individuals may at times be ignorant of their contributing role, they often display significant psychopathology.

The mechanisms of environmental-neurophysiologic interaction remain speculative. The role of environmental influences on brain maturation is noted by Elliot in his discussion of antisocial behavior.[22] The attention deficit syndrome (at times associated with learning disabilities and hyperactivity) is likely to involve complex interactions of constitutional and environmental factors. Elliot noted a past history of this syndrome in a significant percentage of his adult patients with episodic dyscontrol.[21,24] Although retrospective diagnosis of this syndrome may be difficult, studies of children and adolescents with clearly recognized attention deficit syndrome have suggested an increased frequency of aggressive behavior.[13] The role of secondary factors such as frustration due to poor school performance, and rejection by peers and family must also be taken into account.

The characterization of aggressive behavior in humans remains controversial on the question of whether it is innate or acquired. Involvement of limbic structures in the production of aggressive behavior has been demonstrated, but the question of whether the substrate is genetically "wired" in this fashion or whether the necessary connections result from organic and social-environmental influences remains unanswered. Montague argues strongly for the acquired position and contends that experience organizes "prefunctionally developed" neural systems in a fashion that permits the expression of aggressive behavior.[68] Montague does acknowledge a variable contribution from genetic factors, but emphasizes the role of experience in organizing and eliciting aggressive behavior. Although primarily confined to semantic and philosophic concerns at this time, such discussion is not without practical implications. The converse of Montague's position involves speculation about whether environmental influences might be involved in the development of inhibitory neuronal systems that modulate innately organized, genetically determined brain loci associated with aggressive behavior. Such speculations could conceivably affect the design of future treatment programs at the biologic and social levels.

EVALUATION

The evaluation of patients with explosive behavior demands a multidisciplinary approach. The pooled expertise of medical, psychiatric, social, and basic science personnel permit a thorough diagnostic investigation and the formulation of a treatment program; awareness of the problem is clearly of tantamount importance. Questions concerning the patient's impulse control must be asked of both the patient and family members. Complete neurologic and psychiatric histories are essential with particular inquiry into seizures, head injuries, developmental delay, learning disabilities, and difficulties with attention, concentration, and hyperactivity. Inquiry into endocrinologic and metabolic abnormalities should also be made. A thorough search for the use/abuse of ethanol, street drugs, and prescribed medications is indicated. Environmental precipitating factors and review of family history with regard to social and psychodynamic factors, intrafamily violence, and child abuse should also be undertaken.

Many patients do not give complete histories on the initial visit and information must often be acquired over several visits. Review of academic, employment, and military records may provide useful information. Questionnaires such as the Monroe Dyscontrol Scale[66] and the Patient Aggression Rating Form (PARF)[39] may provide diagnostically useful data. A complete mental status assessment as well as a thorough basic neurologic examination are essential.

Additional laboratory information may include basic thyroid screening tests, A.M. cortisol levels, serum testosterone levels, and, when clinically indicated, a dexamethasone suppression test, progesterone levels, and a 5-hour postprandial glucose or a glucose tolerance test. An initial EEG with sleep activation may be followed by repeat study with naso-pharyngeal (NP) leads. Computerized axial tomography often is also indicated. Assessment of personality factors and a thorough neuropsychologic evaluation are helpful. A clinic staff meeting following the individual evaluations often reveals historic information from one team member that was not presented to others.

TREATMENT

As noted, an integrated diagnostic approach is preferred with one individual assuming responsibility for integrating all facets. Although treatment is often multimodal and provided by different specialists, one clinician should retain overall control. Treatment approaches will be discussed in separate sections but overlap will be necessary in many patients.

Pharmacologic Treatment

Anticonvulsants

Anticonvulsants represent one major area of emphasis in treatment of intermittent explosive behavior. A number of workers advocate the use of anticonvulsants, even in the absence of any clear-cut seizure history.[6,65,67,92] Many anticonvulsants have been tried including primidone, diphenylhydantoin, carbamazepine, and ethosuximide[2] with diphenylhydantoin and carbamazepine receiving most emphasis in recent years. A significant body of anecdotal and case reports suggest that anticonvulsants reduce the incidence of episodic rage in some patients. The mechanism by which anticonvulsants are presumed to work is by reducing irritability in populations of neurons. Subcortical recordings lend some credence to this concept but classic epileptic after discharge potentials are infrequently noted in most studies.

Carbamazepine's affective properties are being explored for use in the treatment of bipolar illness,[4] but the extent to which its affective actions depend on anticonvulsant mechanisms is unclear. The design of effective controlled studies is extremely difficult and has serious ethical implications; it is also difficult to control environmental factors while patients are either institutionalized or seen as outpatients. Thus, it is difficult to make generalizations and each case must be considered individually. Anticonvulsants may produce significant toxicity and patients must be monitored closely for side effects, particularly leukopenia in patients on carbamazepine. At present, it is not known whether such treatment must be carried on indefinitely or whether it may be discontinued eventually without recurrence of violent episodes.

Antianxiety Agents and Neuroleptics

Antianxiety agents represent another effective pharmacotherapy for impulse control. Studies suggest that chlordiazepoxide and oxazepain may be among the most effective antianxiety agents.[33,51] Paradoxical responses to longer acting benzodiazepines have been reported,[52] but Bond and Lader suggest that such responses may represent unrecognized drug toxicity.[11] Neuroleptics alone, particularly in high doses, may actually worsen dyscontrol.[40,65,66] The presence of psychotic content, even subtle paranoid ideation, may provide a clinical clue to the usefulness of these drugs. Except for chronically high levels of agitation, less sedating agents such as thiothixene or trifluoperazine are better tolerated. Combinations of a low-dose of a neuroleptic with an anticonvulsant may be successful. A variety of complications may occur with the chronic use of neuroleptics so they must be prescribed thoughtfully with periodic re-evaluation.

Antidepressants and Stimulants

Antidepressants have been suggested for impulse dyscontrol, even in the absence of clearly demarcated affective illness.[32] It would be of interest to study a population of such patients with a dexamethasone suppression screening test and correlate the effect of treatment. Recent studies suggest a correlation of low cerebrospinal fluid serotonin metabolite levels and aggressive behavior.[12] Therefore, if a tricyclic antidepressant is selected, one with greater serotonergic activity such as amitriptyline would be appropriate. Antidepressants are sometimes employed to treat children and younger adolescents with attention-deficit syndromes who are refractory to treatment with stimulant drugs. Considering the possible etiologic relationship between attention-deficit syndromes and impulse dyscontrol, there may be further rationale for the use of tricyclic agents.

The use of stimulants such as D-amphetamine have also been advocated for improving inhibitory functions and impulse control.[79,87] The possibility of drug abuse raises serious questions about the appropriateness of prescribing stimulants to outpatients. Nonetheless, dramatic results have been reported with stimulants and they should be considered in dyscontrol patients with a history that suggests possible attention deficit. It should be noted that improvement in behavior may require higher doses than improvement in attention.[87]

Lithium

The use of lithium to treat impulse dyscontrol has been advocated.[48,96] Positive responses have occasionally been interpreted to indicate undiagnosed affective disorder,[15] but this point has not been proved. Problems with compliance, significant side effects, and lowered seizure threshold require that patients be carefully selected for lithium therapy. A history of seizures or paroxysmal sharp activity on EEG favors use of carbamazepine over lithium.

Propranolol

Elliot reported improvement in impulse control in a few patients with the use of propranolol.[23] Yudofsky et al. recently reported improvement in violent behavior associated with chronic brain syndromes following the use of this agent.[97] No clear guidelines for dosage have been established, and past or current depressive symptoms would be a relative contraindication as would some cardiopulmonary conditions.

Hormonal Control

The use of diuretics and moderate doses of pyridoxine (50 mg/day) have been advocated for premenstrual irritability.[90] Elliot noted decreased edema with diuretic treatment but no significant change in impulse control.[21] The successful use of progesterone for premenstrual aggression has been described by Dalton.[16,17] She points out that use of synthetic progestins may actually worsen dyscontrol.

Antitestosterone agents, including medroxyprogestrone acetate and cyproterone acetate have been successfully employed in the treatment of sexually aggressive male offenders.[47,71] Blumer and Migeon reported a reduction in nonsexual aggressive behavior in a small acetate number of temporal lobe epileptics following treatment with medroxyprogestrone.[10]

Few generalizations, if any, can be made about the pharmacologic treatment of episodic dyscontrol. Multiple problems including compliance, control of environmental factors, and a poor understanding of the pathophysiology demand individualization of pharmacotherapy, often with sequential long-term trials. At times, the results are rewarding. The treatment of underlying conditions such as endocrine abnormalities, hypoglycemia, and tumors, etc. should remain a primary concern. Identifiable (and treatable) conditions constituted slightly more than 7 percent of Elliot's cases.[24]

Surgical Treatment

Temporal lobectomy may decrease the incidence of aggressive behavior associated with a well-lateralized temporal lobe seizure focus.[28,94] Falconer reported that those cases associated with mesial temporal sclerosis had the best results from this procedure.[28] There appears to be general agreement that well-established personality disorders and/or psychosis are not significantly altered.

Patients without a known underlying disorder who respond poorly to pharmacotherapy have occasionally been referred for psychosurgery. This treatment remains controversial,[21,27,93] but despite the complex legal and ethical issues that surround it, psychosurgery may occasionally represent a reasonable step, particularly if the alternative is a lifetime of institutionalization. The prodecure(s) must be selected on an individual basis with respect to both the possible pathophysiologic mechanisms and the skills of the neurosurgeon. The work of Heath[35] using chronic cerebellar stimulation to control intractable explosive behavior may represent a less invasive form of psychosurgery, but the possible production of neuronal damage with chronic use must be considered.[5]

Psychotherapy

Regardless of other therapies chosen, psychotherapy remains an essential part of the treatment of impulse dyscontrol. Even when a previous experience with extended psychotherapy was unsuccessful (a common history), the benefits of continuing this modality are multiple. These include opportunities for ventilation and for positive reinforcement of adaptive responses as well as improvement in compliance to medical treatment and exploration of techniques that may enhance the process of reflective delay. Family therapy or individual therapy for the patient's partner may be indicated. Psychotherapy combined with medical therapy is often more successful than either method alone.

FORENSIC AND ETHICAL CONCERNS

Many social, legal, and ethical issues arise in the management of individuals with episodic dyscontrol.[27,53,78] Application of neurobehavioral methodology to individuals accused of criminal acts demands an assessment of several complex issues. The question of criminal responsibility is often raised.[76] The potential for abuse of brain dysfunction as a reason for exculpability is rather great, but the solution demands a broad perspective.

The position of the expert witness in such cases was recently discussed by Beresford.[7] It is wise to emphasize the speculative nature of our knowledge in the field; reliance should be placed on observed clinical behavior rather than "secondary" evidence of brain dysfunction such as the EEG findings. Legal maneuvering often attempts to exploit speculations about causal relationships. Access to depth electrode monitoring during a violent episode may assist in determining causal factors. The information available from this laboratory procedure would differ substantially from an amnestic defendant's reconstruction of an antisocial act of violence. Despite the differences, actual causal relationships are difficult to prove in both cases and it would seem prudent to acknowledge speculation in these matters during courtroom testimony.

A number of issues arise from questions relating to criminal responsibility. The determination of dangerousness is complex and almost invariably controversial.[3,64,89] Some clinicians suggest that such determinations should be the responsibility of jurists, not mental health workers. Others argue that specialists in the management of abnormal behavior are better equipped to make such decisions. It must be remembered that objective evidence of organic brain dysfunction is not necessarily relevant in determining dangerousness.

Invasive techniques might provide better characterization of causal factors, but the application of such methodologies to individuals suspected of criminal acts is unlikely in the near future. There are many legal and ethical restraints on the use of such techniques in a noncriminal population, and concern about possible coercion increases the opposition to their forensic application. Nonetheless, the inability to provide satisfactory forensic classification of such individuals either as "sick" or "bad" interferes with choice of appropriate place and type of treatment. Clinicians engaged in the management of patients prone to episodic dyscontrol must struggle against a pervasive moral indictment of these individuals and this endeavor requires the constant re-examination of clinical values against the background of wider sociolegal and philosophic concerns.

REFERENCES

1. Adler G: Psychodynamics of Impulsive Behavior, in Wishnie HA, Nevis-Olesen J (eds): Working with the Impulsive Person. New York, Plenum, 1979
2. Andrulonis, PA, Donnelly J, Glueck BC, et al: Preliminary data on ethosuximide and the episodic dyscontrol syndrome. Am J Psychiat 137:1455–1456, 1980
3. APA Task Force on Clinical Aspects of the Violent Individual. Washington DC, American Psychiatric Association, 1974
4. Ayd FA: carbamazepine: A potential alternative for lithium therapy for affective disorders. International Drug Therapy Newsletter, 14, No. 8, 1979
5. Babb TL et al: Electrophysiological studies of long-term electrical stimulation of the cerebellum in monkeys. J Neurosurg 47:353–365, 1971
6. Bach-Y-Rita G, Lion JR, Climent CE, Ervin FR: Episodic dyscontrol: A study of 130 violent patients. Amer J Psychiat 127:1473–1478, 1971
7. Beresford HR: Letter to the Editor. Neurol 30:1339–1340, 1980
8. Blanchard RJ, Blanchard DC: Animal aggression and the dyscontrol syndrome, in Girgis M, Kiloh LG (eds): Limbic Epilepsy and the Dyscontrol Syndrome. Amesterdam, Elsevier, 1980
9. Blumer D: Epilepsy and violence, in Madden DJ, Lion JR: Rage, Hate, Assault and Other Forms of Violence. Spectrum, New York, 1976
10. Blumer D, Migeon C: Hormone and hormonal agents in the treatment of aggression. J Neur and Ment Dis 160:127–137, 1975
11. Bond A, Lader M: Benzodiazepines and aggression, in Sandler M (ed): Psychopharmacology of Aggression. Raven Press, New York, 1979
12. Brown GL, Ballanger JC, Minichiello MD, Goodwin FK: Human Aggression and Its Relationship to Cerebrospinal Fluid 5-Hydroxyindoleacetic Acid, 3-Methoxy-4Hydroxyphenyglycol, and Homovanillic Acid, in Sandler M: Psychopharmacology of Aggression. New York, Raven Press, 1979
13. Cantwell DP: Hyperactivity and Antisocial Behavior. J Am Acad Child Psychiatry 17:252–262, 1978
14. Crowell R, Tew J, Mark V: Aggressive dementia associated with normal pressure hydrocephalus. Report of two unusual cases. Neurology 23:461–464, 1973
15. Cutler N, Heiser JF: Retrospective diagnosis of hypomania following successful treatment of episodic violence with lithium: A case report. Am J Psychiatry 135:753–754, 1978
16. Dalton K: Criminal Aggression and the Pre-Menstrual Syndrome. Presented at International Society for Research and Aggression Conference, Haren, Netherlands, July, 1980
17. Dalton K: The Premenstrual Syndrome and Progesterone Therapy. Chicago, Year Book Medical Publishers, 1977
18. Diagnostic and Statistical Manual of Mental Disorders III. American Psychiatric Association, 1980
19. Ehlers CL, Rickler KC, Hovey JE: A possible relationship between plasma, testosterone, and aggressive behavior in a female out-patient population, in

Girgis M, Kiloh LG (eds): Limbic Epilepsy and the Dyscontrol Syndrome. Amsterdam, Elsevier, 1980
20. Ehrenkranz J, Bliss E, Sheard, M: plasma testosterone: Correlation with aggressive behavior and social dominance in man. Psychosom Med 36:469-475, 1974
21. Elliott FA: Neurological factors in violent behavior (the dyscontrol syndrome), in Sadoff, RL. (ed): Violence and Responsibility. New York, Spectrum, 1978
22. Elliott FA: Neurological aspects of antisocial behavior, in Reid W (ed): The Psychopath: A Comprehensive Study of Anti-Social Disorders and Behaviors. New York, Brunner/Mazel, 1978
23. Elliott FA: Propranolol for the control of belligerent behavior following acute brain damage. Ann Neurol 1:489-491, 1977
24. Elliott FA: Episodic Dyscontrol, Neurological Findings in 190 Cases. Presented at Byberry State Hospital, Philadelphia, March 1980
25. Elliott F: Personal Communication, 1981
26. Ervin FR, Lion JR: Clinical Evaluation of the Violent Patient. National Commission on Causes and Prevention of Violence. 1969
27. Ervin FR, Mark VH: Violence and the Brain. New York, Harper and Row, 1970
28. Falconer MA: Reversibility by temporal lobe resection of the behavioral abnormalities of temporal lobe epilepsy. New Eng J Med 289:451, 1973
29. Felthous AR, Bernard H: Enuresis, fire setting and cruelty to animals: The significance of two-thirds of this triad. J Forensic Sci 24:240-246, 1979
30. Gloor P: Electrophysiological studies of the amegdla, in Fields WS, Sweet WH (eds): Neural Bases of Violence and Aggression. St. Louis, Warren Green, 1975
31. Goddard GV: The kindling model of limbic epilepsy, in Girgis M, Kiloh LG (eds): Limbic Epilepsy and the Dyscontrol Syndrome. Amsterdam, Elsevier, 1980
32. Goldstein M: Brain Research and Violent Behavior, Arch Neurol 30:1-23, 1974
33. Gunn J: Drugs in the violence clinic, in Sandler M, (ed): Psychopharmacology of Aggression. New York, Raven Press, 1979
34. Halgren E, Walter RD, Cherlow D, Crandall PH: Mental phenomena evoked by electrical stimulation of the human hippocampal formation and amygdala. Brain, 101:83-117, 1978
35. Heath RG: Modulation of emotion with a brain pacemaker. J Nerv Ment Dis 165:300, 1977
36. Hirose S: Long-Term Follow-Up of Psychosurgical Operation in Epilepsy with Explosive Behavior and Episodic Confusional States in Atypical Psychoses, in Girgis M, Kiloh LG (eds): Limbic Epilepsy and the Dyscontrol Syndrome. Amsterdam, Elsevier, 1980
37. Hollender MH: Pathological intoxication—is there such an entity? J Clin Psychiatry 40:424-426, 1979
38. Hook EB: Behavioral implication of the human XYY genotype. Science 179:139-150, 1973

39. Hovey JE, Rickler, KC: Neurobehavioral evaluation of aggressive patients in an out-patient clinic, abstracted in: Aggressive Behavior 6:276, 1980
40. Itil, TM, Mukhopadhyay, S: Pharmacological management of human violence. Mod Probl Pharmacopsychiatry 13:139-158, 1978
41. Jaffee R: Letter to the Editor. Neurology 30:1337, 1980
42. Justice B, Justice R, Kraft, I: Early-warning signs of violence: Is a triad enough? Am J Psychiatry 131:457,459, 1974
43. Kelley D: Psychosurgery and the Limbic system. Postgrad Med J 49:825-833, 1973
44. King DW, Ajmone-Narson C: Clinical features and ictal patterns in epileptic patients with temporal lobe foci. Ann Neurol 2:138-147, 1977
45. Klingman D, and Goldberg DA: Temporal lobe epilepsy and aggression. J Nerv and Ment. Dis. 160:324-341, 1975
46. Krynicki, VE: Cerebral dysfunction in repetitively assaultive adolescents. J Nerv Ment Dis 166:59-67, 1978
47. Laschet U: Antiandrogen in the treatment of sex offenders: Mode of action and therapeutic outcome, in Zubin J, Money J (eds): Contemporary Sexual Behavior: Critical Issues in the 1970's. Baltimore, Johns Hopkins University Press, 1973
48. Lena B: Lithium therapy in hyperaggressive behavior in adolescents, in Sandler M: Psychopharmacology of Aggression, New York, Raven Press, 1979
49. Lewis DO: Delinquency, psychomotor epilepsy symptoms, and paranoid ideation: A triad. Am J Psychiatry 133:1395,1398, 1976
50. Lion JR: Evaluation and Management of the Violent Patient. Springfield, CC Thomas, 1972
51. Lion JR: Benzodiazepines in the treatment of aggressive patients. J Clin Psychiatry 40:70-71, 1979
52. Lion JR, Azcarate CL, Koepke HH: Paradoxical rage reactions during psychotropic medication. Dis Nerv Syst 36:557-558, 1975
53. Lion JR, Penna MW: Scientific, clinical and ethical issues in the treatment of aggressive patients, in Madden DJ, Lion JR (eds): Rage, Hate, Assault and Other Forms of Violence. New York, Spectrum, 1976
54. Livingston KE: Limbic Mechanisms. New York, Plenum, 1978
55. Livingston KE: Limbic connections: The limbic system as a substrate for epileptic disorder, in Girgis M, Kiloh LG: (eds): Limbic Epilepsy and the Dyscontrol syndrome. Amsterdam, L Severe, 1980
56. Lloyd CW, Weiss J: Hormones and aggression, in Fields WS, Sweet WH (eds): Neural Bases of Violence and Aggression. St. Louis, Warren Green, 1975
57. Lorimer FM: Violent behavior and the electroencephalogram. Clin Electroencephalography 3:193, 1972
58. Madden DJ: Psychological approaches to violence, in Madden DJ, Lion JR: Rage, Hate, Assault and Other Forms of Violence. New York, Spectrum, 1976
59. Malamud, N: Psychiatric disorder with intracranial tumors of limbic system. Arch Neurol 17:113-123

60. Maletzky, BM: The episodic dyscontrol syndrome. Dis Nerv Syst 36: 178-185, 1973
61. Mark VH, Sweet W, Ervin F: Deep temporal lobe stimulation and destructive lesions in episodically violent temporal lobe epileptics, in Fields WS, Sweet WH (eds): Neural Bases of Violence and Aggression. St. Louis, Warren Green, 1975
62. Matthews R: Testosterone levels in aggressive offenders, in Sandler M (ed): Psychopharmacology of Aggression. New York, Raven Press, 1979
63. Meyer-Bahlburg HF, Nat R, Boon DA et al: Aggressiveness and testosterone measures in man. Psychosom Med 36:269-274, 1974
64. Monahan J: The Clinical Prediction of Violent Behavior. Crime and Delinquency Issues: Monograph Series. U.S. Department of Health and Human Services, Washington, D.C., 1981
65. Monroe RR: Episodic Behavioral Disorders. Cambridge, Harvard University Press, 1970
66. Monroe RR: Brain Dysfunction in Aggressive Criminals. Toronto, Lexington Books, 1978
67. Monroe R: Anticonvulsants in the treatment of aggression. J Nerv Ment Dis 160:119-126, 1975
68. Montague A: Is man innately aggressive? in Fields WS, Sweet WH (eds): Neural Bases of Violence and Aggression. St. Louis, Warren Green, 1975
69. Moyer KE: Kinds of aggression and their physiological basis, in Communications in Behavioral Biology. Part A,2(z):65-87, 1968
70. Narabayshi H, Uno, M: Long-range results of stereotaxic amygdalatomy for behavior disorders. Confina Neural 27:168-172, 1966
71. Neumann F: Pharmacology and potential use of cyproterone acetate. Horm Metab Res 9:1-13, 1977
72. Owen DR: The 47, XYY male: A review. Psychol Bull 78:209-233, 1972
73. Papez JW: A proposed mechanism of emotion. Arch Neurol Psychiatry 38:725-743, 1937
74. Pincus JH: Can violence be a manifestation of epilepsy? Neurology 30:304-307, 1980
75. Pincus JH: Author's Reply. Neurology 30:1340-1341, 1980
76. Ratner RA, Shapiro D: The episodic dyscontrol syndrome and criminal responsibility. Am Acad Psychiatry Law 7:422-431, 1979
77. Reis DJ: Central neurotransmitters in aggressive behavior, in Fields WS, Sweet WH: Neural Bases of Violence and Aggression, St. Louis, Warren Green, 1975
78. Reisen D: Law, mental health, and impulsive patients, in Wishnie HA, Nevis-Olesen J: Working with the Impulsive Person. New York, Plenum, 1979
79. Richmond JS, Young JR, Groves JE: Violent dyscontrol responsive to d-amphetamine. Am J Psychiatry 135:365-366, 1978
80. Riley T, Niedermeyer E: Rage attacks and episodic violent behavior: Electroencephlographic findings in general consideration. Clin Electroencephalography 9:131-139, 1978
81. Rodin EA: Psychomotor epilepsy and aggressive behavior. Arch Gen Psy-

chiatry 28:210,214, 1973
82. Rotenberg M, Mordechai, MI: Impulsiveness and aggression among Israeli delinquents. Brit J Soc Clin Psychol 18:59–63, 1979
83. Sano K: Posterior hypothalmic lesions in the treatment of violent behavior, in Fields WS, Sweet WH (ed): Neural Bases of Violence and Aggression. St. Louis, Warren Green, 1975
84. Serafetinides EA: Epilepsy, cerebral dominance, and behavior, in Girgis M, Kiloh LG (eds): Limbic Epilepsy and the Dyscontrol Syndrome. Amsterdam, Elsevier, 1980
85. Sheard MH: Testosterone and aggression, in Sandler M (ed): Psychopharmacology of Aggression. Raven Press, New York, 1979
86. Smith JS: Episodic rage, in Girgis M, Kiloh LG (eds): Limbic Epilepsy and the Dyscontrol Syndrome. Amsterdam, Elsevier, 1980
87. Sprague RL, Slater EK: Effect of psychopharmacological agents in learning disorders. Pediatr Clin N Am 20:719–735, 1973
88. St. Hilaire JM, Gilbert M, Bouvier, G: Aggression as an epileptic manifestation: 2 cases with depth electrodes studies. Proceedings of the Am Epilepsy Society, Epilepsia 21:184, 1980
89. Steadman HJ: Predicting dangerousness, in Madden DJ, Lion JR (eds): Rage, Hate, Assault and Other Forms of Violence. New York, Spectrum, 1976
90. Stokes J, Mendels J: Pyridoxine and premenstrual tension. Lancet 1(761); 1177–1178, May, 1972
91. Stevens JR, Hermann BP: Temporal Lobe Epilepsy, Psychopathology and Violence: The State of the Evidence. Neurology 31:1127–1132, 1981
92. Tunks EP, Dermer, SW: Carbamazepine in the dyscontrol syndrome associated with limbic system dysfunction. J Nerv Ment Dis 164:156, 1977
93. Valenstein ES: Brain control. New York, Wiley, 1973
94. Walker AE, Blumer D: Long term behavioral effects of temporal lobectomy for temporal lobe epilepsy, in Blumer, Levin K (eds): Psychiatric complications in the epilepsies: Current research and treatment. McLean Hospital Journal, June, 1977
95. Weideking C, Money J, Walker P: Follow-up of 11 XYY males with impulsive and/or sex-offending behavior. Psychol Med 9:287,292, 1979
96. Worral EP: The antiaggressive effects of lithium, in Johnson FN, Johnson S: Lithium in Medical Practice. Baltimore, University Park Press, 1978
97. Yudofsky S, Williams D, Gorman J: Propranolol in the treatment of rage and violent behavior in patients with chronic brain syndromes. Am J Psychiatry 138:218–220, 1981

Commentary

As Chapter 3 so clearly demonstrated, episodic violence is neither a single nor a simple entity. That many individuals with episodic dyscontrol have basic biologic malfunction is quite apparent from the review of the literature and the description of cases presented by Dr. Rickler. On the other hand, it also seems apparent that social factors and environmental stresses may be of considerable significance in individual cases of paroxysmal aggressive behavior and deserve recognition and management. It is unreasonable to expect the practicing neurologist or psychiatrist to understand and appropriately manage all cases of violence. Episodic dyscontrol is not a single disease process but a syndrome that encompasses a number of distinctly different disorders. Only with acceptance of this actuality will it be possible for future studies of episodic dyscontrol to provide sharper diagnostic criteria and better management techniques. While considerable information for handling the paroxysmally violent patient has been offered, the most valuable function of Dr. Rickler's review was the provision of a basic structure with which to cope with these difficult and dangerous patients.

Another important but largely unexplored area involving both psychiatric disorder and epilepsy concerns the psychotic states that develop in some chronic epileptic patients. While such disturbances were clearly noted over a century ago,[2] there was little definition of the problem until about 20 years ago.[1] For most practicing psychiatrists and neurologists, these disorders have remained poorly understood and controversial. Are they merely the chance occurrence of two common disorders (psychosis and epilepsy) in the same individual? Or do they represent a distinct and potentially remediable form of psychosis? And, even more enticing, do they offer a royal road toward the understanding of psychosis? The answers to these questions, pertinent to both psychiatrists and neurologists, will demand a great deal of careful investigation.

While no one would claim that the psychotic complications of epilepsy are common, most would agree that if they do exist as specific disorders many currently go unrecognized. It would follow that if a rational treatment is available, even for just a few of these patients, then most epileptic psychoses are currently being mismanaged. The psychotic complications of epilepsy are a significant medical problem, not so much because of their frequency but because almost all are unrecognized and, therefore, deprived of appropriate therapy. In the following chapter Dr. Trimble presents a review of the background leading to a better understanding of the relationship of epilepsy and psychosis and adds material from his own studies to augment and illustrate these problems.

REFERENCES

1. Hill D: The schizophrenia-like psychoses of epilepsy. Pro Roy Soc 55:315–316, 1962
2. Samt P: Epileptische Irreseinformen. Arch Psychiat 6:110–216, 1876

Michael R. Trimble, M.R.C.P, F.R.C. Psych.

4
The Interictal Psychoses of Epilepsy

HISTORICAL INTRODUCTION

The relationship between psychosis and epilepsy has been commented on since antiquity, and early suggestions of chronic psychotic disorders go back to Willis in the 17th century.[5] In the 19th century, the growth of mental hospitals caused an increasing number of patients with epilepsy to come under the care of neuropsychiatrists, several of whom provided figures specifically on this relationship. Griesinger noted that "a very great number of epileptics are in a state of chronic mental disease even during the intervals between their attacks",[17] and Esquirol reported that of 385 epileptic women, 12 were monomaniacs, 30 were manic, and 34 were furious.[9] Morel introduced the term "larval epilepsy" for those cases in which automatic activity, without a necessarily clear loss of consciousness, included behavioral disturbances such as anger, violence, and emotional outbursts.[31] Falret drew attention to the more immediate mental prodromes of epilepsy, and distinguished them from folie épileptique, which could follow epileptic attacks in some patients and substitute for them in others.[10] He classified psychiatric disorders of epilepsy into three types: peri-ictal, interictal, and long-term insanities, the latter being "those phenomena of longer duration constituting true madness, whose onset should be described as either associated with or independent of any seizural manifestations." Echeverria reported that nocturnal epilepsy was more likely to be complicated by insanity than daytime epilepsy, and that hallucinations occurred in 86 percent of cases, 62 percent of which were auditory.[7] He divided psychiatric illness into three types: intermittent, remittent, and continuous.

Comprehensive accounts of mental states found in epilepsy were given by Maudsley[30] and Turner.[50] Maudsley noted the development of states of insanity in chronic cases—which often progressed to dementia—in which "exaggerated development of the religious sentiment" occurred and was associated with visions and revelations from on high. Turner commented on paroxysmal psychoses which either precede, succeed, or replace the convulsive episodes and included hallucinatory, delusional, maniacal, melancholic, or psychasthenic states. He also noted that a number of epileptic patients passed "eventually into a state of continued delusional insanity, requiring asylum treatment. . . ."

Thus, by 1900 many authors had commented on the interparoxysmal mental state in epilepsy and had noted the development of psychosis. Several reports then appeared that specifically examined these psychoses, referring in particular to the schizophreniform variety. Gruhle quoted 23 authors who described individual cases, and commented particularly on the gradual development of a chronic paranoid psychosis in established epileptic patients.[18] He felt that these cases did not represent combinations of two different diseases, but that they were truly symptomatic schizophrenias. Glaus documented eight cases in detail in which schizophrenia and, particularly, paranoid syndromes, occured.[15] In seven of these cases, the epilepsy antedated the psychosis, and in the majority the schizophrenia developed at a time when the epileptic seizures decreased or disappeared altogether.

The increasing use of the EEG and the identification of temporal lobe lesions in association with epilepsy led to the recognition that psychiatric disorders were more common in cases with focal temporal lobe epilepsy than in other forms of epilepsy.[13] Pond referred to the chronic paranoid-hallucinatory state in epilepsy as a definitive entity, and noted that all patients with this condition had temporal lobe epilepsy with typical complex auras.[35] Again he noted that the epileptic attacks began some years before the psychotic symptoms, and that the latter often appeared when the epileptic fits were diminishing in frequency. Hill also commented on this clinical condition, again noting the relationship to temporal lobe seizures.[21]

Since these descriptions, a number of more comprehensive studies have been carried out including those of Slater and Beard,[40] Flor-Henry,[11,12] Bruens,[3] Taylor,[46] Kristensen and Sindrup,[26] Jensen and Larsen,[22] Perez and Trimble,[33] and Sherwin,[39] and will be discussed further.

Although one conclusion to be drawn from this literature is that a relationship between psychosis and epilepsy exists, an alternative view has been expressed, namely that epilepsy and psychosis are biologically antagonistic.[28] This idea seems to have originated in the 1920s with observations of a low prevalence of epilepsy in schizophrenia[15,25] and the introduction of convulsive therapy by von Meduna in the 1930s that was based on a theory of antagonism between fits and psychosis.[51] This apparent paradox was resolved by Davison and Bagley, who suggested that while there is an affinity between the two disorders, there are some individual cases in which an antagonism can be noted between schizophrenic symptoms and convulsions, whether spontaneous or induced.[4]

THE ANTAGONISM HYPOTHESIS

The relationship between psychosis and epilepsy can be subdivided into peri-ictal conditions in which a clear neurophysiologic relationship exists between the epileptic seizure and the mental state, and interictal states which are the chronic disorders described in this chapter.

A different phenomenon was described by Landolt.[27] He recorded changes in the EEG during both preseizure dysphoric episodes and limited periods of frank psychosis which sometimes lasted days or weeks. During these episodes he noted improvement in previously abnormal EEGs; he termed this "forced normalization." At the end of psychotic episodes the EEGs were again abnormal. Dongier collected information on 536 psychotic episodes that occurred in 516 epileptic patients.[6] Consciousness was disturbed in 69 percent, and delusions occurred in 54 percent; 40 percent had centrencephalic epilepsy; and 44 percent had psychomotor epilepsy. Patients with clouding of consciousness were more likely to have centrencephalic epilepsy than focal or psychomotor epilepsy. A relationship was observed between disturbance of consciousness and the presence of diffuse delta waves or continuous bisynchronous spike-wave discharges on the EEG. EEG abnormalities disappeared during the psychosis in 78 cases, and 53 percent of these showed no clouding of consciousness. Delusions were particularly frequent in patients in whom a preexisting focal discharge disappeared, and in these patients the episode lasted a particularly long time, sometimes several weeks. These observations, in addition to a number of other documented clinical cases in the literature,[4] indicate that it is possible to define a group of patients in whom there is a well-defined antagonism between psychotic symptoms and EEG abnormalities. The later work of Landolt indicated that such alternations were more common following the suppression of spike-wave discharges with anticonvulsant drugs. Ethosuximide seems particularly related to this sequence of events, and the psychosis in some cases may be prolonged if the state is not recognized.[52]

Both Landolt[27] and Dongier[6] suggested that paranoid and schizophreniform states were more likely to be seen after the suppression of focal, particularly temporal focal, as opposed to generalized, discharges. Several explanations have been put forward to explain these phenomena. Landolt regarded the EEG changes as causal to the development of the psychosis. Reynolds drew attention to biochemical explanations; he noted that anti-epileptic drugs could precipitate a psychosis and that epileptic fits could be induced by antipsychotic drugs in schizophrenic patients.[37] He particularly highlighted the relationship between folic acid and both the mental state and seizures and the ability of anti-epileptic drugs to lower folic acid levels. An alternative hypothesis has been suggested involving dopamine.[49] The most efficacious antipsychotic drugs block dopamine, and drugs such as amphetamine, which are dopamine agonists, can lead to a psychosis that is indistinguishable from schizophrenia. A number of clinical observations and laboratory experiments have shown that dopamine agonists raise the seizure threshold and that dopamine antagonism decreases it, often provoking seizures.[29] There thus appears to be a relationship between psychosis, epilepsy, and dopamine such that dopamine antagonism resolves a psychosis but lowers the seizure threshold, whereas dopamine agonism increases the seizure threshold but may provoke or exacerbate psychosis. Alterations of dopamine activity, which can occur spontaneously or result from the administration of anti-epileptic or antipsychotic drugs, could thus underlie these clinical observations of antagonism.

ON THE AFFINITY BETWEEN EPILEPSY AND PSYCHOSIS

Neither schizophrenia nor epilepsy are rare disorders, and the appearance of both conditions in the same person may be the result of chance. Slater and Beard estimated the expectation of this coincidence and statistically predicted the number of new cases each year in the greater London area.[40] In their studies, they easily documented 69 cases of epilepsy and schizophrenia which they considered to be far in excess of chance. They criticized earlier papers that had suggested a low prevalence of epilepsy existed in schizophrenic populations[2] and suggested on statistical grounds, that patients who suffered from epilepsy developed a schizophrenia-like illness with increased frequency. A number of other authors have reported an increased prevalence of epilepsy among schizophrenic patients. Kraepelin suggested that epilepsy occurred as a precursor to dementia praecox, and noted it in about 16 percent of his cases.[24] Yde et al. noted that epilepsy was twice as common in 715 patients with schizophrenia as it was in a general population.[53] Results such as these, however, have been questioned by Stevens,[42] who noted that the calculation of the probability that epilepsy and schizophrenia will occur in the same individual in the general population does not apply when dealing with referred populations. In her own studies, she found schizophrenia to be underrepresented in referred psychiatric populations.[43]

Two studies are of most importance here. In the first, Gudmundsson surveyed the epileptic population of Iceland and noted that 5.5 percent of the men and 9.1 percent of the women were psychotic.[19] The second study is the recently published follow-up report of Ounsted and Lindsay.[32] In 1964, these authors took a continuous, unselected sample of 100 children with clinically diagnosed temporal lobe epilepsy who demonstrated an EEG focus in one or both temporal regions. In 1977, these children were re-examined and nine were found to be psychotic showing schizophrenic signs or symptoms. In both of these studies, the development of psychosis was far higher than expected for a nonepileptic population.

The first comprehensive study of the relationship between epilepsy and psychosis was that of Slater and Beard.[40] Of the 69 patients they examined, 11 had chronic psychoses that had been preceded by recurrent, short-lived confusional states, 46 had a psychosis that was highly typical of paranoid schizophrenia, and 12 had hebephrenic schizophrenia. In all these patients, little evidence existed of abnormal premorbid personality or family history of psychiatric disturbance that would suggest a predisposition to schizophrenia. The mean age of onset of the psychosis was 29.8 years, and it occurred after the epilepsy had been present for a mean of 14.1 years. Although it was not possible to relate the onset of the mental illness to any change in the quantity or quality of the fits in most patients, in some 25 percent of cases the psychotic symptoms appeared when the frequency of generalized seizures was decreasing. They were unable to document any relationship between the anticonvulsant drugs that the patients received and the subsequent psychotic illness, but noted that the most common form of epilepsy was temporal lobe epilepsy. Although clinical neurologic findings were usually negative, air encephalography, which was carried out in 56 cases, showed abnormalities in 39, usually that of atrophy. In 19 cases there was dilatation of one or both temporal horns.

That these sort of observations are not confined to Western cultures is indicated from the studies of Asunti and Pillutla who found a schizophrenia-like psychosis in 11 out of 42 epileptic patients in Western Nigeria.[1] These patients had many of the characteristics described by Slater and Beard, including the preservation of affect and a correlation between duration of the epilepsy and the onset of the psychosis.

Bruens studied 19 epileptic patients with psychotic states, the duration of which varied from 2.5 months to 29 years.[3] Nine cases had a paranoid syndrome with systematized delusions and two had a schizophrenia-like psychoses. Hallucinations and delusions were particularly marked in the symptomatology, and religious coloration was common. In 16 of the patients, temporal lobe epilepsy was noted. He reaffirmed Slater's suggestion that a fairly constant interval existed between the onset of the epilepsy and the onset of the psychosis, and assumed a causal relationship between the two disorders. In contrast to Slater, he commented that none of the psychoses noted filled the strict criteria for a diagnosis of schizophrenia, the quality of phenomenology not being typical.

Jensen and Larsen presented data on 20 Danish patients with psychosis and temporal lobe epilepsy who were drug-resistant and had undergone anterior temporal lobe resection.[22] Eleven of the 20 patients had developed their psychosis preoperatively, but in 9 the psychopathology developed after surgery and apparent relief from their seizures. Thirteen were said to have schizophrenia-like psychosis. More focal neurophysiologic abnormalities were noted in the psychotic group, although in those who were preoperatively psychotic, the lobectomy did not influence the course of the psychosis.

Despite reservations by certain authors,[23,42] a number of other studies have emphasized the relationship between temporal lobe abnormalities and psychosis. In a study of 275 cases, Gibbs noted that 17 percent of patients with anterior temporal spike activity had features of psychosis. Ervin et al. noted that in a group of 42 patients with temporal spikes, 34 had received a clinical diagnosis of schizophrenia.[8] The most severe psychiatric disturbances were noted in those with psychomotor seizures. Rodin et al. presented six cases in detail in which psychomotor epilepsy was associated with schizophrenic symptomatology.[38] Glaser evaluated 37 patients with psychomotor temporal lobe seizure states who had psychotic episodes lasting from 1 to many days.[14] He emphasized the disturbed thought processes, interrupted or broken flow of association, and word-finding difficulties that occur in these patients.

LATERALITY OF FOCUS AND PSYCHOSIS

A significant advance was made by Flor-Henry in a comprehensive but retrospective study of 50 cases of temporal lobe epilepsy who had formerly been classified as psychotic.[11] A nonpsychotic control group was also examined. When compared with the controls, the schizophreniform psychotics were found to have fewer psychomotor seizures and to have epilepsy lateralised particularly to the dominant hemisphere, while patients with nondominant foci tended to be manic-depressive. These laterality effects were confirmed by Gregoriadis et al.[16] in a group of 52 hospitalised psychotic-epileptic patients, although no details of this study have ever been published.

Another controlled investigation has recently been undertaken on 192 patients with complex partial seizures and psychosis by Kristensen and Sindrup.[26] They noted that the fit frequency for complex partial seizures was lower in the psychotic group, and that an interval with a median of 18 years occurred between the onset of the epilepsy and the psychosis. They subdivided their patients depending on whether the seizures were accompanied by automatisms, epigastric aura, or were superficially initiated (psychic seizures). There was a significantly greater number of patients with automatisms in the psychotic group. Clinical neurologic and otoneurologic examination showed a greater proportion of psychotic patients to have findings indicative of an organic brain lesion, and EEGs demonstrated that psychotic patients have maximal focal spike activity at the mediobasal temporal lobe surface. They were unable however to confirm the laterality differences noted by Flor-Henry.

Jensen and Larsen were unable to confirm or refute the laterality findings,[22] and Bruens did not comment on it.[3] Further evidence, however, has come from the work of Taylor,[46] Sherwin,[39] Toone and Driver,[48] Perez and Trimble,[34] and Ounsted and Lindsay.[32] Taylor examined patients who had undergone unilateral temporal lobectomy for uncontrolled complex partial seizures. The psychotic patients, diagnosed as schizophrenia-like, tended to have hamartomatous lesions, as opposed to medial temporal sclerosis, and there was an excess of left-sided lesions (69 percent). Sherwin used stereo-encephalography with implanted temporal electrodes to establish laterality in seven cases whose histories suggested schizophreniform-like psychosis. Five had left-sided lesions. Toone and Driver reported a retrospective study of 56 patients in which schizophreniform states were associated with EEG foci and CAT scan abnormalities of the left side. Perez and Trimble, in a prospective study, noted a high incidence of left temporal EEG abnormalities in patients diagnosed by standardised and validated rating scales as schizophrenia-like. Finally, seven of the nine cases in Ounsted and Lindsay's series who developed a schizophreniform illness on follow-up had left-sided temporal lobe epilepsy, the other two having bilateral abnormalities. This latter study is especially important since the laterality had been decided in 1964, leaving little possibility for bias. None of the above authors has confirmed Flor-Henry's suggestion that manic-depressive psychosis is linked to nondominant hemisphere lesions.

PHENOMENOLOGY OF PSYCHOSIS

One difficulty with many of the above studies is the lack of consistency regarding terms such as psychosis and schizophrenia-like, etc. This may explain some of the contradictory findings. Pond, in his early paper, described a paranoid hallucinatory psychotic state in association with temporal lobe epilepsy, and agreed with Marchand and Ajuriaguerra that manic-depressive psychoses were quite rare in epilepsy.

Pond described the symptoms of the epileptic psychotic state as "paranoid ideas which may become systematized, ideas of influence, auditory hallucinations often of a menacing quality, and occasionally frank thought disorders with neologisms, condensed words, and inconsequential sentences." Religious coloring of these paranoid ideas was common, and he commented on the warm affect of such patients in contrast to the affective changes of process schizophrenia. The symptomatology of Slater's patients included delusions in clear consciousness; this was noted in all patients but two, although primary delusional experiences, supposedly characteristic of schizophrenia, were seldom observed. Mystical delusions with religious overtones were very common. Passive feelings were a prominent finding and were often closely connected with systematized ideas of persecution. Special powers were claimed by many patients, such as the ability to heal people by looking at them, or being able to see through walls or split atoms.

The majority of patients also had hallucinatory experiences, often visual and complex. The most common hallucinations, however, were auditory and frequently comprised persecutory voices. Voices talking about the patient in the third person and those which commented on the patient's actions or repeated their own thoughts were likewise relatively common. Thought disorder was shown in half the patients, usually as a relative incapacity to handle abstract concepts. Thought blocking and neologisms were also commented upon as were sentences that were never finished or showed disturbed syntax.

Affective disturbances of some kind were shown by all his patients, usually in the form of periodic moods of depression or irritability. This was often short-lived and severe. Seventeen patients had attempted suicide on one or more occasions. The so-called flattened affect was noted in 28 patients, but more commonly affect remained warm, in contrast to process schizophrenic patients. Manneristic behavior was noted in many, although catatonic phenomena were rare.

Flor-Henry used Kraepelinian categories, the diagnosis of schizophrenia being related to the presence of thought disorder and disturbances of affect with or without symptoms such as hallucinations. In contrast, manic-depressive states were characterised by euphoric or depressive alterations of mood exhibiting periodicity and leaving the personality intact between phases. Bruens noted the symptomatology in his 19 patients to be as follows: 9 had paranoid syndromes with delusions that were more or less systematized, 5 had psychosis with marked mental regression and transient paranoid symptoms, 2 had schizophrenia-like psychosis with thought disorder and affective disturbance, and 3 had relatively short-lived confusional states. Hallucinations occurred in 15 out of the 19 patients and were auditory in 12. The hallucinations usually consisted of voices which were heard almost continuously, without clouding of consciousness. Religious and sexual themes were common in these phenomena, and visual hallucinations were reported in 7. Delusions were seen in 15 cases, 9 of which were delusions of reference, with grandiose delusions the second most frequently recorded. Manic-depressive symptomatology was not a predominant syndrome in any of his cases, although it is important to note that delusions of guilt occurred in 4 patients. Kristensen and Sindrup examined patients with paranoid hallucinatory psychosis and epilepsy, although they did not discuss the phenomenology preferring to use the term epileptic psychosis. Jensen and Larsen did not clearly define the phenomenology of their group either,[22] being characterised as psychosis with paranoid delusions.

Perez and Trimble have recently assessed the precise phenomenology of the psychoses of epilepsy using a standardised and validated rating scale,[33] the Present State Examination (PSE) of Wing. The results from the PSE schedule were analysed using the Catego computer program, in which the original items noted during the interview pass through a progressive series of condensations in which decisions about the actual diagnostic category of patients are postponed until the final stage. This method is known to be reliable in the diagnosis of schizophrenia, particularly for the identification of nuclear schizophrenia, based on Schneider's first rank symptoms. Twenty-four consecutively referred psychotic patients with epilepsy were compared with 11 nonepileptic patients who were clinically diagnosed as suffering from schizophrenia. Half of the patients in the epileptic group had identical symptom profiles to those in the schizophrenia control group, and the majority received a dignosis of nuclear schizophrenia. All the latter had temporal lobe epilepsy, the majority having bilateral or left-sided lesions. The other patients showed a variety of other psychoses, although in this series manic pictures were frequent and paranoid psychosis rare.

MECHANISMS OF CHRONIC INTERICTAL PSYCHOSIS

The evidence presented suggests that the chronic interictal psychoses of epilepsy occur with increased frequency in patients with temporal lobe epilepsy. The work of Kristensen and Sindrup suggests that patients with complex partial seizures seem most prone and that dysfunction of medial temporal structures are important in the pathogenesis. Several authors have implied an association between left temporal lobe abnormality and schizophreniform illness, and the work of Perez and Trimble indicates that phenomenologically this is identical to schizophrenia in nonepileptic populations. The link between the nondominant hemisphere and manic-depressive psychosis has yet to be substantiated. Other factors that may be of importance are a diminishing seizure frequency with the onset of the psychosis (another manifestation of antagonism), structural lesions, and a development of the abnormality before puberty. While several authors have reiterated Slater's point about there being a standard time interval between the epilepsy and the psychosis,[26,22] this has been criticised by Stevens,[41] partly on the grounds that the average age of onset of temporal lobe epilepsy is earlier than schizophrenia when they occur independently. As Toone pointed out, however, temporal lobe epilepsy actually has a wide range of age of onset, the peak epoch being between 25 and 50 years, while first admission for schizophrenia is between 20 and 40 years in the majority of subjects.[47] In most cases reported in the above studies, the epilepsy precedes the psychosis, and not vice versa.[47] The lack of a genetic predisposition to schizophrenia and the absence of premorbid schizoid personality traits in these patients implies that lesional factors are of prime importance in their pathogenesis.[40]

There are two main hypotheses. The first is that the schizophrenia-like illnesses are epileptic in origin and should be referred to as epileptic psychoses. The second is that they are a manifestation of organic neurologic damage and thus not specific for epilepsy.[40] The former view has been most strongly expressed by Flor-Henry.[11] He criticized the absence of a control population in some of the older studies, noted the constant observation of an inverse relationship between frequency of psychomotor seizures and the onset of the psychosis, commented on the laterality effect he had noted, and suggested that it was not structural damage, but the characteristics of the seizures that lead to the clinical picture. Continuing abnormal epileptic neuronal activity was thought to be responsible, therefore, for the schizophrenic syndrome. Support for this suggestion comes from depth electrode studies in psychotic patients who do not have epilepsy. Abnormal activity in the deep temporal structures is associated with suppression of surface cortical activity, and when patients are psychotic abnormal spike-wave activity may be detected in these areas, which is not seen on conventional surface electrodes.[20]

Bruens put forward the idea that both organic and psychodynamic events potentiate each other.[3] The patient is unable to protect himself against the vicissitudes of life except by using pathologic defence mechanisms, which result in psychosis. Pond suggested it was the abnormal experiences associated with temporal lobe epilepsy which gradually became integrated into a person's psychic life that led to the development of the psychosis.[36] These explanations do not account for the laterality findings, however, and as Slater and Beard point out, do not take into account the volitional disturbances, thought disorders, and hebephrenic symptoms noted in some of these patients.

Symonds pointed to the epileptic disorder of function.[45] He suggested that the loss of balance between excitation and inhibition at synaptic junctions leads not only to the paroxysmal phenomena of epilepsy, but also that the continuous disorder of neuronal function leads to interictal symptoms, the nature of which will be related to the site of the focal activity. It was, he suggested, not the loss of neurones in the temporal lobe that was responsible for the psychosis but the disordered activity of those that remain.

The most important changes, however, cannot reside in the affected temporal lobe since several authors have reported cases of psychosis occurring after temporal lobectomy.[46,22,39] In addition, if a number of years do exist between the beginning of the epilepsy and the onset of the psychosis, as some of the studies suggest, modification of Symonds' ideas may be necessary. The discovery in experimental neurophysiology of kindling may provide an important link here. Thus it is extremely difficult to kindle epileptic seizures in certain parts of the limbic system, particularly those that are catecholaminergic. Kindling of the mesolimbic dopamine system leads not to seizures, but to marked behaviour changes that persist after the kindling has ceased.[44] The possibility arises that similar mechanisms may exist in man, such that chronic abnormal activity in the medial temporal limbic system in some forms of epilepsy leads to a kindling process resulting in the development of abnormal behavior patterns and psychosis. The neuroanatomic connections between amygdala and hippocampus and the midline septal nuclei are well established, as are the links between the latter and dopamine-rich areas of the limbic midbrain circuit such as the nucleus accumbens (this features predominently in recent work on the pathogenesis of schizophrenia in nonepileptic populations). Because the behavior changes associated with kindling of the mesolimbic dopamine system are enhanced by the administration of dopamine agonists, it is probable that kindling is associated with altered postsynaptic function of dopamine receptors. As noted, increased dopamine activity tends to increase the seizure threshold. As with the mechanism of antagonism discussed above, these observations may be invoked to explain the clinical findings of an association between persistent abnormal temporal lobe activity and psychosis, and the tendency of its development to be associated with declining seizure frequency.

While kindling may not be the ultimate mechanism of synaptic changes in such patients, and denervation supersensitivity, or altered neurotransmitter harmony by synaptic sprouting may seem better candidates to explain the clinical phenomena, future studies should seek further clarification of the precise phenomenology of the psychotic states associated with epilepsy. Evidence for abnormalities should be investigated by seeking neurophysiologic and neurochemical changes, especially in mesolimbic and mesocortical areas of the brain.

REFERENCES

1. Asunti T, Pillutla VS: Schizophrenia-like psychoses in Nigerian epileptics. Br J Psychiatry 113:1375-1379, 1967
2. Bartlet JEA: Chronic psychosis following epilepsy. Am J Psychiatry 114:338-343, 1957
3. Bruens JH: Psychosis in epilepsy. Psychiatria Neurologia Neurochiurgia 74:175-192, 1971
4. Davison K, Bagley CR: Schizophrenia-like psychoses associated with organic disorders of the central nervous system, in Herrington RN (ed): Current Problems in Neuropsychiatry. Kent, Headley, 1969, p 113
5. Dewhurst H: Thomas Willis' Oxford Lectures. Oxford, Sandford, 1980
6. Dongier S: Statistical study of clinical and electroencephalographic manifestations of 536 psychotic episodes occurring in 516 epileptics between clinical seizures. Epilepsia 1:117-142, 1959
7. Echeverria MG: On epileptic insanity. American Journal of Insanity 30:1-51, 1873
8. Ervin F, Epstein AW, King HE: Behavior of epileptic and nonepileptic patients with temporal spikes. Arch Neurol Psychiatry 74:488-497, 1955
9. Esquirol JED: Des maladies mentales considérées sous les rapports medical, hygiénique et medico-legal. Paris, Baillière, 1838
10. Falret J: De L'état mental des épileptiques. Archives générales de medicine 16:661-679, 1860
11. Flor-Henry P: Psychosis and temporal lobe epilepsy. Epilepsia 10:363-395, 1969
12. Flor-Henry P: Epilepsy and psychopathology, in Granville-Grossman K (ed): Recent Advances in Clinical Psychiatry, vol 2. Edinburgh, Churchill Livingstone, 1976

13. Gibbs FA: Ictal and non-ictal psychiatric disorders in temporal lobe epilepsy. J Nerv Ment Dis 113:522-528, 1951
14. Glaser GH: The problem of psychosis in psychomotor temporal lobe epileptics. Epilepsia 5:271-278, 1964
15. Glaus A: Ueber Cominationen von Schizophrenie und Epilepsie. Z diegesante neurol psychiat 135:450, 1931
16. Gregoriadis A et al: A correlation between mental disorders and EEG and AEG findings in temporal lobe epilepsy, in de la Fuente, Ramon, Weisman, MN (eds): World Congress of Psychiatry, 5th, Mexico City, 1971. Amsterdam, Excerpta Medica, 1973
17. Griesinger W: Mental Pathology and Therapeutics. Robertson CL, Rutherford J (trans), London, New Sydenham Society, 1867
18. Gruhle HW: Ueber den Wahn bei Epilepsie. Zeitschrift ges Neurol Psychiat 154:395-399, 1936
19. Gudmundsson G: Epilepsy in Iceland. Acta Neurol Scand 43 (Suppl 25):1-124, 1966
20. Heath RG: Subcortical brain function correlates of psychopathology and epilepsy, in Shagass C, Gershon S, Friedhoff AJ (eds): Psychopathology and Brain Dysfunction. New York, Raven Press, 1977
21. Hill D: Psychiatric disorders of epilepsy. Med Press 229:473-475, 1953
22. Jensen I, Larsen JK: Psychoses in drug-resistant temporal lobe epilepsy. J Neurol Neurosurg Psychiatry 42:948-954, 1979
23. Kiloh LG: Psychiatric aspects of epilepsy, in Winton RR (ed): Geigy Symposium on Epilepsy. Australia, Geigy, 1971
24. Kraepelin E: Dementia Praecox and Paraphrenia. Edinburgh, Livingstone, 1919
25. Krapf E: Epilepsie und Schizophrenie. Arch Psychiat Nervenkr 83:547-586, 1928
26. Kristensen O, Sindrup EH: Psychomotor epilepsy and psychosis. Acta Neurol Scand 57:361-370, 1978
27. Landolt H: Serial encephalographic investigations during psychotic episodes in epileptic patients and during schizophrenic attacks, in Lorentz de Haas (ed): Lectures on Epilepsy. London, Elsevier, 1958
28. Marchand L, De Ajuriaguerra J: Epilepsies: Leurs formes Cliniques, Leur traitements. Paris, Desclée de Brouwer, 1948
29. Meldrum B, Anlezark A, Trimble M: Drugs modifying dopamine activity and behaviour, the EEG and epilepsy in *Papio papio*. Eur Pharmacol 32:203-213, 1975
30. Maudsley H: Responsibility in Mental Disease. London, Henry S King, 1874
31. Morel BA: D'une forme de délire, suite d'une surexcitation nerveuse se rattachant á une variété non ecore décrite d'epilepsie. Gazette Hebdoma daire de medecine et de Chirurgie 7:773-775, 1860
32. Ounsted C, Lindsay J: The long-term outcome of temporal lobe epilepsy in childhood, in Reynolds EH, Trimble MR (eds): Psychiatry and Epilepsy. London, Churchill Livingstone, 1982, p 185-215
33. Perez MM, Trimble MR: Epileptic psychosis—diagnostic comparison with

process schizophrenia. Br J Psychiatry 137:245-249, 1980
34. Perez MM, Trimble MR: The phenomenology of the chronic phychoses of epilepsy. Adv Biol Psychiatry 8 (in press)
35. Pond DA: Psychiatric aspects of epilepsy. Journal of the Indian Medical Profession 3:1441-1451, 1957
36. Pond D: The schizophrenia-like psychoses of epilepsy—Discussion, in Proceedings of the Royal Society of Medicine 55:311, 1962
37. Reynolds EH: Epilepsy and schizophrenia. Relationship and biochemistry. Lancet i:398-401, 1968
38. Rodin EA, De Jong RN, Waggoner RW, Bagchi BK: Relationship between certain forms of psychomotor epilepsy and schizophrenia. Arch Neurol Psychiatry 77:449-463, 1957
39. Sherwin I: Specificity of psychopathology in epilepsy, significance of lesion laterality, in Girgis M, Kiloh LG (eds): Limbic Epilepsy and the Dyscontrol Syndrome. Amsterdam, Elsevier, 1980
40. Slater E, Beard AW: The schizophrenia-like psychoses of epilepsy. Br J Psychiatry 109:95-150, 1963
41. Stevens JR: Psychiatric implications of psychomotor epilepsy. Arch Gen Psychiatry 14:461-471, 1966
42. Stevens JR: Interictal clinical manifestations of complex partial seizures, in Penry JK, Daly DD (eds): Advances in Neurology, vol II. New York, Raven Press, 1975
43. Stevens JR: Biologic background of psychoses in epilepsy, in Carger R, Angeleri F, Penry JK (eds): Advances in Epileptology: XI Epilepsy International Symposium. New York, Raven Press, 1980, pp 167-172
44. Stevens JR, Livermore A: Kindling in the mesolimbic dopamine system: Animal model of psychosis. Neurology 28:36-46, 1978
45. Symonds C: The schizophrenia-like psychoses of epilepsy—Discussion, in: Proceedings of the Royal Society of Medicine. 55:311, 1962
46. Taylor DC: Factors influencing the occurrence of schizophrenia-like psychosis in patients with temporal lobe epilepsy. Psychol Med 5:249-254, 1975
47. Toone B: Psychoses of epilepsy, in Reynolds EH, Trimble MR (eds): Psychiatry and Epilepsy. London, Churchill Livingstone, 1982, p 113-137
48. Toone B, Driver MV: Psychosis and epilepsy, Res Clin Forum 2(2):121-128, 1980
49. Trimble MR: The relationship between epilepsy and schizophrenia: A biochemical hypothesis. Biol Psychiatry 12:299-304, 1977
50. Turner WA: Epilepsy: A Study of the Idiopathic Disease. New York, Macmillan, 1907
51. Von Meduna L: Die Konvulsiontherapie der Schizophrenie. Halle Marhold, 1937
52. Wolf P: Personal communication
53. Yde A, Lohse E, Faurbye A: On the relationship between schizophrenia, epilepsy and induced convulsions. Acta Psychiatr Scand 16:325-388, 1941

The Interictal Psychoses of Epilepsy

Commentary

As Dr. Trimble's discussion clearly notes, the presence of psychosis as a complication of epilepsy has long been controversial. Attempts to demonstrate phenomenologic differences between the epileptic and nonepileptic psychoses have not been consistently successful. Some suggest that the psychotic break caused by epilepsy has a shorter duration than the similar nonepileptic psychosis. Some look for a seizure disorder as the underlying disease in the so-called alternating psychosis.[2] Differences in basic affect and/or personality are more commonly cited. Sir Denis Hill noted that the ability to establish a warm rapport was easier with the epileptic with schizophrenia-like psychosis than with the schizophrenic,[3] but this is a difficult phenomenon to quantitate. The effect of long-term epilepsy on personality has also proved difficult to substantiate. Many investigators are adamant that at least some chronic epileptics do undergo a change of personality. Thus, one textbook categorically states that "it is however certain that personality changes may take place after the onset of epilepsy."[6] This apparently reasonable statement has not been easy to document.

It seems probable that many individuals currently diagnosed and treated as schizophrenic actually have a history of a seizure disorder that was mild, occurred many years before the onset of psychosis, and has long been forgotten. The onset of psychosis in a patient with a long history of epilepsy who maintains a warm and interested affect and/or has undergone an alteration in personality can suggest that the psychosis is a complication of epilepsy. This diagnosis is rarely made but if such a possibility is accepted, the schizophrenia-like psychoses must be considerably more frequent than currently recognized.

Just as the entity itself is controversial, the question of treatment for the psychotic complications of seizures is also difficult. Response to anticonvulsant medication may or may not be helpful (and anticonvulsants may be a cause of increased behavioral problems). The antipsychotic drugs appear to act more as symptomatic than specifically therapeutic treatment for these psychoses. It is now suggested that some psychotic complications may stem from sensitivity to a particular anticonvulsant and that onset of psychosis in the long-standing epileptic may be an indication for a change of medication.[2] A number of more radical treatments have been tried, some with at least partial success. For instance, it has been suggested that decreasing the anticonvulsant drug levels (even to the point of removing anticonvulsants and allowing occasional seizures) can lead to improved behavior.[4] Some even suggest that electroshock therapy can be used successfully to treat the schizophreniform complications of epilepsy.[6] None of the above treatment suggestions has been widely used or put to any controlled study but, at least in some clinical situations, each has proved helpful. Any schizophrenia-like complication in a known epileptic should be scrutinized carefully as a quite different therapeutic approach may be indicated.

The subject of acquired intellectual impairment is a different but equally common and difficult topic as that of epileptic behavioral complications. At the present time, dementia represents one of the most frequent and devastating of all neurobehavioral problems. With a surprising suddenness, dementia has come to be a crucial clinical and investigative topic. The current interest in dementia is predicated in large part by the fact that serious mental deterioration is much more common among the elderly. The vast increase in the number of older-age individuals over the past several decades (it is estimated that half of all the humans in the history of mankind who have lived for more than 65 years are alive at the present time) coupled with projections indicating further increase in this population, makes dementia one of the more serious of all current public health problems.

One of the important contributions from the first volume of *Psychiatric Aspects of Neurologic Disease* was a strong rebuttal of the use of the word "irreversible" in the definition of dementia.[5] This position has become widely accepted, at least as a definition,[1] but among practitioners a tendency to consider dementia an irreversible and therefore untreatable disorder remains firmly entrenched. Most current research studies on dementia focus on Alzheimer's disease, the most common form of dementia caused by cortical degeneration: Unfortunately, Alzheimer's disease is presently an untreatable disorder. Other forms of dementia are acknowledged and are of admitted importance because at least some respond favorably to appropriate treatment. These treatable disorders have received relatively little emphasis even though many of the cases of dementia seen by psychiatrists and neurologists are strikingly different. Several disorders, such as the mental deterioration of severe alcoholism and the mental deterioration seen with severe depression, are notoriously difficult problems in neurobehavior. Dementia is far too vast a problem to be handled in the four chapters devoted to the topic in this book; attention will be focused on new and/or controversial points that, hopefully, will aid the clinician. The first of the four chapters presents an up-dated discussion of the cortical dementias with particular emphasis given to the Alzheimer and Pick's varieties of degeneration and includes both a review of the neuropathologic characteristics and an outline of clinical information which allows differentiation of these two insidious dementing disorders.

REFERENCES

1. American Psychiatric Association: Diagnostic and Statistical Manual of Mental Disorders—III. Washington, Am Psychiat Assoc 1980
2. Helmchen VH: Psychiatrische Prognose bei Epilepsien. Schweizer Archiv fuer Neurologie, Neurochiurgie und Psychiatrie 124:71-88, 1979
3. Hill D: The schizophrenia-like psychoses of epilepsy. Pro Roy Soc 55:315-316, 1962
4. Landolt H: Die Temperalloppenepilepsie und ihre Psychopathologie. Bibl Psychiat Neurol (Basel) 112:451, 454, 459, 462, 1960
5. Lipowski ZJ: Organic brain syndromes: Overview and classification, in Benson DF, Blumer D (eds): Psychiatric Aspects of Neurologic Disease. New York, Grune & Stratton, 1975, pp 11-35
6. Mayer-Gross W, Slater E, Roth M: Clinical Psychiatry (ed 3). London, Balliere, Tindall and Cassell, 1969
7. Plum F: Dementia: An approaching epidemic. Nature 279:372-373, 1979

Jeffrey L. Cummings, M.D.

5
Cortical Dementias

Dementia is a clinical syndrome defined as an acquired persistent deterioration in mental function involving at least three of the following areas of neuropsychologic activity: language, memory, visuo-spatial skills, personality or emotion, and cognition (abstraction, calculation).[31] There are two clinical varieties of dementia: a subcortical type arising from disturbances of basal ganglia, thalamus, and rostral brainstem structures, and a cortical type produced by cerebral cortical degeneration.[11] Subcortical dementias are characterized by slowing of cognition, memory disturbances, affective changes, and "dilapidation" of cognition (see Chapter 6). The cardinal manifestations of cortical dementias are aphasia, amnesia, agnosia, and apraxia. The subcortical conditions associated with dementia have a prominent movement disorder as part of their clinical symptomatology, whereas primary cortical dementias lack motor system abnormalities until late in their clinical courses. Extrapyramidal disorders such as Parkinson's disease, Huntington's disease, progressive supranuclear palsy, lacunar state, normal pressure hydrocephalus, and Wilson's disease account for most of the primary subcortical dementias; Alzheimer's disease and Pick's disease produce most of the cortical dementias. Conditions such as Jakob Creutzfeldt disease and multi-infarct dementia may exhibit both cortical and subcortical characteristics. In this chapter, Alzheimer's and Pick's disease will be described in detail and the features that may distinguish them will be emphasized. Other diseases that produce a cortical type dementia will also be discussed and their differentiating features noted. No distinction will be made between Alzheimer's disease with onset before age 65 and senile dementia beginning after age 65. The pathologic findings are identical, and the clinical manifestations in the two age groups are sufficiently similar to justify combined discussion.

ALZHEIMER'S DISEASE

Alzheimer first described the disease that bears his name in 1907.[153] He reported a 51-year-old woman who became excessively jealous of her husband, had memory difficulties, and got lost in her own apartment. Her spontaneous speech included paraphasic errors, her comprehension of language was impaired, and she was unable to demonstrate the use of common objects. Her gait was normal and no other neurologic abnormalities were found. Histologic examination of the brain revealed that many neurons contained neurofibrillary tangles and there were abundant senile plaques (miliary foci) in the cerebral cortex. In 1910, Kraepelin began the tradition of applying Alzheimer's name to the dementing process characterized by these distinctive histologic alterations.[27.]

Alzheimer's disease accounts for between 3 and 20 percent of autopsies in chronic mental hospitals[51,61,157] and the disease is two to three times more common in women than in men.[81] Most cases begin between the ages of 50 and 70 with death occurring in 1 to 10 years.[51,133] Several patients presenting with the disease in their early forties have been reported.[42,85] Alzheimer's disease is usually sporadic but occasionally occurs on a familial basis[20,25,37,40,85,95,151] and inheritance then follows an autosomal dominant pattern.[115] There is an increased incidence of Alzheimer's disease, senile dementia, Down's syndrome, and hematologic malignancies among relatives of patients with Alzheimer's disease[25,63] and nearly all elderly Down's syndrome patients develop Alzheimer's disease.[108]

Clinical Course

The clinical course of the disease can be divided into three stages. The pattern of temporal evolution and progression of the clinical features is useful in the diagnosis of Alzheimer's disease and may be crucial in differentiating it from other dementing illnesses. Memory disturbance is nearly always the earliest feature noted by the patient or his family. Carelessness in work habits and personal appearance and spatial and temporal disorientation also occur early. Paranoia often contributes to the initial symptomatology. With progression into the second stage of the disease, aphasic, apractic, and agnosic disturbances occur as well as increasing disorientation and motor restlessness. Terminally, the intellectual deficits are exaggerated and combined with progressive immobility, incontinence, and the appearance of primitive reflexes.[21,61,135]

Amnesia, a deficit in the ability to learn new information, is present nearly universally in the early stages of Alzheimer's disease.[81,134,135,139] It regularly precedes other changes in mood and behavior. Confabulation may accompany the amnesia but typically appears later in the course of the illness.[114,138,149] Experimental investigation of the memory defect suggests that patients are unable to encode auditory information successfully. Coding for short-term memory is inefficient and storage for eventual recall is seriously compromised.[98,99] Other factors such as impaired concentration, interference effects, and failure to recognize auditory signals may also contribute. Rarely, difficulties in naming have antedated the amnesia,[51] but the diagnosis of Alzheimer's disease should be regarded as dubious if recent memory loss is not among the earliest intellectual changes.

Visuo-spatial functions are also impaired early in the course of Alzheimer's disease.[1,132,133,135] The patients become lost in familiar surroundings and may be spatially disoriented in their own homes. Dressing disturbances are common. On examination, the patients are unable to copy three-dimensional representations such as a cube and may do poorly when attempting to copy two-dimensional figures. As the disease progresses, spatial disorientation and loss of visuo-spatial skills become more profound.

Personality and social behavior of Alzheimer's disease patients are usually remarkably well preserved even in the face of gross intellectual deterioration.[133] Personality changes occur in some patients, however, and several varieties of character alterations have been described. Larson et al. found that 69 percent of their 377 patients had "simple" dementia without major personality changes, 18 percent became paranoid, and 10 percent had affective disturbances.[80] Sim and Sussman found depression in 12 of their 22 patients.[132] When paranoia is present, the delusions are poorly systematized and loosely held.[51] In addition to the psychiatric alterations, the general activity levels of the patients may change. Apathy or restlessness occur[81,96,134] and, in some cases, an initial loss of spontaneity is followed by a period of restless hyperactivity.[68,124,136] Terminally, the patients are profoundly akinetic, bed-ridden, and rigid.[1,81,134]

Language changes are among the most useful clinical signs in detecting cortical dementing processes, and the pattern of linguistic deterioration may aid in the differential diagnosis of Alzheimer's disease. Word-finding difficulty in spontaneous speech is the earliest sign of language impairment.[51,61,124] Testing at this time reveals preserved confrontation naming but impaired ability to generate lists of words in a given category.[9,10] As the disease progresses, spontaneous speech becomes empty and a frank anomia is apparent.[45,55,88,125] At this stage, patients may become overly talkative and develop a fluent paraphasic logorrhea similar to Wernicke's aphasia or transcortical sensory aphasia[51,85,124] or they may manifest a markedly diminished verbal output.[62,135,151] Language comprehension is also increasingly compromised as the disease progresses.[135] In the middle and late phases of the illness, a variety of reiterative speech disturbances emerge. Echolalia,[78,104,134] the tendency to repeat words and sentences addressed to the patient, palilalia,[58,134,151] the tendency to repeat words and phrases initiated by the patient, and/or logclonia,[45,75,124,134] the repetition of the final syllable of a word, have been noted. Terminally, the vocal output takes the form of repetitive sounds that are unrecognizable as language.[73,140] Complete mutism is uncommon.

Speech, the mechanical act of language production, is normal early in Alzheimer's disease but may become abnormal as other motor system abnormalities appear. Stuttering[6,37,55] and a slurring dysarthria[16,36,55,62,100,135] have been described.

Agnosias and apraxias in Alzheimer's disease patients are difficult to interpret in view of coexisting deficits in language and memory. Despite these difficulties, some information is available. Of 18 cases of Alzheimer's disease verified histologically, Sjogren et al. found that 5 had visual agnosia.[135] Polatin et al. considered agnosias to be characteristic of Alzheimer's disease[114]; and Rochford found that in some demented patients impairment of confrontation naming was secondary to disturbed visual recognition.[121] Ideational apraxia, defined as a failure to correctly manipulate objects in the absence of obvious sensory or motor deficits, and ideomotor apraxia, the inability to do on command an act that can be done spontaneously, occur in many Alzheimer's disease patients; they usually appear in the middle stage of the illness after language and memory disturbances are firmly established and before terminal motor changes are present.[1,68,81] One study found that 21 of 24 patients in the second stage of the illness were markedly apractic,[134] and Sjogren et al. found that 72 percent of their patients were apractic in stage two.[135]

A variety of other behavioral and cognitive alterations occur as the disease advances. Adams and Victor[1] and Lishman[81] noted that acalculia becomes apparent by the second stage of the illness; and several observers reported the presence of a "mirror sign" in which the patients sit in front of a mirror and talk to their own images.[61,135,139] Poor judgement, loss of abstraction capabilities, distractability, right-left confusion, and lack of concentration may begin early and become prominent as the disease advances. The Klüver-Bucy syndrome may appear in the terminal phase of the disease.[81,138]

Neurologic signs, conspicuously absent during the early and middle phases of Alzheimer's disease, appear in the last stage of the illness. Extrapyramidal rigidity, gegenhalten, or spasticity may be found on motor system examination.[75,77,81,132,133] The terminal position is frequently one of paraplegia or quadriplegia in flexion.[1,135,158] Seizures may occur as the illness progresses to the final stage.[68,75,81,114,132,133] Myoclonic jerks, sudden unsustained muscular contractions sometimes gross enough to move a limb, are not uncommon in the later stages of Alzheimer's disease.[39,48,71] Jacob noted that myoclonus was more common among heredofamilial cases.[71] Terminally, urinary and fecal incontinence occur and primitive reflexes, including grasp and suck responses, become evident.[1,81,109] The patient eventually succumbs to a urinary tract infection or aspiration pneumonia.

Neuropsychologic assessment in Alzheimer's disease aids in the identification and quantitation of cognitive and memory deficits; it does little to help in diagnosing the etiology of the impairments. Perez et al. found that Alzheimer's disease patients and patients with multiinfarct dementias had qualitatively similar performances on the Wechsler Adult Intelligence Scale, though the Alzheimer's patients consistently performed more poorly.[110] Their worst performance was on the block design subtest. Gainotti et al. constructed a dementia battery of verbal, visuo-spatial, and memory tests and found that Alzheimer's disease patients did significantly more poorly on tests of constructional abilities and verbal and visuo-spatial memory than depressed patients or patients with subcortical dementias.[46]

Laboratory Findings

Laboratory investigation of patients with Alzheimer's disease is primarily concerned with detecting diseases that resemble Alzheimer's disease but may be reversible if detected and treated.[31] The electroencephalogram (EEG) and computerized tomography (CT) are the two most useful diagnostic tools. Harner emphasizes that most treatable causes of dementia produce prominent EEG abnormalities, whereas the degenerative dementias show few EEG changes in the initial stages of development.[59] Early in the course of Alzheimer's disease there may be minimal slowing of posterior alpha activity or slight excess of theta activity. As the disease advances, progressive slowing occurs and in the final stages there is diffuse slow wave activity. Focal abnormalities are rare.[52,53]

Computerized tomography is a reliable means of detecting structural alterations such as subdural hematomas, hydrocephalus, brain tumors, abcesses, and cerebral infarctions that may simulate Alzheimer's disease. The CT scan is less helpful in establishing a diagnosis of Alzheimer's disease. Most cases have dilated ventricles and enlarged cortical sulci, but atrophy without dementia and dementia without atrophy have been reported.[67] The absence of atrophy should stimulate a search for treatable causes of dementia,[43] but the presence of atrophy should not be the sole basis for a diagnosis of dementia.[150] As Alzheimer's disease progresses, there is a rough correlation between advancing dementia and increasing atrophy on the CT scan.[35]

Research techniques measuring regional cerebral blood flow and cerebral glucose metabolism are available in some institutions. Cerebral blood flow studies have shown that flow in gray matter is significantly reduced and that the usual augmentation of flow induced by intellectual activity is less in Alzheimer's disease patients than in normal controls.[69] Gustafson et al. correlated reduced cerebral blood flow in parietal and frontal regions with language disturbances in demented patients.[55] Metabolic scans measuring the pattern of ^{18}F-deoxyglucose utilization also show disturbances of the metabolic activity of posterior parietal and frontal association cortices, whereas subcortical structures and primary motor and sensory cortex have normal or near normal metabolism.[11]

Routine blood, serum, and urine studies are normal in Alzheimer's disease, and the cerebrospinal fluid is normal or shows only a mild elevation of protein content. Research investigations have demonstrated impaired cellular immune function involving T-cell lymphocytes,[7] elevated levels of antibodies against brain tissue,[101] and abnormalities of serum protein electrophoresis.[8] Aneuploidy, an abnormal number of chromosomes, is found in the lymphocytes of some patients.[25,72]

Histopathologic Alterations

Pathologic alterations in Alzheimer's disease involve changes at the macroscopic level, the light and electronmicroscopic levels, and in the neurochemical composition of affected tissues.[27] Grossly, the brains are atrophic, often weighing less than 1000 g.[145] The atrophy involves temporal, frontal, and parietal regions. Sparing of occipital cortex and the primary motor and sensory cortices may be evident.[73,94]

Histologic changes involving the neurons of the cortex are the most striking pathologic findings of the disease. The classic neuronal alterations include neurofibrillary tangles, senile plaques, and granulovacuolar degeneration. Identical changes occur in the aging brain unaccompanied by dementia, although the changes are less abundant.[145] The diagnosis of Alzheimer's disease thus depends on an identifiable clinical pattern combined with the characteristic neuropathologic changes. Neurofibrillary tangles consist of irregular thickening, contortions, and conglutination of

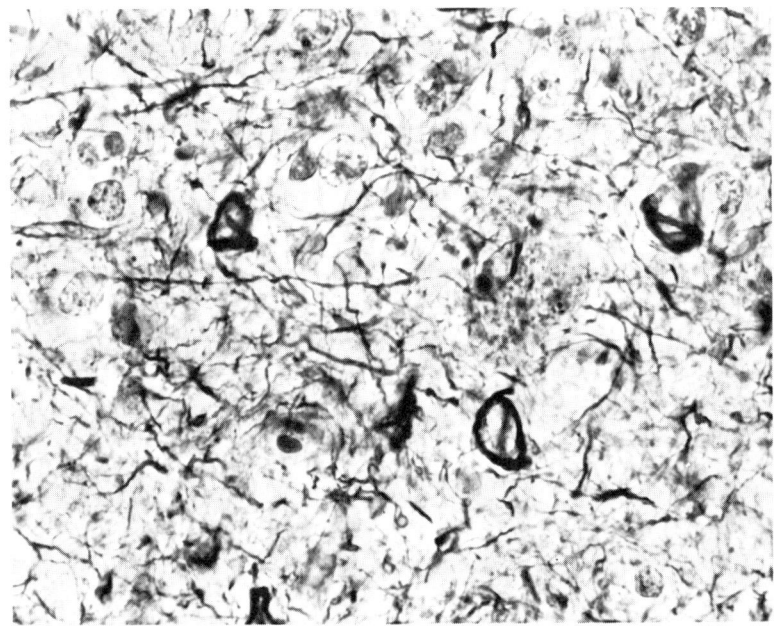

Fig. 5-1. Alzheimer's neurofibrillary tangles in neurons of the frontal cortex (Glees stain, × 480)

intraneuronal extranuclear neurofibrils.[74] They form bizarre triangle and loop shapes in the cells and are best demonstrated by silver stains (Fig. 5-1). The tangles occur preferentially in the pyramidal cells of the neocortex, the hippocampus, and the amygdala. They also occur in the raphe nuclei of the brain stem and the locus coeruleus.[65,70] Electron microscopy reveals that the tangles are composed of neurofilaments arranged in bifilar helices. Each helix strand is 100 Å wide and the helix has a twist every 800 Å.[79,143]

Senile plaques are areas of tissue degeneration containing abnormal unmyelinated neuronal processes and measuring from 5 to 150 μ in size.[74] They show an affinity for silver stains (Fig. 5-2) and consist of an outer zone of degenerating neuritic processes, a middle zone of swollen axons and dendrites, and a central amyloid core.[79] Hypertrophy of astrocytes is visible near the plaques and microglial cells invade in the final phases of plaque formation.[44] The plaques occur primarily in the gray matter of the cerebral cortex, but are found in smaller numbers in the basal ganglia, thalamus, hypothalamus, and midbrain. By electron microscopy the plaques appear to be composed of thickened axis cylinders, abnormal dendritic processes, altered boutons termineaux, and neuronal processes packed with thickened neurofibrils.[60,86]

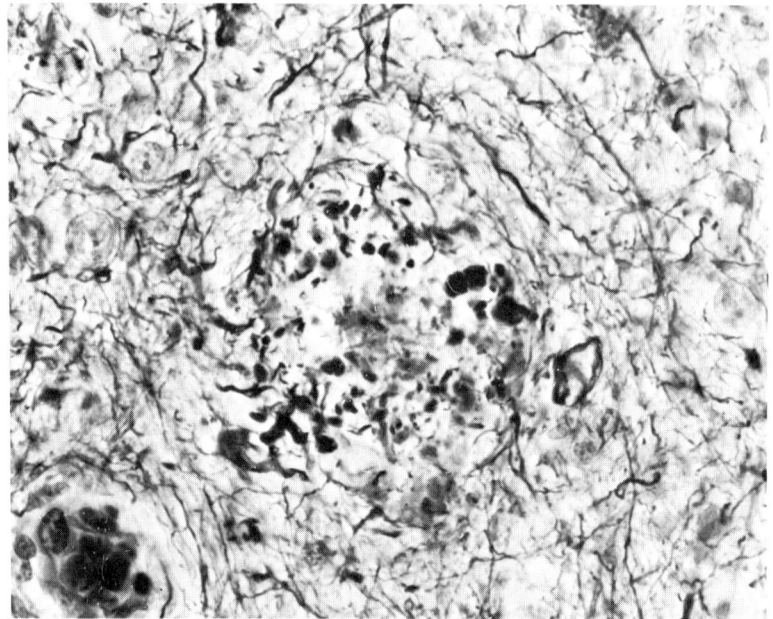

Fig. 5-2. Senile plaque comprised of degenerating neuronal proceses surrounding an amyloid core (Glees stain, × 480)

Granulovacuolar degeneration consists of clusters of intracytoplasmic vacuoles up to 5 μ in diameter, each containing a granule 0.5–1.5 μ in size. In Alzheimer's disease the change is highly selective for the pyramidal neurons of the hippocampal formation and is rarely found outside of the hippocampus.[157] There is a gradual increase in granulovacuolar degeneration in normals from 60 to 90 years of age, but few patients without dementia have severe changes.[147]

In addition to the neurofibrillary tangles, senile plaques, and granulovacuolar degeneration, there are other less unique histopathologic changes in Alzheimer's disease. Neuronal loss occurs, particularly in the third and fifth cortical layers, and there is astrocytic hyperplasia in the areas of degeneration.[22,27]

A few cases of Alzheimer's disease are found to have amyloidosis of the small vessels of the cerebral cortex.[28,90,103,107] In these patients, senile plaques tend to be much more abundant than neurofibrillary tangles; multiple small vascular infarcts may be present, and massive cerebral hemorrhage may occur terminally.

Investigators have attempted to define a quantitative relation between the degree of dementia exhibited by the patient during life and the intensity or abundance of the neuropathologic changes. Blessed,

Tomlinson, and Roth found a significant correlation between increasing numbers of senile plaques in the cerebral cortex and increasing dementia.[13,123] In a later study, the same investigators showed that Alzheimer's neurofibrillary changes were present in severe degree in the hippocampus and in large numbers throughout the cortex in a significantly larger proportion of the demented patients than in a control group.[146] The widespread occurrence of neurofibrillary tangles was the factor which best distinguished the demented from the control patients. They noted that severe changes of either neurofibrillary, senile plaque, or granulovacuolar type were seen only in demented patients.

Neurochemical Studies

Neurochemical studies of Alzheimer's disease brains have provided new insights into the pathophysiology of this dementia. The most striking finding is a preferential loss of choline acetyltransferase activity from assayed cortical regions.[15,33,112] Postsynaptic muscarinic cholinergic receptor binding remains normal, indicating that there is a selective loss of presynaptic cholinergic neurons or nerve terminals. Correlation studies demonstrate a roughly linear relationship between increased senile plaque count, decreased choline acetyltransferase activity, and more profound intellectual impairment.[111]

Pathogenesis

The pathogenesis of Alzheimer's disease is unknown, but there are several current theories regarding its etiology. Aluminum intoxication, disordered immune function, viral infection, and defects in formation of cellular filaments have each been proposed and supportive evidence for each etiologic theory adduced. Crapper et al. assayed brains of Alzheimer's disease patients and found elevated levels of aluminum.[29] The elevations were not large, however, and the toxicity of relatively small increases in aluminum concentrations is unknown. Other investigators have failed to find any differences in aluminum content between normal brains and brains of demented patients.[92] Experimentally, aluminum induces neurofilamentous changes similar to Alzheimer's neurofibrillary tangles, but the filaments are straight rather than twisted into helices as in Alzheimer's disease, and they tend to occur in the brain stem and spinal cord rather than cortically.[159] Current evidence offers little support for a significant role for aluminum in the pathogenesis of Alzheimer's disease.

Serum Protein abnormalities,[8] elevated brain antibody levels,[101] and impaired cellular immune functions[7] of Alzheimer's disease patients suggest that alterations in immunologic activity play a role in the pathogenesis of the disease. Disturbed immune function could also account for the amyloid in the senile plaques and the amyloid occasionally found in the cerebral vessels.[49] Whether those immunologic alterations are primary or secondary to some other more basic process remains to be determined.

A viral etiology for Alzheimer's disease has also been suggested. Kidd postulated that the senile plaques form in reaction to accumulations of viral particles in the neuronal processes,[79] and De Boni and Crapper found that they could induce neurofibrillary tangles in cultured fetal cortical neurons by exposing them to an extract prepared from the brain of an Alzheimer's disease patient.[14] This observation suggested the presence of a transmissable (viral) agent. Against this hypothesis is the information from Gajdusek's laboratory (Goudsmit et al.) demonstrating that despite many attempts, it has not been possible to reliably transmit Alzheimer's disease to experimental animals.[54] Animals innoculated with brain tissue from two familial cases of Alzheimer's disease developed a spongiform encephalopathy like Creutzfeldt-Jakob disease, but other animals innoculated with the same tissue showed no neurologic deterioration, and the possibility of contamination or laboratory error was not excluded. Innocula from many other cases produced no neurologic disease. At present, the viral etiology of Alzheimer's disease remains an unconfirmed possibility.

The observation that Alzheimer's disease, Down's syndrome, hemotologic malignancies, and chromosomal aneuploidy occur more frequently than expected in the families of patients with Alzheimer's disease has led to the suggestion that there is an underlying defect in microtubule organization.[25,63] Each condition has an abnormality of microtubular function, and they could represent different expressions of a common microtubular defect. Like the other theories of the etiology of Alzheimer's disease, more information is needed to confirm or deny this hypothesis, but any causal explanation will have to take these epidemiologic observations into account.

Management

Treatment of Alzheimer's disease is still largely symptomatic. The discovery of selectively decreased levels of choline acetyltransferase in the brains of Alzheimer's disease patients[15,33,112] led to attempts to treat patients with acetylcholine precursors such as lecithin and choline.[17,116,137] The results have not been encouraging, but a few patients treated early in their clinical course have shown modest improvement.[38] Until better ways of intervening in the pathophysiologic process are found, the management of Alzheimer's disease patients will continue to be on a symptomatic basis. Minor tranquilizers should be avoided in demented patients because they produce confusion and increase intellectual compromise. When aggression or combativeness are a problem, low doses of major tranquilizers should be used. Side effects, particularly postural hypotension, must be monitored carefully. When antidepressants are indicated, a tricyclic agent with few anticholinergic side effects should be chosen. Vasodilators are of no proven benefit in the treatment of demented patients.[64]

PICK'S DISEASE

In 1892, Arnold Pick first described a unique dementing disorder associated with prominent lobar atrophy of the brain. He reported a 71-year-old man with a 3-year history of progressive dementia. On examination, the patient was aphasic, made many verbal paraphasic errors, and had difficulty recognizing objects. The patient died several months later, and an autopsy performed by Chiari revealed marked atrophy involving the frontal and temporal lobes. The striking histologic characteristics of the process were described in 1911 by Alzheimer, and in 1926, Onari and Spatz suggested the eponym "Pick's disease" for the illness.[102]

Pick's disease usually begins between the ages of 40 and 60,[56,136] though cases beginning as early as 21[84] and as late as 80[12] have been described. Death occurs in 2 to 15 years[18,77] with most patients dying 6 to 12 years after onset of the disease.[32,136] Women are affected slightly more frequently than men.[18,77,136] Jervis found that the disease accounted for 0.2 to 1.6 percent of mental hospital populations and was 10 to 15 times less common than Alzheimer's disease.[74] Eighty percent of cases of Pick's disease are sporadic and 20 percent are of hereditary origin.[41] Autosomal dominant inheritance is the pattern of hereditary transmission in the familial cases.[89,126,128]

Clinical Course

Like Alzheimer's disease, the clinical course of Pick's disease can be divided into three stages.[74,106,120,135] The initial stage consists of changes in emotion, affect, and behavior with impaired judgment and loss of insight. During the middle phase of the illness, progressive intellectual deterioration occurs and aphasia often dominates the clinical picture. In the final stage, an extrapyramidal disorder may appear, and the patient becomes mute and incontinent. Death results from an aspiration pneumonia or a urinary tract infection.

Lishman emphasized that it is chiefly in the mode of onset that Pick's disease differs from other dementing illnesses.[81] The disorder is most easily recognized in the initial stage before distinctive behavioral features are submerged in the progressive dementia and advancing intellectual deterioration. Personality and emotional alterations precede obvious intellectual decline. The character changes include emotional blunting, apathy, and a restriction in the field of interest to immediate personal concerns.[19,76,120] The resulting behavior is tactless, lacks propriety, and may be frankly antisocial.

The Klüver-Bucy syndrome may be among the first behavioral disturbances heralding the onset of Pick's disease. This complex of behavioral changes includes hyperorality, loss of affective responses, hypermetamorphosis (the tendency to compulsively explore all objects as soon as they are seen), hypersexuality, dietary changes, and sensory agnosias. Partial or complete manifestations of the syndrome occur early in the course of Pick's disease[3,4,32,55,113] with the patients exhibiting various combinations of affective disturbances, hypersexuality, "gluttony," hyperorality, hypermetamorphosis, and visual or auditory agnosia.[2,34,126,128,141]

Agnosias may occur without other aspects of the Klüver-Bucy syndrome. Visual object agnosia,[32,89,117] prosopagnosia,[32,41,87,131] and auditory agnosia[32,76] have been described. The agnosias appear in the early or middle phases of the disease process.

While emotional and affective changes dominate the early stages of Pick's disease, cognitive and intellectual compromise become obvious as the disease progresses. Aphasia spans the clinical course of Pick's disease but tends to dominate the middle phases. The earliest abnormalities are word-finding difficulties in spontaneous speech and anomia on naming tasks.[4,12,32,34,84,126] Verbal paraphasia is prominent in some cases. One patient reported by Cummings and Duchen[32] called glasses "clocks" and a wrist watch a "hand watch." Robertson, le Roux, and Brown observed that their Pick's disease patients with anomic aphasia were circumlocutory, used many generic terms such as "thing," relied on single words to convey several meanings, and substituted from their restricted vocabularies an available word for other unrecalled terms.[120] Impaired comprehension becomes evident concurrently with other language disturbances. As the disease progresses, echolalia and excessive use of stereotyped phrases and sentences become prominent.[12,32,41,60,102,139,144] Mayer-Gross described an exaggerated form of this stereotyped speech that he called the "gramophone syndrome."[91] It consists of the reiteration of a single anecdote told in the same way nearly every time the patient is required to speak. Terminally, many patients become completely mute.[32,55,83,84,89,102,130,139]

Memory disturbances are difficult to assess in Pick's disease because of the presence of aphasic and agnosic impairments. Cummings and Duchen found that patients often demonstrated relatively intact memory in their general behavior even when formal memory testing was impossible.[32] One patient arrived punctually for tea long after emotional and language disturbances became evident. As the disease progresses into the terminal stages, mnestic abilities deteriorate.

Visuo-spatial skills also may be preserved until relatively late in the disease. Patients may be able to copy figures and find their way around in hospitals even when language and emotional abilities are obviously compromised.[19,32,120,135] In the final phases of the illness, spatial orientation is lost.

Elementary neurologic abnormalities of motor and sensory systems are absent during most of the course of Pick's disease. As the illness progresses into the last stages, motor abnormalities of an extrapyramidal type frequently appear,[2,32,84,89,113,126] and myoclonus has occasionally been observed.[3,89,126] Seizures are uncommon in Pick's disease. Terminally, the patients are mute and immobile with urinary and fecal incontinence.

Laboratory Findings

Laboratory studies usually provide little help in the diagnosis of Pick's disease. Routine blood, serum, urine, and cerebrospinal fluid are unremarkable. In preliminary studies, Constantinidis found increased urinary zinc excretion in Pick's disease patients.[23] Electroencephalograms tend to remain normal until late in the course of the illness.[53,141] When EEG abnormalities appear, they are usually diffuse, though focal frontal or temporal slow-wave activity has been reported occasionally.[32] Few patients with confirmed Pick's disease have been studied by computerized tomography, but the few available observations suggest that pronounced lobar atrophy is demonstrable in some cases.[32,93] The presence of frontal and/or temporal lobar atrophy in a demented patient is supportive but not definitive evidence for the diagnosis of Pick's disease.

Histopathologic Alterations

Pathologic alterations of the brains of Pick's disease patients are obvious on gross inspection. The brains are reduced in size and many weigh less than 1000 gm.[32,102,119,144] In most cases, the atrophy has a decidedly lobar distribution (Fig. 5-3). The anterior hemispheric regions show the most profound changes. Seventeen to 22 percent have primarily temporal atrophy; 22 to 27 percent show mainly frontal involvement; 38 to 56

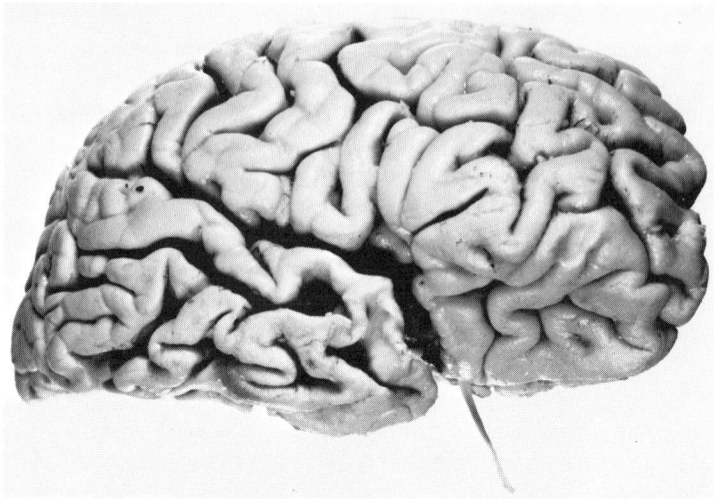

Fig. 5-3. Macroscopic appearance of brain in Pick's disease. Temporal lobar atrophy is apparent, with relative sparing of other cortical regions. (Appreciation is expressed to Dr. Richard Hunter of the Friern's Hospital, London, for providing this specimen.)

percent have mixed frontal and temporal atrophy; and a small number have atrophy involving the posterior hemispheric regions or show generalized atrophy.[27,41,135] Corsellis found that the atrophy was bilaterally symmetric in only one third of cases; one half showed a left-sided predominance; and one-fifth had more atrophy on the right.[27]

The atrophy in anterior temporal and inferior frontal regions may be sufficiently severe to produce deep sulci and "knife-edged" gyri.[27,32,74,83,84,89] An abrupt transition is sometimes evident between involved and uninvolved cerebral cortical regions.[27,126,131] The precentral gyrus and the posterior third of the superior temporal gyrus tend to be selectively spared, whereas the anterior and medial temporal areas and the orbitofrontal cortex show the most severe atrophic changes.[27,32,126,129]

Cellular Alterations

The distinctive cellular alterations of Pick's disease are highly characteristic, do not overlap with the changes of normal aging, and are virtually pathognomonic of the disease. The two unique cellular alterations are the occurrence of Pick bodies in many neurons and the presence of "inflated" neurons. The abnormal cells are found in atrophic cerebral cortical areas and are accompanied by neuronal loss, astrocytic gliosis, and occasional microglial cell proliferation. White matter in the atrophic areas is also altered. Extensive gliosis is evident and loss of myelin occurs where gliosis is severe.[27,32,74,102] In areas of profound cortical involvement, spongiform changes are evident.[32,84,89] Neurofibrillary tangles, senile plaques, granulovacuolar degeneration, and vascular changes are found only to the extent expected for the patient's age.

Pick bodies are dense intracellular structures occurring in the neuronal cytoplasm (Fig. 5-4). They are the size of the nucleus and stain deeply in silver preparations. They tend to be single within the cell although compound structures have occasionally been noted.[27,74,127,130] Inflated cells are enlarged neurons with highly argyrophilic cytoplasm but without discrete structures. The nucleus is displaced to the edge of the cell.[27,74,127] Cummings and Duchen identified abnormal argyrophilic neurons similar to inflated cells but the cells were not greatly enlarged.[32]

Electron microscopic study of Pick cells reveals that the Pick bodies and the inflated cells are composed of 100 Å neurofilaments and 240 Å neurotubules. The filaments and tubules are distributed throughout the cytoplasm of the inflated cells and condensed into aggregates in the cells with Pick bodies. The bodies are not membrane bound and bear no resemblance to viral inclusions.[27,117,131,148,156]

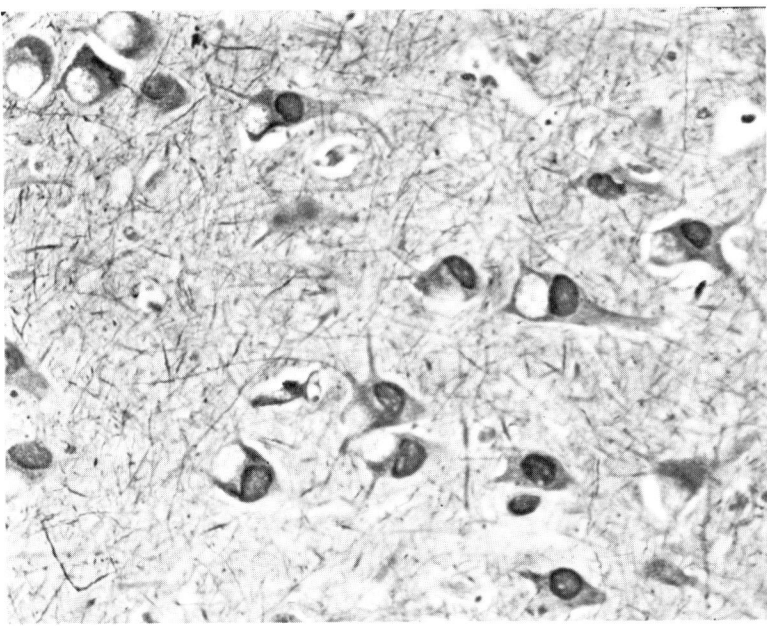

Fig. 5-4. Pick bodies. Neurons from medial temporal cortex contain a dense, argyrophilic structure. The nucleus is unstained and displaced to the side of the cell. (von Braunmuhl, × 400)

The topographic distribution of the Pick cells is confined to the cerebral cortex. The more superficial cortical layers are maximally involved.[27,74,83] Within the medial temporal lobe the parahippocampal and adjacent hippocampal areas and the entire amygdaloid complex contain the greatest abundance of Pick cells.[5,32] Neurons of the orbitofrontal and prefrontal cortex are also involved. Neuronal loss and astrocytic gliosis occur to a variable extent in the basal ganglia and thalamus, but the characteristic Pick cells are not found in these subcortical structures.[2,27,32,74,155]

An unresolved problem in the nosology of Pick's disease concerns the cases that have marked lobar atrophy but lack Pick cells. Jervis found that Pick cells occur in only one third of cases that otherwise had pathologic findings typical of Pick's disease.[74] Constantinidis et al. were able to find Pick bodies in 20 percent of their cases and inflated cells in 59 percent.[24] This leaves a substantial number of cases without characteristic neuronal alterations. Neumann originally proposed that Pick's disease be divided into two types indicating the presence or absence of Pick's cells respectively.[102] Later, she and Cohn suggested that the two types might represent different disease entities and called the second group "progressive subcortical gliosis."[105] This classification has not been widely applied, but the issue will not be resolved until clinical and pathologic information is available on a larger number of cases.

The neurochemistry of Pick's disease has been studied little. Postsynaptic muscarinic cholinergic receptors have been assayed and found to be decreased[152,160] but further characterization of the disease remains to be done.

Pathogenesis

The etiology and pathogenesis of Pick's disease is unknown. Most investigators consider it a neuronal degenerative process originating in the cell body,[30,155] but others consider the changes in the neuronal soma to be secondary. Williams emphasized the similarity of the neuronal changes to those following axonal injury and suggested that the disease was an axonal disorder.[154] Wisniewski et al. also supported this concept on the basis of their electron microscopic observations.[156] At present, there is insufficient evidence to decide between these alternative hypotheses.

Management

The treatment of Pick's disease is primarily symptomatic. Based on their studies suggesting abnormal zinc metabolism in Pick's disease, Constantinidis and colleagues have treated a few patients with heavy metal chelating agents and noted clinical improvement.[24] These promising findings need confirmation. Treatment with major tranquilizers for aggression and combativeness, along with preventive measures to avoid urinary tract infections, aspiration pneumonia, and decubitus ulcers continue to be the principal means of management.

DIFFERENTIATION OF ALZHEIMER'S DISEASE AND PICK'S DISEASE

Alzheimer's disease and Pick's disease share many clinical features. Both are idiopathic dementing disorders arising in late middle age and progressing slowly and relentlessly to death. They affect women more than men. Language disturbances are prominent in both diseases and motor abnormalities do not appear until late in the illnesses. EEG and CT scanning help exclude other causes of dementia, but may not differentiate Alzheimer's from Pick's disease. Some clinicians believe clinical differentiation of the two illnesses is impossible, while others have suggested they can be separated on the basis of characteristic clinical features. It may not be possible to distinguish all cases, but there are a sufficient number of differences in the course and expression of the two diseases to allow at least tentative separation of some cases on clinical grounds.

Table 5-1 summarizes the principal features that distinguish the two conditions. The differential value of many of the characteristics depends on when they appear in the temporal course of the illness. The diseases are more readily separated on the basis of early clinical alterations before progressive deterioration obliterates differentiating features.[81] The clinical

Table 5-1
Clinical Features That Distinguish Alzheimer's Disease and Pick's Disease

Alzheimer's Disease	Pick's Disease
Amnesia, early	Amnesia, late
Visuo-spatial disturbances, early	Visuo-spatial disturbances, late
Personality changes, late	Personality changes, early
Klüver-Bucy syndrome, late	Klüver-Bucy syndrome, early
Language disturbances	Language disturbances
Palilalia and logoclonia, common	Palilalia and logoclonia, rare
Stereotyped speech, not frequent	Stereotyped speech, characteristic
Terminal mutism, uncommon	Terminal mutism, common
Seizures, not uncommon, late	Seizures, uncommon
CT scan, shows widespread atrophy	CT scan, shows lobar atrophy

sign most often noted to separate the two diseases is the early appearance of amnesia in Alzheimer's disease contrasted with the relative preservation of memory in the early stages of Pick's disease.[19,32,41,81,106,114,133,136,139] Haase[56] and Cummings and Duchen[32] noted that, like memory, spatial orientation was compromised early in Alzheimer's disease and preserved until late in Pick's disease.

Another feature consistently noted to distinguish the two cortical dementias was the preservation of personality and social graces in Alzheimer's disease compared with the early loss of tact, sensitivity, and personal propriety in Pick's disease.[19,53,81,114] Cummings and Duchen found that the early appearance of the Klüver-Bucy syndrome in Pick's disease contrasted with its late occurrence in Alzheimer's disease.[32]

Language disturbances are a prominent part of both Alzheimer's disease and Pick's disease. In each condition the earliest features are word-finding difficulties in spontaneous speech and anomia. As the diseases progress, different patterns of linguistic deterioration occur. At least one subgroup of Alzheimer's disease develops a fluent paraphasic logorrhea similar to Wernicke's aphasia.[51,85,124] A fluent aphasic output of this type is uncommon in Pick's disease. As Alzheimer's disease progresses, palilalia and logoclonia become prominent, while advancing Pick's disease is more likely to result in excessive use of verbal stereotypes, auditory agnosia, and marked echolalia.[32,41,76] Terminal mutism is more common in Pick's disease than Alzheimer's disease.

Seizures occur in the late phases of cortical dementias and are reported more often in Alzheimer's than in Pick's disease.[41,56,106,114,139]

Among diagnostic studies, the CT scan may provide information that aids in distinguishing the two diseases. CT scans of Alzheimer's disease patients may show wide-spread atrophy, while scans of Pick's disease patients reveal lobar atrophy affecting frontal and/or temporal lobes.[32,93] Lobar atrophy should not be regarded as pathognomonic of Pick's disease, however, since atrophy affecting primarily the frontal and temporal lobes has occasionally been reported in Alzheimer's disease.[142]

Polatin et al.[114] and Sjogren et al.[135] reported that agnosias were found more commonly in Alzheimer's disease than in Pick's disease; but visual object agnosia,[32,89,117] prosopagnosia,[32,41,87,131] and auditory agnosia[32,76] have been reported in Pick's disease sufficiently commonly to indicate that they do not differentiate the two conditions.

Clinical differences between Alzheimer's and Pick's disease reflect differences in the topographic pattern of cerebral involvement in the two processes. The relative preservation of personality, early loss of spatial orientation, and tendency to develop a fluent aphasia in Alzheimer's disease correlate with the propensity of the disease to involve posterior hemispheric regions.[19,32,91] In Pick's disease the early deterioration of personality and relative preservation of visuo-spatial skills reflects the anterior hemispheric and limbic system degeneration. The early appearance of the Klüver-Bucy syndrome in some cases of Pick's disease correlates with severe medial temporal and diffuse amygdaloid involvement in that disease[32] contrasting with limited amygdaloid complex changes in Alzheimer's disease.[26,66]

OTHER CORTICAL DEMENTIAS

Alzheimer's and Pick's diseases are the two principal degenerative dementias affecting the cerebral cortex. A variety of other processes—particularly vascular and infectious diseases—also can involve the cortex and produce aphasia, agnosia, amnesia, and apraxia similar to those seen in the degenerative conditions. In nearly all cases, however, these processes are accompanied by motor, somatosensory, or visual abnormalities which distinguish them from the degenerations primarily affecting cortical structures.

Multi-infarct Dementia

Multi-infarct dementia can involve the cerebral cortex and affect cognition and memory. Hachinski et al. found the following features to characterize dementias produced by cerebrovascular disease: abrupt onset, step-wise progression, fluctuating course, nocturnal confusion, relative preservation of personality, depression, somatic complaints, emotional lability, history of hypertension, history of strokes, evidence of associated atherosclerosis, focal neurologic symptoms, and focal neurologic signs.[57] CT scanning supports the diagnosis when ischemic lesions are visualized.[82]

Infectious Processes

Infectious processes that cause dementias with cortical features include Creutzfeldt-Jakob disease, progressive multifocal leukoencephalopathy, and general paresis. Creutzfeldt-Jakob disease is caused by a transmissible slow virus which may invade any level of the neuraxis.[47] When the cerebral cortex is involved, a cortical type dementia will be evident but is nearly always accompanied by pyramidal or extrapyramidal motor signs and myoclonus.[122] Progressive multifocal leukoencephalopathy is a viral disease of the nervous system which occurs in individuals with chronic myeloproliferative, lymphoproliferative, or granulomatous diseases. Personality changes, aphasia, and amnesia may occur and are accompanied by focal motor and sensory signs.[118] General paresis, a syphilitic spirochetal infection of the brain, causes personality changes, amnesia, and cognitive impairment. Focal neurologic signs and tremor are common.[97]

SUMMARY

Alzheimer's disease and Pick's disease are the two primary cortical dementing illnesses. The major neurologic impairments they produce are aphasia, agnosia, apraxia, and amnesia. Signs of motor disturbance do not appear until the final phase of the illnesses. Clinical differentiation of Alzheimer's and Pick's disease is difficult but the pattern of evolution can help distinguish them. Early amnesia and visuo-spatial disorientation characterize Alzheimer's disease, whereas early emotional and personality deterioration are more indicative of Pick's disease. Vascular and infectious illnesses that cause similar dementias can be differentiated by the concurrence of focal motor or sensory signs.

ACKNOWLEDGMENT

The author gratefully acknowledges Professor Leo Duchen and his staff at the Department of Neuropathology, Institute of Neurology, National Hospital for Nervous Diseases, Queen Square, London, for guiding the preparation and study of the pathologic material used in this chapter.

REFERENCES

1. Adams RD, VictorM: Principles of Neurology. New York, McGraw-Hill, 1977, pp 401-405
2. Akelaitis AJ: Atrophy of basal ganglia in Pick's disease. Arch Neurol Psychiatry 51:27-34, 1944
3. Aronson SM, Aronson BE: Clinical neuropathological conference. Dis Nerv Syst 34:124-130, 1973
4. Balajthy B: Symptomatology of the temporal lobe in Pick's convolutional atrophy. Acta Med Acad Sci Hung 20:301-316, 1964
5. Ball MJ: Topography of Pick inclusion bodies in hippocampi of demented patients. J Neuropathol Exp Neurol 38:614-620, 1979
6. Barrett AM: A case of Alzheimer's disease with unusual neurological disturbances. J Nerv Ment Dis 40:361-374, 1913
7. Behan PO, Behan WMH: Possible immunological factors in Alzheimer's

disease, in Glen AIM, Whalley LJ (eds): Alzheimer's Disease. Early Recognition of Potentially Reversible Deficits. London, Churchill Livingstone, 1979, pp 33-35
8. Behan PO, Feldman RG: Serum proteins, amyloid and Alzheimer's disease. J Am Geriatr Soc 18:792-797, 1970
9. Benson DF: Aphasia, alexia, and agraphia. London, Churchill Livingstone, 1979, pp 169-170
10. Benson DF: Neurologic correlates of anomia, in Whitaker H, Whitaker HA (eds): Studies in Neurolinguistics, vol 4. New York, Academic Press, 1979, 295-328
11. Benson DF, Cummings JL, Kuhl DE: Dementia: Cortical and subcortical. Presented at the 33rd Annual Meeting, Am Acad Neurol, Toronto. April 1981
12. Binns JK, Robertson EE: Pick's disease in old age. J Ment Sci 108:804-810, 1962
13. Blessed G, Tomlinson BE, Roth M: The association between quantitative measures of dementia and of senile change in the cerebral grey matter of elderly subjects. Br J Psychiatry 114:797-811, 1968
14. de Boni U, Crapper DR: Paired helical filaments of the Alzheimer's type in cultured neurons. Nature 271:566-568, 1978
15. Bowen DM, Smith CB, White P, Davison AN: Neurotransmitter-related enzymes and indices of hypoxia in senile dementia and other abiotrophies. Brain 99:459-496, 1976
16. Boyd DA: A contribution to the psychopathology of Alzheimer's disease. Am J Psychiatry 93:155-175, 1936-1937
17. Boyd WD, Graham-White J, Blackwood G et al: Clinical effects of choline in Alzheimer senile dementia. Lancet 2:711, 1977
18. Brain R, Walton JN. Brain's Diseases of the Nervous System, 7th ed. London, Oxford University Press, 1969, p 992
19. Brun A, Gustafson L: Limbic lobe involvement in presenile dementia. Arch Psychiat Nervenkrank 228:79-93, 1978
20. Bucci L: A familial organic psychosis of Alzheimer type in six kinship of three generations. Am J Psychiatry 119:863-866, 1963
21. Coblentz JM, Mattis S, Zingesser LH et al: Presenile dementia. Arch Neurol 29:299-308, 1973
22. Colon EJ: The cerebral cortex in presenile dementia. Acta Neuropath. [Suppl] (Berl) 23:281-290, 1973
23. Constantinidis J: Zinc metabolism in presenile dementias, in Glen AIM, Whalley LJ (eds): Alzheimer's Disease. Early Recognition of Potentially Reversible Deficits. London, Churchill Livingstone, 1979, pp 48-49
24. Constantinidis J, Richard J, Tissot R: Pick's disease. Histological and clinical correlations. Eur Neurol 11:208-217, 1974
25. Cook RH, Ward BE, Austin JH: Studies in aging of the brain: IV. Familial Azheimer disease: Relation to transmissible dementia, aneuploidy, and microtubular defects. Neurology 29:1402-1412, 1979
26. Corsellis JAN: The limbic areas in Alzheimer's disease and in other condi-

tions associated with dementia, in Wolstenholme GEW, O'Connor M (eds): Alzheimer's Disease and Related Conditions. London, J and A Churchill, 1970, pp 37–45
27. Corsellis JAN: Ageing and the dementias, in Blackwood W, Corsellis JAN (eds): Greenfield's Neuropathology. London, Edward Arnold, 1976, pp 796–848
28. Corsellis JAN, Brierly JB: An unusual type of presenile dementia. Brain 77:571–587, 1954
29. Crapper DR, Krishnan SS, Quittkat S: Aluminum, neurofibillary degeneration and Alzheimer's disease. Brain 99:67–80, 1976
30. Critchley M: The neurology of old age. Lancet 1:1119–1127, 1221–1230, 1331–1336, 1931
31. Cummings JL, Benson DF, LoVerme S Jr: Reversible dementia. JAMA 243:2434–2439, 1980
32. Cummings JL, Duchen LW: The Klüver-Bucy syndrome in Pick's disease: Clinical and pathological correlations. Neurology, 31:1415–1422, 1981
33. Davies P, Maloney AJF: Selective loss of central cholinergic neurons in Alzheimer's disease. Lancet 2:1403, 1976
34. Davison C: Circumscribed cortical atrophy in the presenile psychoses—Pick's disease. Am J Psychiatry 94:801–818, 1938
35. Donaldson AA: CT Scan in Alzheimer presenile dementia, in Glen AIM, Whalley LJ (eds): Alzheimer's Disease. Early Recognition of Potentially Reversible Deficits. London, Churchill Livingstone, 1979, pp 97–101
36. English WH: Alzheimer's disease. Psychiatr Q 16:91–106, 1942
37. Essen-Moller E: A family with Alzheimer's disease. Acta Psychiat Neurol Scand 21:233–244, 1946
38. Etienne P, Gauthier S, Dastoor D et al: Alzheimer's disease: Clinical effect of lecithin treatment, in Glen AIM, Whalley LJ (eds): Alzheimer's Disease. Early Recognition of Potentially Reversible Deficits. London, Churchill Livingstone, 1979, pp 173–178
39. Faden AI, Townsend JJ: Myoclonus in Alzheimer Disease. Arch Neurol 33:278–280, 1976
40. Feldman RG, Chandler KA, Levy LL, Glaser GH: Familial Alzheimer's disease. Neurology 13:811–824, 1963
41. Ferraro A, Jervis GA: Pick's disease. Clinicopathologic study and report of two cases. Arch Neurol Psychiatry 36:739–767, 1936
42. Ferraro A, Jervis GA: Alzheimer's disease. Psychiat Q 15:3–16, 1941
43. Fox, JH, Topel JL, Huckman MS: Use of computerized tomography in senile dementia. J Neurol Neurosurg Psychiat 38:948–953, 1975
44. Friede RL, Magee KR: Alzheimer's disease. Neurology 12:213–222, 1962
45. Fuller SC: Alzheimer's disease (senium praecox): The report of a case and review of published cases. J Nerv Ment Dis 39:440–455, 536–557, 1912
46. Gianotti G, Caltagirone C, Masullo C, Miceli G: Patterns of Neuropsychologic impairment in various diagnostic groups of dementia, in Amaducci L, Davison AN, Antuono P (eds): Aging of the Brain and Dementia. New York, Raven Press, 1980, pp 245–250

47. Gajdusek DC: Unconventional viruses and the origin and disappearance of kuru. Science 197:943-960, 1977
48. Gimenez-Roldan S, Peraita P, Lopez Agreda JM et al: Myoclonus and photic-induced seizures in Alzheimer's disease. Eur Neurol 5:215-224, 1971
49. Glenner GG: Current knowledge of amyloid deposits as applied to senile plaques and congophilic angiopathy, in Katzman R, Terry RD, Bick KL (eds): Alzheimer's Disease: Senile Dementia and Related Disorders. New York, Raven Press, 1978, pp 493-501
50. Gonatas NK, Anderson W, Evangelista I: The contribution of altered synapses in the senile plaque: An electron microscopic study in Alzheimer's dementia. J Neuropathol Exp Neurol 26:25-39, 1967
51. Goodman L: Alzheimer's disease. J Nerv Ment Dis 117:97-130, 1953
52. Gordon EB: Serial EEG studies in presenile dementia. Br J Psychiatry 114:779-780, 1968
53. Gordon EB, Sim M: The EEG in presenile dementia. J Neurol Neurosurg Psychiat 30:285-291, 1967
54. Goudsmit J, Morrow CH, Asher DM et al: Evidence for and against the transmissibility of Alzheimer disease. Neurology 30:945-950, 1980
55. Gustafson L, Hagberg B, Ingvar DH: Speech disturbances in presenile dementia related to local cerebral blood flow abnormalities in the dominant hemisphere. Brain Lang 5:103-118, 1978
56. Haase GR: Diseases presenting as dementia, in Wells CE (ed): Dementia, 2nd ed. Philadelphia, FA Davis Company, 1977, pp 27-67
57. Hachinski VC, Iliff LD, Zilhka E et al: Cerebral blood flow in dementia. Arch Neurol 32:632-637, 1975
58. Hannah JA: A case of Alzheimer's disease with neuropathological findings. Canad Med Assoc J 35:351-366, 1936
59. Harner RN: EEG evaluation of the patient with dementia, in Benson DF, Blumer D (eds): Psychiatric Aspects of Neurologic Disease. New York, Grune & Stratton, 1975, pp 63-82
60. Hassin GB, Levitin D: Pick's disease. Clinicopathologic study and report of a case. Arch Neurol Psychiatry 45:814-833, 1941
61. Henderson DK, Maclachlan SH: Alzheimer's disease. J Ment Sci 76:646-661, 1930
62. Heston LL, Lowther DLW, Leventhal CM: Alzheimer's disease. Arch Neurol 15:225-233, 1966
63. Heston LL, Mastri AR: The genetics of Alzheimer's disease. Arch Gen Psychiatry 34:976-981, 1977
64. Hier DB, Caplan LR: Drugs for senile dementia. Drugs 20:74-80, 1980
65. Hirano A, Zimmerman HM: Alzheimer's neurofibrillary changes. Arch Neurol 7:227-242, 1962
66. Hooper MW, Vogel FS: The limbic system in Alzheimer's disease: A neuropathologic investigation. Am J Pathol 85:1-20, 1976
67. Huckman MS, Fox J, Topel J: The validity of criteria for the evaluation of cerebral atrophy by computerized tomography. Radiology 116:85-92, 1975
68. Hughes W: Alzheimer's disease. Gerontol Clin 12:129-148, 1970

69. Ingvar DH, Risberg J, Schwartz MS: Evidence of subnormal function of association cortex in presenile dementia. Neurology 25:964-974, 1975
70. Ishii T: Distribution of Alzheimer's neurofibrillary changes in the brain stem and hypothalamus of senile dementia. Acta Neuropathol 6:181-187, 1966
71. Jacob H: Muscular twitchings in Alzheimer's disease, in Wolstenholme GEW, O'Connor M (eds): Alzheimer's Disease and Related Conditions. London, J and A Churchill, 1970, pp 75-89
72. Jarvik LF: Genetic factors and chromosomal aberrations in Alzheimer's disease, in Katzman R, Terry RD, Bick KL (eds): Alzheimer's disease: Senile Dementia and Related Disorders. New York, Raven Press, 1978, pp 273-277
73. Jervis GA: Alzheimer's disease. Psychiat Q 11:5-18, 1937
74. Jervis GA: Alzheimer's disease. Pick's disease, in Minckler J (ed): Pathology of the Nervous System, vol 2. New York, McGraw-Hill, 1971, pp 1385-1395, 1395-1404
75. Jervis GA, Soltz SE: Alzheimer's disease—the so-called juvenile type. Am J Psychiatry 93:39-56, 1936
76. Kahn E, Thompson LT: Concerning Pick's disease: Am J Psychiatry 13:937-946, 1933-1934
77. Karp H: Dementia in adults, in Baker AB, Baker LH (eds): Clinical Neurology vol 2. New York, Harper and Row, 1976, pp 5-13
78. Kasanin J, Crank RP: Alzheimer's disease. Arch Neurol Psychiatry 30:1180-1183, 1933
79. Kidd M: Alzheimer's disease—An electron microscopical study. Brain 87:307-320, 1964
80. Larson T, Sjogren T, Jacobson G: Senile dementia. Acta Psychiat Scand [Suppl 167] 39:1-259, 1963
81. Lishman WA: Organic Psychiatry. London, Blackwell, 1978, pp 540-549
82. Loeb C: Clinical diagnosis of multi-infarct dementia, in Amaducci L, Davison AN, Antuono P (eds): Aging of the Brain and Dementia. New York, Raven Press, 1980, pp 251-260
83. Lowenberg K: Pick's disease. A clinicopathologic contribution. Arch Neurol Psychiatry 36:768-789, 1936
84. Lowenberg K, Boyd DA Jr, Salon DD: Occurrence of Pick's disease in early adult years. Arch Neurol Psychiatry 41:1004-1020, 1939
85. Lowenberg K, Waggoner RW: Familial organic psychosis (Alzheimer's type). Arch Neurol Psychiatry 31:737-754, 1934
86. Luse SA, Smith KR Jr: The ultrastructure of senile plaques. Am J Pathol 44:553-563, 1964
87. Malamud N, Boyd DA Jr: Pick's disease with atrophy of the temporal lobes. Arch Neurol Psychiatry 43:210-222, 1940
88. Malamud W, Lowenberg K: Alzheimer's disease. Arch Neurol Psychiatry 21:805-827, 1929
89. Malamud N, Waggoner R.W: Genealogic and clinicopathologic study of Pick's disease. Arch Neurol Psychiatry 50:288-303, 1943

90. Mandybur TI: The incidence of cerebral amyloid angiopathy in Alzheimer's disease. Neurology 25:120–126, 1975
91. Mayer-Gross W, Critchley M, Greenfield JG, Meyer A: Discussion on the presenile dementias: Symptomatology, pathology, and differential diagnosis. Proc Roy Soc Med 31:1443–1454, 1937–1938
92. McDermott JR, Smith AI, Igbal K, Wisniewski HM: Aluminum and Alzheimer's disease. Lancet 2:710–711, 1977
93. McGeachie RE, Felming JO, Sharer LR, Hyman RA: Diagnosis of Pick's disease by computed tomography. J Comput Assist Tomog 3:113–115, 1979
94. McMenemy WH: Alzheimer's disease. J Neurol Psychiatry 3:211–240, 1940
95. McMenemy WH, Worster-Drought C, Flind J, Williams HG: Familial presenile dementia. J Neurol Psychiatry 2:293–303, 1939
96. Merritt HH: A textbook of Neurology, 5th ed. Philadelphia, Lea and Febiger, 1973, pp 442–445
97. Merritt HH, Springlova M: Lissauer's dementia paralytica. Arch Neurol Psychiatry 27:987–1030, 1932
98. Miller E: Efficiency of coding and the short-term memory defect in presenile dementia. Neuropsychologia 10:133–136, 1972
99. Miller E: On the nature of the memory disorder in presenile dementia. Neuropsychologia 9:75–81, 1971
100. Miller E, Hague F: Some characteristics of verbal behaviour in presenile dementia. Psychol Med 5:255–259, 1975
101. Nandy K: Brain-reactive antibodies in aging and senile dementia, in Katzman R, Terry RD, Bick KL, (eds): Alzheimer's Disease: Senile Dementia and Related Disorders. New York, Raven Press, 1978, pp 503–512
102. Neumann MA: Pick's disease. J Neuropathol Exp Neurol 8:255–282, 1949
103. Neumann MA: Combined amyloid vascular changes and argyrophilic plaques in the central nervous system. J Neuropathol Exp Neurol 19:370–382, 1960
104. Neumann MA, Cohn R: Incidence of Alzheimer's disease in a large mental hospital. Arch Neurol Psychiatry 69:615–636, 1953
105. Neumann MA, Cohn R: Progressive subcortical gliosis; a rare form of presenile dementia. Brain 90:405–418, 1967
106. Nichols IC, Weigner WC: Pick's disease—a specific type of dementia. Brain 61:237–249, 1938
107. Okazaki H, Reagen TJ, Campbell RJ: Clinicopathologic studies of primary cerebral amyloid angiopathy. Mayo Clin Proc 54:22–31, 1979
108. Olson MI, Shaw C-M: Presenile dementia and Alzheimer's disease in mongolism. Brain 92:147–156, 1969
109. Paulson GW: The neurological examination in dementia, in Wells CE (ed): Dementia, 2nd ed. Philadelphia, FA Davis, 1977, pp 169–188
110. Perez FI, Rivera VM, Meyer JS et al: Analysis of intellectual and cognitive performance in patients with multi-infarct dementia, vertebro-basilar insufficiency with dementia, and Alzheimer's disease. J Neurol Neurosurg Psychiat 38:533–540, 1975
111. Perry EK. Correlations between psychiatric neuropathological and bio-

chemical findings in Alzheimer's disease, in Glen AIM and Whalley LJ (eds): Alzheimer's Disease. Early Recognition of Potentially Reversible Deficits. London, Churchill Livingstone, 1979, pp 27-32

112. Perry EK, Perry RH, Blessed G, Tomlinson BE: Necropsy evidence of central cholinergic deficits in senile dementia. Lancet 1:189, 1977
113. Pilleri G: The Klüver-Bucy syndrome in man. Psychiat Neurol (Basel) 152:65-103, 1966
114. Polatin P, Hoch PH, Horwitz WA, Roizin L: Presenile psychosis. Am J Psychiatry 105:96-101, 1948
115. Pratt RTC: The genetics of Alzheimer's disease, in Wolstenholme GEW, O'Connor M (eds): Alzheimer's Disease and Related Conditions. London, J and A Churchill, 1970, pp 137-143
116. Renvoize EB Jerram T: Choline in Alzheimer's disease. N Engl J Med 301:330, 1979
117. Rewcastle MB, Ball MJ: Electron microscopic structure of the "inclusion bodies" in Pick's disease. Neurology 18:1205-1213, 1968
118. Richardson EP Jr: Progressive multifocal leukoencephalopathy, in Vinken PJ, Bruyn GW (eds): Handbook of Clinical Neurology, vol 9, Multiple Sclerosis and Other Demyelinating Diseases. New York, Elsevier, 1970, pp 485-499
119. Riese W: Senility. Proc First Int Cong Neuropathol 2:437-443, 1952
120. Robertson EE, le Roux A, Brown JH: The clinical differentiation of Pick's disease. J Ment Sci 104:1000-1024, 1958
121. Rochford G: A study of naming errors in dysphasic and in demented patients. Neuropsychol 9:437-443, 1971
122. Roos R, Gajdusek DC, Gibbs CJ Jr: The clinical characteristics of transmissible Creutzfeldt-Jakob disease. Brain 96:1-20, 1973
123. Roth M, Tomlinson BE, Blessed G: Correlation between scores for dementia and counts of 'senile plaques' in cerebral grey matter of elderly subjects. Nature 209:109-110, 1966
124. Rothschild D: Alzheimer's disease. Am J Psychiatry 91:485-518, 1934
125. Rothschild D, Kasanin J: Clinicopathologic study of Alzheimer's disease. Arch Neurol Psychiatry 36:293-321, 1936
126. Sanders J, Schenk VWD, Van Veen P: A family with Pick's disease. Amsterdam, Uitgave van de N.V. Noord-Hollandsche, 1939
127. Scharenberg K: The histologic structure of the "inclusion bodies" of the neurons in Pick's disease. J Neuropathol Exp Neurol 17:346-351, 1958
128. Schenk VWD: Reexamination of a family with Pick's disease. Ann Hum Genet 23:325-333, 1958-1959
129. Schenk VWD, van Mansvelt T: The cortical degeneration in Pick's syndrome. Folia Psychiat Neurol Neurochir Neerland 58:42-62, 1955
130. Schochet SS Jr, Earle KM: Pick's disease with compound intraneuronal inclusion bodies. Acta Neuropathol (Berlin) 15:293-297, 1970
131. Schochet SS Jr, Lampert PW, Lindenberg R: Fine structure of the Pick and Hirano bodies in a case of Pick's disease. Acta Neuropathol 11:330-337, 1968

132. Sim M, Sussman I: Alzheimer's disease: Its natural history and differential diagnosis. J Nerv Ment Dis 135:489-499, 1962
133. Sim M, Turner E, Smith WT: Cerebral biopsy in the investigation of presenile dementia. Br J Psychiatry 112:119-125, 1966
134. Sjogren H: Twenty-four cases of Alzheimer's disease. Acta Med Scand [Suppl 246]:225-233, 1950
135. Sjogren T, Sjogren H, Lindgren AGH: Morbus Alzheimer and morbus Pick. Acta Psychiat Neurol Scand [Suppl 82]:1-152, 1952
136. Slaby AE, Wyatt RJ: Dementia in the presenium. Springfield, Illinois, Thomas, 1974, pp 42-68, 69-76
137. Smith CM, Swash M, Exton-Smith AN et al: Choline therapy in Alzheimer's disease. Lancet 2:318, 1968
138. Sourander P, Sjogren H: The concept of Alzheimer's disease and its clinical implications, in Wolstenholme GEW, O'Connor M (eds): Alzheimer's Disease and Related Conditions. London, J and A Churchill, 1970, pp 11-32
139. Stengel E: A study of the symptomatology and differential diagnosis of Alzheimer's disease and Pick's disease. J Ment Sci 89:1-20, 1943
140. Stern K, Reed GE: Presenile dementia (Alzheimer's disease) Am J Psychiatry 102:191-197, 1945
141. Swain JM: Electroencephalographic abnormalities in presenile atrophy. Neurology 9:722-727, 1959
142. Tariska I: Circumscribed cerebral atrophy in Alzheimer's disease: A pathological study, in Wolstenholme GEW, O'Connor M (eds): Alzheimer's Disease and Related Conditions. London, J and A Churchill, 1970, pp 51-69
143. Terry RD: Ultrastructural alterations in senile dementia, in Katzmann R, Terry RD, Bick KL (eds): Alzheimer's Disease: Senile Dementia and Related Disorders. New York, Raven Press, 1978, pp 375-382
144. Thorpe FT: Pick's disease (circumscribed senile atrophy) and Alzheimer's disease. J Ment Sci 78:302-314, 1932
145. Tomlinson BE: The pathology of dementia, in Wells CE (ed): Philadelphia, FA Davis, 1977, pp 113-153
146. Tomlinson BE, Blessed G, Roth M: Observations on the brains of demented old people. J Neurol Sci 11:205-242, 1970
147. Tomlinson BE, Kitchner D: Granulovacuolar degeneration of hippocampal pyramidal cells. J Pathol 106:165-185, 1972
148. Towfighi J: Early Pick's disease. A light and ultrastructural study. Acta Neuropathol (Berlin) 21:224-231, 1972
149. Uyematsu S: On the pathology of senile psychosis. J Nerv Ment Dis 57:1-25, 131-156, 237-260, 1923
150. Wells CE, Duncan GW: Danger of over reliance on computerized cranial tomography. Am J Psychiatry 134:811-813, 1977
151. Wheelan L: Familial Alzheimer's disease. Ann Hum Genet 23:300-310, 1958-1959
152. White P, Goodhardt MJ, Keet JP et al: Neocortical cholinergic neurons in

elderly people. Lancet 1:668-671, 1977
153. Wilkins RH, Brody IA: Alzheimer's disease. Arch Neurol 21:109-110, 1969
154. Williams HW: The peculiar cells of Pick's disease. Arch Neurol Psychiatry 34:508-519, 1935
155. Winkleman NW, Book MH: Asymptomatic extrapyramidal involvement in Pick's disease. J Neuropathol Exp Neurol 8:30-42, 1949
156. Wisniewski HM, Coblentz, JM, Terry RD: Pick's disease. A clinical and ultrastructural study. Arch Neurol 26:97-108, 1972
157. Woodard JS: Clinicopathologic significance of granulovacuolar degeneration in Alzheimer's disease. J Neuropathol Exp Neurol 21:85-91, 1962
158. Yakovlev PI: Paraplegia in flexion of cerebral origin. J Neuropathol Exp Neurol 13:267-296, 1954
159. Yates CM: Aluminum and Alzheimer's disease, in Glen AIM, Whalley LJ (eds): Alzheimer's Disease. Early Recognition of Potentially Reversible Deficits. London, Churchill Livingstone, 1979, pp 53-56.
160. Yates CM, Simpson J, Maloney AFJ et al: Biochemical studies on postmortem brain in dementia, in Amaducci L, Davison AN, Antuono P, (eds): Aging of the brain in dementia. New York, Raven, 1980

Commentary

For generations, neurologists have been taught (and most have subsequently taught) that so few cases of Pick's disease have ever been recognized in life that it is virtually impossible for the clinician to distinguish between Pick's and Alzheimer's diseases in the living patient; only the neuropathologist could confidently separate the two. Dr. Cummings has not only carefully reviewed and clarified the neuropathologic differences between the Alzheimer and Pick varieties of cortical dementia but he has also provided new clinical observations on Pick's disease—most notably the presence of findings characteristic of the Klüver-Bucy syndrome. Most startingly, though, he has provided a solid means for differentiating the Alzheimer and Pick disorders on purely clinical grounds. Using these features, we should be able to separate the Alzheimer and Pick types of dementia seen in clinical practice. When this clinical approach is coupled with the growing recognition that the Alzheimer neuropathologic changes are present in many patients without serious mental deterioration[2] and that many patients with the gross neuropathologic characteristics of Pick's disease do not have the pathognomonic cellular changes, a totally different picture emerges. While there is good evidence that Alzheimer neuropathologic changes are seen in greatest quantity in patients with severe dementia,[1] it is equally clear that identical neuropathologic stigmata are present in most aging individuals, even those who were never demented. It would appear that the clinician, using the clinical guides outlined by Dr. Cummings, may be the only one who can properly distinguish the varieties of cortical dementia and separate them from the normal aging population. The neuropathologist can confirm the clinical impression.

The importance of learning and utilizing a clinical approach to dementia is further stressed in the following chapter. This chapter discusses the status of dementia as a public health menace, the possibility that diagnoses are commonly incorrect, (particularly overdiagnosis of Alzheimer's disease), and the hope that many individuals with dementia actually have treatable disorders. Chapters 5 and 6 present an overview of this neurobehavioral disorder and can be used as an initial guide by the clinician who evaluates and treats patients with these disorders. Chapters 7 and 8 will examine in more detail several areas of the dementia problem that are particularly troublesome, demanding careful diagnosis and appropriate treatment.

REFERENCES

1. Blessed G, Tomlinson BE, Roth M: The association between quantitative measures of dementia and of senile change in the cerebral grey matter of elderly subjects. Br J Psychiatry 114:797–811, 1968
2. Tomlinson BE: The pathology of dementia, in Wells CE (ed): Dementia, ed 2. Philadelphia, Davis, 1977

D. Frank Benson, M.D.

6
The Treatable Dementias

THE PROBLEM

While far from uncommon, dementia has consistently been a difficult and confusing problem for physicians. In fact, the term dementia was declared obsolete many years ago,[32] primarily because of the disorderly diagnostic chaos that it represented. The problem has not disappeared, however, and dementia is currently recognized as a serious challenge to both clinicians and researchers. For many years dementia was defined as irreversible,[9,27] a status that discouraged efforts in both research and clinical management. This definition has been attacked in recent years[22] and the current official nomenclature (DSM-III) no longer demands an irreversible status;[3] the definition of dementia remains an elusive problem, however, without meaningful or helpful divisions.

While estimates of frequency vary widely, dependent upon the definition, the incidence of dementia must be considered enormous. The occurence of dementia increases sharply with advancing years and the growth in the portion of the population over age 65 is creating an increasing population of dements. Several estimates of the occurrence of dementia have been offered in recent years. For instance, it has been stated that 4.5 percent of all individuals over age 65 have severe dementia while another 8–10 percent in that age group have a milder but significant degree of mental deterioration.[31] From a different approach, it has been estimated that almost half of all patients currently resident in nursing homes in the United States are there because of dementia.[28] It is suggested that the cost for supporting these individuals amounts to 12 billion dollars a year[28] and projections based on the increasing size of the aged population are truly alarming. Dementia presently is the fourth or fifth leading cause of major medical disability in the United States[19] and it must be acknowledged as one of the most formidable of current public health problems.[17]

For many years dementia was discussed as a unitary entity. Thus, a review of the literature reveals that most current research articles discuss work on "Dementia." This holistic, "big D" approach to dementia has tended to confound an already confusing topic. While most investigators and many clinicians recognize that many different causes of dementia can be listed, the unitary, "big D" approach limits advances in understanding. Until research can be focused on the separate causes underlying dementia the problem will remain insoluble.

While the unitary approach to dementia is ancient, several comparatively recent factors have engrained it further. One such factor has been the tendency for contemporary psychiatrists to include all mental deterioration under the rubric of organic brain syndrome. While this conveniently indicates that organic mental disorders are separate from more psychodynamically generated mental problems, this classification lumps all organically derived mental disorders, including the dementias, into a single diagnostic category. This produces severe diagnostic limitations; it is analagous to labeling all psychiatric patients crazy. Even worse, this diagnostic lumping of many severe problems has supported the widely believed dictum that dementia is irreversible and cannot be treated.

A second current influence stems from the investigative work of Blessed, Tomlinson, and Roth who emphasized the importance of the Alzheimer type of neuropathologic changes in the overall picture of dementia[5,30,35] (see Chapter 5 for further discussion). Current writings state "recent studies make it evident that most dementia reflects Alzheimer-senile disease, a primary cellular abnormality of the brain observed predominately in persons in their later decades.[28]" On this basis research has been focused on the genetic, neurochemical, viral, immune, and toxic disorders that might underlie cortical cellular changes of the type seen in Alzheimer's disease. To date these efforts have not provided specific understanding or treatment for Alzheimer's disease, much less any other types of dementia.

In 1965, a radically different idea was suggested by demonstration that an occult hydrocephalus with communication between the ventricular system and the subtentorial subarachnoid space (now called normal pressure hydrocephalus) often produced a severe dementia that could be reversed with appropriate surgery.[1] The presence of a "reversible dementia" stimulated interest in other disorders capable of producing dementia that would respond to appropriate management. While usually considered only a small portion of the total dementia problem,[10,23] the varieties of reversible dementia have become a subject of growing interest in recent years.[8]

This chapter will discuss not only the fully reversible dementias but also the many types of dementia that will respond in some degree to treatment—the treatable dementias. To study these disorders it is necessary to outline parameters separating them from the cortical degenerative disorders.

THE DIFFERENTIAL DIAGNOSIS OF DEMENTIA

Although some definition of dementia is needed, this has proved to be a remarkably difficult task. Most definitions suggest that dementia is an acquired disturbance of intellectual function, an accurate statement but far too broad and vague. For this discussion dementia will be defined as a sustained loss of intellectual capacity that includes disturbance in at least three of the following parameters:

1. cognitive function (manipulation of old knowledge)
2. memory (the ability to learn new information or retrieve old information)
3. visuo-spatial functions (construction and topographic capabilities)
4. communication ability (speech and language disturbances)
5. personality (alterations in personal behavior)

Abnormality in all five parameters is not necessary to consider dementia but if only a single ability is severely compromised while the others are relatively preserved, another term is appropriate. Severe language or memory disturbances occurring alone, for instance, are better called aphasia and amnesia, respectively. One important facet of this definition is the implication that the mental capabilities have been lost or seriously impaired and that they were normal previously. The mental abnormalities of chronic mental retardation, then, should also be separated from dementia.[36]

While dementing disorders that feature severe cortical degeneration (primarily Alzheimers and Pick's diseases) have been recognized for years (as described in Chapter 5), dementing disorders with primary pathology in the subcortical regions have only recently been recognized.[2,24] These so-

Table 6-1
Differential Diagnosis—Cortical versus Subcortical Dementia

	Cortical (Alzheimer, Pick)	Subcortical (Huntington, Wilson, PSP, Parkinson)
Appearance	Alert, healthy (often appear younger than stated age)	Abnormal (infirm, disheveled, perplexed)
Activity	Normal	Abnormal (slow)
Stance	Erect	Abnormal (stooped, hyperextended, twisted)
Gait	Normal (pacing is common)	Abnormal (dancing, ataxic, festinating, unsteady)
Movements	Normal	Abnormal (tremor, chorea, dystonia)
Verbal Output (speech)	Normal	Abnormal (dysarthric, hypophonic, mute)
Language	Abnormal (anomia, paraphasia)	Normal
Cognition	Abnormal (unable to manipulate knowledge)	Dilapidated (less than normal)
Memory	Abnormal (unable to learn)	Forgetful (problem with retrieval)
Visuospatial skill	Abnormal (constructional disturbance)	Sloppy (due to movement problem)
Emotional state	Abnormal (unaware, unconcerned)	Abnormal (apathetic, lacking drive)

called subcortical dementias are readily differentiated from the cortical type of dementias by comparison of clinical features (Table 6-1). Some of these differentiating features deserve emphasis because of their crucial role in understanding dementia.

The best recognized causes of subcortical dementia (Huntington's disease, Wilson's disease, Parkinson's disease, and progressive supranuclear palsy) all feature striking movement disorder, a primary neurologic abnormality. In contrast, primary neurologic deficit is either absent or occurs only in the very advanced stages of the cortical dementias, thus providing one basic difference. Severe memory disturbance, best described as an inability to learn, is a characteristic of Alzheimer's disease and occurs early in the course. The memory disturbance in the subcortical dementias, on the other hand, is better described as a problem in retrieving information already learned. These patients continue to learn new information well into the course of their disease but have significant problems initiating retrieval of the information. Given an appropriate structure these individuals can remember many recently learned details.[7] This common memory disturbance has been called forgetting to remember[2] and is discussed further in Chapter 12.

One of the more characteristic differences between the cortical and the subcortical types of dementia concerns verbal communication. Both groups show serious problems but the problems involve entirely different aspects. In both Pick's and Alzheimer's disease there is an early and significant *language* disturbance with word-finding problems, paraphasias, decreased comprehension and other aphasic disturbances. Until very late in the disease, individuals with these disorders will not have problems with speech (dysarthria, slurring, hypophonia, etc.). In subcortical dementia, in contrast, there is no language disturbance until very late in the course, but difficulties with *speech* such as significant slowness, decreased volume (hypophonia), and lack of articulatory crispness (dysarthria) occur early and in most of these disorders progress until mutism occurs.

Of all the features separating the two types of dementia, the most striking is the slowness of individuals with subcortical dementia. This slowness involves not only motor activity but also comprehension of stimuli, thought processing, and language formulation—features that are absent in the cortical dementias until very late in the course. The generalized slowness of the subcortical dementias is well-defined by the single term "psychomotor retardation," reflecting the retardation of both psychic and motor functions. Psychomotor retardation, however, has traditionally been used to designate other problems, most particularly the affective disorder known as depression. If one accepts psychomotor retardation as an indication of subcortical dementia, then many additional mental disorders can be included within this framework and subcortical dementia can be elevated to a common and important mental disturbance. These disorders make up most of the group of disorders that can be called the treatable dementias.

The mental alterations of severe depression are well-characterized as psychomotor retardation, and most of the features of subcortical dementia listed in Table 6-1 are routinely present in severely depressed patients. In this light, depression may be considered a form of dementia, an overlap most notably present in the entity known as depressive pseudodementia,[20,29] although even lesser degrees of depression show characteristics of dementia. This aspect of depression is discussed more fully in Chapter 5.

Another disorder capable of producing dementia and psychomotor retardation is multi-infarct dementia.[14] Two varieties of this disorder can be described. In one, the patient has suffered several or many separate strokes involving large volumes of cortical and subcortical structures in both hemispheres and shows dementia along with many other neurologic disabilities. The second, more subtle, variety is most often seen in individuals with severe hypertension who have suffered multiple tiny infarcts (lacunes), most of which involve deep subcortical structures; there may be no neurologic residue except for a progressive dementia featuring psychomotor retardation.

The most common variety of severe psychomotor retardation is the chronic confusional state, the vast clinical diversity indicated in Table 6-2. Many extrinsic and intrinsic disorders can affect brain function. If acute, they are referred to as acute confusional states (see Chapter 1) or acute exogenous reactions.[6] Many disorders are chronic, however, and if sufficiently severe will produce a dementia, almost always with the features of psychomotor retardation. Among the sources of a dementia clinical

Table 6-2
Etiologic Categories of Dementia

Systemic disease
Endocrine disease
Vascular disease
Deficiency states
Infectious diseases
Chemical poisonings
Drug poisonings
Intracranial tumors
Chronic neurologic states
Psychogenic disorders
Miscellaneous disorders

The Treatable Dementias

picture, the chronic confusional states must be ranked high in both frequency and importance (see Tables 6-3 to 6-11).

By recognizing that there are many causes of psychomotor retardation, most of which produce a dementia-like clinical state, the number of disorders that cause dementia becomes immense with far more individuals showing subcortical than cortical dementia. For the clinician, differentiation of the two types is a useful starting point for the management of dementia.

In addition to the clinical observations outlined in Table 6-1, diagnostic aid can come from the laboratory. Vast improvements have been made in laboratory techniques for the study of dementia in recent years and, although these still remain deficient, considerable progress in diagnostic aids can be anticipated in the next decade. The laboratory presently provides many valuable confirmations of clinical suspicions but relatively few specific diagnoses.

One of the laboratory tools commonly used to study dementia is psychologic testing. Altogether too often the clinician merely recognizes deficient mentation and refers the patient to a psychologist with the expectation that psychometric evaluation will define the problem. At the current state of the art, psychologic testing cannot differentiate the many varieties of dementia. Many psychologic tests give excellent quantitative estimates of the overall mental state but fail to qualitatively separate the varieties of dementia. Several investigators have produced psychometric batteries that they suggest can detect Alzheimer's disease[11,13]; to date, however, this work is still investigational—not the level of a clinical diagnosis—and even these investigators make no claim that their batteries can distinguish the many varieties of treatable dementia. The physician, therefore, must use clinical skills, not neuropsychologic tests, to diagnose the varieties of dementia.

The clinical laboratory may demonstrate the etiology underlying a treatable dementia but, unfortunately, this only occurs if the appropriate question is asked. Dementia batteries of clinical lab tests usually include multichannel blood chemistries plus blood counts, serology, liver and thyroid function tests, heavy metal screens, B_{12} and folate levels, plus various additional tests. In general, the battery approach is to be condemned. It is expensive and routinely unrewarding; even more dangerous, these batteries can lull the unsophisticated clinician into believing he has adequately sought the causes of dementia. The number of disorders capable of producing dementia is almost countless and batteries can investigate only a small percentage of potential causes. The clinical laboratory, on the other hand, is invaluable for confirmation of a diagnosis suspected from clinical studies. Properly selected laboratory tests often solve the riddle of a mental deterioration.

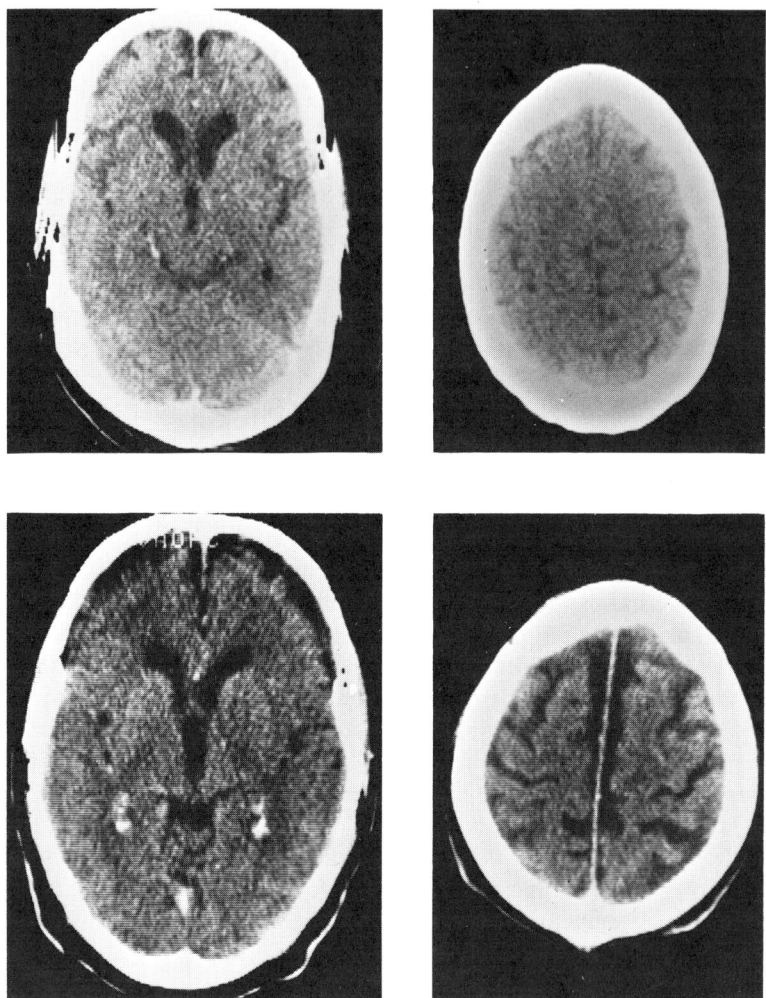

Fig. 6-1. X-ray CT of two patients referred to rule out dementia. The upper two scans are from a 58-year-old man with well advanced dementia and the findings of Alzheimer's disease. The x-ray CT scan was read as within normal limits. The two lower scans are of a 47-year-old man without dementia (IQ of 137 at the time of the scan) but with a history of alcohol abuse. Note the massive cortical atrophy and grossly enlarged third ventricle.

In recent years, x-ray computerized tomography (CT) has proved to be a valuable tool in the evaluation of individuals with dementia. For many clinicians the x-ray CT scan is the primary diagnostic tool for dementia, an unfortunate circumstance. While the x-ray CT scan clearly demonstrates a number of treatable causes of dementia, particularly the

The Treatable Dementias

intracranial mass lesions, it does not provide valid information on many causes of dementia. Recent literature includes many descriptions of the degree of cortical atrophy seen on x-ray CT in cases of dementia.[15,26,33] In general, increased atrophy, both central (ventricular dilatation) and cortical (increased sulcal markings) are said to occur with increased degrees of dementia. Recent studies, however, clearly demonstrate that x-ray CT findings of atrophy do not indicate the degree of dementia.[12,25] Individuals may show severe central and cortical atrophy and yet have no dementia while other individuals with advanced dementia may be within the limits of normal for their age group (see Fig 6-1). When specifically positive, the x-ray CT is an extremely valuable tool in the workup of dementia but, like all other laboratory tests, it functions best as a confirmatory test, not as a screening device.

One laboratory study, however, the electroencephalogram (EEG), can be used as a screening device with considerable usefulness and should be performed on *every* individual undergoing a workup for dementia. The EEG, like the x-ray CT, on occasion produces a diagnosis of the cause of dementia (particularly the presence of seizure activity or demonstration of focal slow wave activity) but even nonspecific EEG findings may be pertinent. The cortical dementias, in general, produce far less EEG abnormality than the subcortical varieties. Stated another way, if the EEG pattern of a dementia patient looks worse than the mental state, there is a high probability of a treatable disorder. The converse, with the mental state appearing much worse than the EEG pattern, is seen with the cortical dementias but also with the psychogenic pseudodementias. If the EEG is seriously abnormal in the early stages of a dementing illness, the probability of a treatable cause is very high, a vital piece of information in the workup of dementia.

In summary, a crucial but currently underemphasized aspect of dementia concerns diagnosis. Differentiation into cortical or subcortical (psychomotor retardation) varieties plus the use of laboratory aids can help the clinician discover those disorders that are treatable. Although these disorders are myriad and considerable ingenuity and deductive ability will be required to make a final diagnosis, the results can be rewarding.

THE TREATABLE DEMENTIAS

The concept that all dementia is irreversible has been discarded[21] but, in truth, there is little or no specific treatment available for many causes of dementia. Nonetheless, many other causes of dementia can be treated and discovery of a treatable variety is an important first step. Treatable and reversible are not necessarily synonymous. While some dementing disorders can be completely reversed (returning the patient to a fully normal mental state), many causes of dementia can be treated successfully without the mental disorder being totally reversed. Thus, in certain diseases (e.g., Wilson's disease) the dementing process is stopped by appropriate treatment but often without return to fully normal status. Early diagnosis with initiation of appropriate management holds the level of mental deterioration to a minimum.

Some of the currently recognized causes of dementia that are considered untreatable (e.g., Jakob-Creutzfeldt disease) may well have specific treatment in the future. Accurate diagnosis of these presently untreatable disorders will provide a better base for future treatments. The many current attempts to alter "Dementia" pharmacologically would seem doomed to failure because of the vast heterogeneity of the disease processes being treated.

It can be seen that the only way to discuss the treatable dementias is through etiology but this produces overwhelming problems. Literally, hundreds of different disease processes can produce dementia. To handle this with any degree of parsimony, some artificial separation is necessary. The inclusion of a disease process in one category or another is open to argument, and any list of causes of dementia is admittedly incomplete. The list presented in Table 6-2 offers only an initial step for the discussion of treatable dementia. Within each category there are many disorders that deserve attention.

Systemic Diseases

It is well-recognized that a variety of systemic illnesses can and do produce serious problems with mentation. Table 6-3 lists a number of such disorders. In many of these disorders insufficient oxygen reaches the brain, usually because of pulmonary or cardiac insufficiency or severe hematologic abnormality. Most often the disease processes are well known to the clinician before the recognition of mental deterioration; it is not uncommon, however, for a dementia picture to be present when the physical abnormality is either unrecognized or inadequately controlled. In such circumstances the dementia can easily be misdiagnosed as an independent (and untreatable) disorder. Recognition that the systemic disease may be the cause of the dementia plus careful re-evaluation of the medical state and initiation of appropriate management may produce a remarkable reversal of the dementia. Chronic systemic disorders represent one of the more common causes of dementia.

Table 6-3
Systemic Diseases

Pulmonary insufficiency (hypoxia)	Severe anemia
Pneumonia	Polycythemia vera
Emphysema	Blood dyscrasias
Atelectasis	Hypertensive encephalopathy
Bronchiectasis	Uremia
Pleural effusion	Hypernatremia
Altitude sickness	Hyperlipidemia
Sleep apnea	Porphyria
Pickwickian syndrome	Portal sytemic encephalopathy
Cardiac insufficiency	Remote effects of carcinoma
Arrythmia	Dialysis dementia
Coarctation	Heat stroke
Aortic/mitral stenosis	Hyponatremia
Cardiac failure	Kuf's disease

Endocrine Diseases

While not as common, mental deterioration may accompany severe endocrinopathy. Table 6-4 lists some of the hormone disturbances known to produce a dementia picture. The endocrine abnormality may go unrecognized and, particularly in the elderly, mental deterioration may be the major problem, leading to a diagnosis of dementia. Again, recognition of the characteristics of the treatable dementias plus a healthy level of suspicion for the endocrinopathies can lead to a proper diagnosis and rewarding management of a treatable cause of dementia.

Table 6-4
Endocrine disease

Addison's disease
Panhypopituitarism
Myxedema (hypothyroidism)
Hypoparathyroidism
Hyperparathyroidism
Recurrent hypoglycemia
Cushing's disease
Steroid therapy
Hyperthyroidism
Hypercalcemia
Hypocalcemia

Table 6-5
Vascular Diseases

Systemic lupus erythematosis
Temporal arteritis
Granulomatous-angiitis
Periarteritis nodosa
Vogt-Koyanagi Haroda disease
Moya-Moya
Takayasu's syndrome
Cogan's syndrome
Carotid artery stenosis/occlusion
Basilar artery stenosis/occlusion
Giant aneurysm
Cortical microinfarction
Binswanger's disease
Embolism
Thrombosis

Vascular Diseases

Vascular disorders were once presumed to underlie much of the mental deterioration seen with advancing age. Careful neuropathologic studies have failed to confirm the presence of arteriosclerotic brain changes in many such individuals, and there has been a reactive tendency to disregard vascular disease as a cause of dementia in the past few years. This is not accurate either as there are many individuals in whom a specific relationship between vascular disease and mental deterioration can be identified. Table 6-5 lists some of the more common vascular diseases known to be associated with dementia. Note that the table includes both the vasculitides and the more prosaic atherosclerotic disturbances of intra- and extra-cranial blood vessels that cause stroke. As noted earlier, two varieties of multi-infarct dementia are recognized, one secondary to multiple large infarcts and the other a product of multiple small subcortical lacunes. A third disorder, called cortical polyinfarction, has recently been described.[18] In this disorder the many punctate infarcts present in the cortex are thought to be due to emboli from cardiac tissues. Mental deterioration can accompany a great many extra- and intra-cerebral vascular diseases.

Infectious Diseases

A broad spectrum of infectious diseases are known to produce serious alterations in mentation. The classic example is neurosyphilis which,

The Treatable Dementias

Table 6-6
Infectious Diseases

Syphilis
Tuberculosis
Chronic fungus infection
Cysticercosis
Whipple's disease
Cerebral abcess
Progressive multifocal leukoencephalopathy
Herpes encephalitis
Inclusion cell encephalitis (Herpes)
Jakob-Creutzfeldt disease
Equine encephalitis
Measles
Chickenpox
Cryptococcosis (torula)
Behcet's syndrome
Kuru
Hydatid cysts
Schistosomiasis
Sarcoidosis
Subacute sclerosing panencephalitis (SSPE)

before the advent of penicillin, was probably the major cause of dementia. While no longer common, neurosyphilis can still be seen and is only one of a large number of systemic and central nervous system (CNS) infections that can cause mental deterioration. Table 6-6 lists some of the infectious disorders known to cause mental deterioration. Although the list is incomplete, it emphasizes the importance of a thorough study of all individuals with progressive mental deterioration. Chronic inflammatory disorders can only be discovered and treated if they are given proper consideration. Appropriate treatment is often available and can not only stop the progression but lead to improvement or even reversal of the mental deterioration.

Chemical Poisoning

In an era that has advertised "better living through chemistry," many medical disturbances are the result of excessive exposure or idiosyncratic sensitivity to the chemicals in the environment. Table 6-7 lists of some of the hundreds of recognized chemical causes of dementia. Many more compounds belong on this list and many, many more will be added in years to come. Included among the chemical poisons are the heavy metals, long

Table 6-7
Chemical Poisoning

Nitrobenzenes
Anilines
Bromated hydrocarbons
Chronic CS_2 exposure
Chronic CCT_4 exposure
Triorthochlorylphosphate
Trichloroethylene
Toluene
Organophosphates
Carbon monoxide
Alcohol, ethyl
Alcohol, methyl
Mercury
Lead
Aluminum
Manganese
Arsenic
Thallium

recognized as causes of mental deterioration, but even more of a problem are the many newly generated chemical compounds that we are exposed to. Some exposure comes through industrial toxins, some through accidental poisoning, but most are purposefully added to our environment. The chemical poisons are almost always difficult to discover and, not infrequently, a diagnosis of psychogenic disorder is made before the chemical cause is recognized. Psychotherapy is understandably ineffective in the management of chemical CNS toxicity. Again, realization that the clinical findings of a treatable dementia are present can direct the clinician to a proper direction for investigation. Most of the chemically caused dementias respond to treatment and many are fully reversible.

Drug Poisoning

A continually increasing source of mental symptomatology in our society stems from the use and abuse of pharmaceuticals. This includes not only drugs that individuals self prescribe, either from the street market or from the shelves of the pharmacy, but also the drugs prescribed for patients by physicians. Table 6-8 lists some of the drugs reported to have caused dementia. It must be recognized that this is a small list and that many, many more drugs in current use are capable of producing a picture of mental deterioration. Demonstration of this possibility demands con-

The Treatable Dementias

Table 6-8
Drug Poisoning

Methyldopa
Haloperidol
Clonidine
Fluphenazine
Disulfram
Lithium carbonate
Phenothiazine
Bromides
Phenytoin
Mephenytoin (Mesanotoin®)
Barbiturates
Propranolol hydrochloride
Atropine
Belladonna
Digitalis
Imipramine
Methotrexate (with cerebral irradiation)

siderable scrutiny of the patient's history. Patients often accept the drugs prescribed by a physician to be correct and normal and do not even report them unless specifically questioned. Even more troublesome is the possibility that the patient has been using drugs from a pharmacy or a nonmedical source and has failed to report this to the clinician. Although some "remedies," such as medicated cough drops, are not even considered to be drugs by many patients, long-term use may produce mental symptoms. Many well-established and vital medications such as digitalis, the phenothiazines, phenytoin, and the barbiturates, etc. are capable of producing serious mental deterioration in susceptible patients, even at nontoxic levels. Drugs are an increasingly frequent cause of dementia—a tenet that must be emphasized. The treatment is simple—usually only cessation or decreased dosage of the medication—and often extremely rewarding.

Deficiency States

While not so common, some specific nutritional deficiency states are known to produce a striking dementing picture (Table 6-9). Best known of these is the dementia that occurs with subacute combined sclerosis, a deficiency of Vitamin B_{12}. Folate and niacin deficiencies are each said to produce dementia, and some of the complications of alcohol, particularly Korsakoff's psychosis, Marchiafava-Bignami disease, and alcoholic en-

Table 6-9
Deficiency States

B_{12} deficiency
Pellagra
Folate deficiency
Marchiafava-Bignami disease
Alcoholic encephalopathy

cephalopathy may actually be based on specific deficiency states. (See Chapter 7 for an additional description of the dementia that can occur with chronic alcoholism.) Among the more consistent signs of a metabolic dementia are psychomotor retardation and the characteristic slowing of the EEG frequency. In fact, the diffusely slow toxic-metabolic pattern of the EEG can be used as a valuable clue in the workup of a mentally deteriorated patient if it is remembered that a similar pattern may be seen in the deficiency states and with chemical or pharmaceutical poisoning.

Intracranial Tumor

Most neurologists are alert to the possibility of intracranial tumor and readily consider this diagnosis. Table 6-10 lists some of the intracranial mass lesions known to produce dementia. In many instances an intracranial tumor will first manifest through specific neurologic findings

Table 6-10
Intracranial Tumor

Glioblastoma
Astrocytoma
Oligodendroglioma
Ependymoma
Medulloblastoma
Metastasis
Granuloma
Meningioma
Pituitary adenoma
Craniopharyngioma
Reticulum cell sarcoma
Carcinomatosis of meninges
Colloid cyst (third ventricle)
Hodgkins disease
Gumma
Tuberculoma

The Treatable Dementias

such as seizures, paresis, and focal headache, etc. It is not at all uncommon, however, for a tumor to be neurologically quiescent for a prolonged period, either through location in a comparatively "silent" area or because the tumor grows slowly and compensation of the surrounding structures permits it to reach tremendous size before producing basic neurologic disturbances. All neurologists have seen individuals who present with a progressive dulling of mentation of long duration which, in retrospect, was caused by a slowly growing intracranial mass lesion. The mental dulling is frequently accompanied by additional alterations in behavior which are sufficient to warrant psychiatric evaluation and, not infrequently, a course of psychotherapy is undertaken. The x-ray CT scan has proved to be a valuable diagnostic aid in ferreting out intracranial tumors although false-negative scans, particularly in early stages of tumor development, are not uncommon. The EEG provides another tool for screening but may also be falsely negative in the very early stages. Often only a well-developed suspicion, persistent concern, and repeated tests will allow the correct diagnosis to be made. The final outcome will be dependent upon the prognosis and intracranial location of the tumor; in many instances the improvement in mentation after treatment of an intracranial tumor mass is gratifying.

Chronic Neurologic States

In addition to the infectious disorders and intracranial tumors that primarily involve the central nervous system, a broad variety of other chronic neurologic states can be the cause of mental deterioration. These are listed together in Table 6-11 but it must be recognized that this list encompasses a broad variety of disorders with distinctly different etiologies. Included are the chronic CNS degenerative disorders, many of which are not treatable at present. These include disorders such as Friedreich's and other forms of hereditary ataxia, the Alzheimer and Pick types of dementia, the Parkinsonian-dementia complex of Guam, and the other progressive degenerative disorders such as Schilder's disease and Hallervorden-Spatz disease. As stressed in all modern neurologic texts, many of the chronic neurologic disorders are treatable. Entities such as epilepsy, multiple sclerosis, and Huntington's and Parkinson's diseases will respond to appropriate treatment and the mental deterioration stopped or reversed. It should never be considered that dementia in the presence of a chronic neurologic disorder precludes treatment. Useful and valuable treatments are available for many of these disorders, and it is suspected that many more of these disorders will have specific treatments in the future.

Table 6-11
Chronic Neurologic States

Epilepsy
Multiple sclerosis
Parkinson's disease
Progressive supranuclear palsy
Huntington's disease
Hereditary ataxia (olivo-ponto-cerebellar degeneration, Friedreich's ataxia, striato-nigral degeneration)
Multiple-infarcts
Pick's disease
Senile dementia
Senility
Wilson's disease
Fahr's disease (idiopathic cerebral calcinosis)
Machado (Azorean) disease
Adult polysaccharoidosis
Adrenoleukodystrophy
Metachromatic leukodystrophy
Parkinson-dementia complex of Guam
Bilateral thalamic degeneration
Schilder's disease
Hallervorden-Spatz disease
Progressive subcortical gliosis
Myoclonic epilepsy
Down's syndrome

Psychogenic States

For a number of years it has been suggested that some psychogenic states could produce a false or pseudodementia. This has been most prominently suggested for depression, but a state of pseudodementia is also said to occur in both schizophrenia and hysteria. One specific diagnostic entity, usually classed as an hysterical pseudodementia, is Ganser's syndrome. Table 6-12 lists the recognized psychogenic sources of a dementia picture. If one accepts the premise developed earlier in this chapter that pscyhomotor retardation is a form of mental deterioration (dementia), then the term pseudodementia would not be correct for these entities, as all can occur in a state of psychomotor retardation similar to that occurring in other varieties of dementia. It would appear more appropriate to accept that these psychiatric disorders are causing true dementia; whether they are based totally or even partially on psychogenic factors is an unresolved question but, in most instances, these are reversible dementias.

The most common of the psychogenic dementing disorders occur with severe (psychotic) depression. With this disorder there is a marked

Table 6-12
The Pseudodementias

Schizophrenia
Hysterical symptoms
Ganser's syndrome
Depression
Malingering

slowing of both motor and mental functions, forgetfulness, a dilapidation of cognitive function, and even the physical manifestations of tremor, shakiness, weakness, and ataxia. While the presence of depression is usually obvious from the history and the course of the illness (see Chapter 8), individual cases may be seen in which the presenting picture of mental deterioration is so strong that the depressive features are hidden and clinically indistinguishable from other forms of dementia. The mental deterioration associated with depression usually clears with appropriate therapy. If the psychogenic mental deteriorations are added to the diagnostic possibilities considered by the clinician evaluating a patient with mental deterioration, recognition and appropriate management of these eminently treatable dementias would result.

Miscellaneous

Despite the many disorders classified above, other problems remain that can affect the brain and produce mental deterioration as a side effect but are not readily placed into any of the etiologic categories mentioned. Table 6-13 lists a number of such disorders and, again, it must be recognized as an incomplete list. Most significant in this group are the effects of trauma. Often lumped together under the term posttraumatic encephalopathy, a multitude of different alterations in mental effec-

Table 6-13
Miscellaneous

Trauma
Dementia pugilistica
Subdural hematoma
Fat embolization
Hydrocephalus
Excessive ECT
Paget's disease
Basilar impression
Arnold-Chiari syndrome
Bends (nitrogen emboli)

tiveness can occur and be sufficiently severe to warrant the term dementia (see Chapter 11). Dementia pugilistica is one of the more dramatic variations of posttraumatic dementia; it is an uncommon, progressive dementia accompanied by seizures that occurs late in the career or following the retirement of some professional boxers. Trauma can also produce syndromes such as the Capgras syndrome, reduplicative paramnesia, and normal pressure hydrocephalus in which dementia can be a significant part of the clinical picture. In addition to trauma, Table 6-13 lists a wide variety of unrelated disturbances that can cause mental deterioration; the clinician must be alert for such disorders as many respond to appropriate management.

TREATMENT OF DEMENTIA

As can be realized from perusal of the lists of disorders recognized as causes of dementia, the treatment for most types of dementia is the treatment appropriate for the underlying etiology. In many instances the treatment for an etiologically produced dementia is specific and often offers good prognosis for the disease process and, secondarily, for improved or return to normal mental function. The etiologies capable of producing dementia are so broad and varied that the treatment of dementia appears to entail most of the treatment modalities available in the field of medicine. The search for a single treatment for all dementias is obviously naive and doomed to failure. Because there are so many different causes of dementia, only a few of the treatments for the more common disorders can be discussed here.

The first and most important principle in the treatment of a demented patient concerns good general health. Many of the disturbances listed above are based on or associated with abnormal general health. This may be a nutritional deficiency, a physical disease, or some type of environmental or dietary poisoning, including the effects of prescribed medications. The first step in the treatment of dementia is a careful screening for body contaminants and removal or replacement of these noxious substances. The patient's return to good dietary habits, good sleeping and exercise habits, and his withdrawal from chemical and pharmaceutical poisons will correct dementia in a sizeable number of individuals. Response to these general measures is often slow, however, and the clinician may be unsure of their usefulness. During the period of intense investigation for possible causes of dementia, a program of good general health practices should be instituted and may, by itself, aid recovery of mental function.

More specific medical treatments are often necessary in individuals with etiologically produced dementias. Thus, the correction of cardiac, pulmonary, hepatic, gastrointestinal, or other disorders which are producing sufficient problems to interfere with mentation often brings about amelioration of the mental deterioration. Internists routinely treat patients with severe mental alterations due to acute or chronic systemic illness and bring about a return to a normal mental state through correction of the medical abnormality. In most such instances the basic medical problem is recognized and treated; dementia, however, is not even considered as a diagnosis. Many such patients, however, have mental findings that fit the definition of dementia and if the medical problem is inadequately treated, will remain mentally disabled. Not all medical problems are obvious. It can be estimated that thousands of the individuals currently residing in nursing homes with the diagnosis of dementia actually have correctable medical abnormalities as the cause of their mental picture. In many more of these patients, in addition, the medical treatment itself is the cause of the mental deterioration. Replacing one treatment modality with another with different side effects may be crucial for the management of a dementia that is complicating systemic disease.

A number of surgical treatments are effective for specific types of dementia. Surgical decompression of an intracranial tumor, abcess, or other mass lesion may dramatically improve the mental state. One specific surgical treatment is the shunting of cerebral spinal fluid into the cardiac atrium or the peritoneum to correct the dementia caused by some forms of hydrocephalus.[4,16] While not as common as the medical treatments of dementia, surgical intervention is certainly useful for some causes of dementia and can produce dramatic alterations in mental function.

Psychiatric therapy can be helpful in the management of dementia in two different ways. First, the psychogenic varieties of dementia often respond to appropriate psychiatric management. Antidepressant drugs and the use of electroshock therapy have both proved effective in correcting depressive pseudodementia. Most such patients show a gratifying if not total improvement in mental activity. Appropriate treatment of schizophrenic and hysterical symptomatology can also alter the disordered mentation. While far less common as causes of dementia, the psychogenic causes deserve consideration and, when present, intense management, as the prognosis for improvement is good.

A very different type of psychologic management may also be beneficial in dementia. This is the social and psychiatric manipulation necessary to provide a supportive environment. Mental deterioration is both aggravated and exaggerated by family and social demands. Appropriate counseling of the patient, the family, and other environmentally important persons can ease the situation and produce smoother functioning, both for the patient and those in the patient's environment. Counseling is particularly important for individuals with treatable but not reversible dementia or an untreatable type of dementia. In such situations, appropriate alteration of the patient's environmental situation can allow the patient to function at optimum. In some instances this may demand custodial care, but more often manipulation of the patient's current living situation can lighten the social demands sufficiently to allow the mildly or moderately demented individual to carry on many familiar activities.

While the treatment of the psychogenic causes of dementia is probably best handled by a specialist experienced in the management of major psychiatric diseases, the counseling and environmental manipulation activities can and should be carried out by all physicians. Counseling of this type, in fact, should always be included with the more specific management of the etiologic varieties of dementia mentioned above. A lack of such counseling often limits the outcome of a successful medical or surgical treatment for dementia.

Finally, mention should be made of the burgeoning search for a pharmacologic remedy for dementia. The past decade has witnessed the excited introduction of many different drugs to treat or cure dementia. Some have biochemical effects deemed advantageous for specific cerebral activity; others have more general attributes. Most have been reported with a flush of success, based on limited trials and an intricate theoretic background. Most have failed abysmally when put to even mildly stringent clinical investigations. Among recent examples are physostigmine, vasopressin, amphetamine, choline, lecithin, hydrozine, methylphenidate, and megavitamin therapies. As noted, most such trials are doomed to fail because of an inability to differentiate varieties of dementia. It would be unlikely that any single pharmacologic substance could successfully correct the vast number of different states underlying dementia.

There is a spark of hope, however. A number of studies have noted that some treated patients did show improvement in some aspects of behavior. It does not seem improbable that a chemical replacement therapy providing a general boost to nervous system activities may be discovered. While not effective against the specific causes of dementia, such a nostrum might provide increased mental activity for many. Also, the behavior altered may not be specific for memory or cognitive function, the modalities usually monitored; alterations in arousal, motivation, selective attention, and sequencing, etc. may greatly aid the individual suffering a deterioration of mental powers. The drug studies will be watched with hopeful anticipation.

FUTURE CONSIDERATIONS

Based on the preceding discussion, some considerations on the future of dementia as a medical problem are warranted. As noted, all current projections indicate that dementia will become one of the most common and most serious of all medical problems in the next several decades. Most of these predictions, however, are made on the basis of a single, essentially untreatable, disorder called dementia—a disorder that increases in frequency with advancing age. Little attention has been given to the treatment of dementia in these predictions; and the possibility that a significant portion of the present incidence may represent unrecognized, treatable dementia is ignored. In addition, it cannot be assumed that current diagnostic and treatment methods are the best that will ever be available. Merely recognizing the treatable varieties of dementia would greatly improve the potential for successful management with present measures, and it can be confidently anticipated that the better treatments for many of the causes of dementia will appear in the future. Obviously, future advances in treatment will alter the outlook for many causes of dementia but, as now, they will still depend on the diagnostic acumen of physicians. All physicians must become better acquainted with the many causes of dementia so they can discover and treat patients with dementing disorders.

Finally, any discussion of the incidence of dementia in the future demands some discussion of the mental deterioration that occurs with normal aging. It is widely recognized that many (in fact, most) otherwise healthy individuals show decreased mental capability as they advance in age. It is presently assumed that this deterioration reflects a dropout of cortical neurones similar to the state in Alzheimer's disease. It is well-documented that this type of cortical change does occur and that it increases with advancing age,[34] and most current research efforts on the neurologic problems of aging focus on disturbed cortical neuronal function. Were this true, a treatment for Alzheimer's disease would also be a treatment for the mental deterioration of aging, a worthy research challenge.

A comparison of the physical and mental attributes of the normal aging popululation with the attributes listed in Table 6-1, however, suggests a radically different picture. In many mental acts the normal aged show forgetfulness (not an inability to learn), dilapidated (but not totally lost) cognitive skills, and softer, less articulate vocal output (rather than aphasia). Physically, they show stooped posture, unsteady gait, and tend to be tremulous; they are not erect, active, and healthy appearing as are patients with Alzheimer's disease. And, of course, the most universal of the signs of aging is a slowing down of all functions, a form of psychomotor retardation. From this comparison it would appear probable that the mental deterioration seen in normal aging is much more closely related to the subcortical dementia picture than to the cortical dementia of Alzheimer's disease. It seems entirely possible that the mental picture in normal aging reflects an alteration of one or several neurotransmitter systems. As such, the mental deterioration of aging may respond to a specific pharmacologic therapy in the manner of dopamine therapy for Parkinsonism. At least the clinical appearance offers sufficient suggestion in this direction to warrant additional research.

In summary, in this chapter a clinical separation of the major types of dementia has been outlined, and it has been suggested that many (possibly a majority) of the causes of dementia can be corrected by appropriate treatment. Recognition of the treatable forms of dementia should lead to better management and improve the outcome for many individuals facing this dread problem.

REFERENCES

1. Adams RD, Fisher CM, Hakim S, et al: Symptomatic occult hydrocephalus with "normal" cerebrospinal-fluid pressure: A treatable syndrome. N Eng J Med 273:117-126, 1965
2. Albert ML, Feldman RG, Willis AL: The sub-cortical dementia of progressive supranuclear palsy. J Neurol Neurosurg Psychiat 37:121-130, 1974
3. American Psychiatric Association: Diagnostic and Statistical Manual of Mental Disorders—III. Washington, Am Psych Assoc, 1980
4. Benson DF: Normal pressure hydrocephalus: A controversial entity. Geriatrics 29:126-132, 1974
5. Blessed G, Tomlinson BE, Roth M: The association between quantitative measures of dementia and of senile change in the cerebral grey matter of elderly subjects. Br J Psychiatry 114:797-811, 1968
6. Bleuler M: Acute mental concomitants of physical diseases, in Benson DF, Blumer D (eds): Psychiatric Aspects of Neurologic Disease. New York, Grune & Stratton 1975, pp 37-61
7. Caine ED, Ebert MA, Weingartner H: An outline for the analysis of dementia. Neurology 27:1087-1092, 1977
8. Cummings J, Benson DF, LoVerme S Jr: Reversible dementia. JAMA 243:2434-2439, 1980
9. Freedman AM, Kaplan HI: Comprehensive Textbook of Psychiatry. Baltimore, Williams & Wilkins, 1967
10. Freemon F: Evaluation of patients with progressive intellectual deterioration. Arch Neurol 33:658-659, 1976

11. Fuld P: Behavioral signs of cholinergic deficiency in Alzheimer dementia. Presented at the 2nd Conference of the International Study Group on the Pharmacology of Memory Disorders Associated with Aging, Zurich, Switzerland, April 3-5, 1981
12. Gado M: CT scanning in dementia. Presented at the 110th Annual Session, California Medical Association, Anaheim, California, March 13, 1981
13. Gainotti G, Caltagirone C, Masullo C, Miceli G: Patterns of neuropsychologic impairment in various diagnostic groups of dementia, in Amaducci L, Davison AN, Antuono P (eds): Aging of the Brain and Dementia. New York, Raven, 1980, pp 245-250
14. Hachinski VC, Lassen NA, Marshall J: Multi-infarct dementia: A cause of mental deterioration in the elderly. Lancet 3:207-210, 1974
15. Huckman MS, Fox J, Topel J: The validity of criteria for the evaluation of cerebral atrophy by computed tomography. Radiology 116:85-92, 1975
16. Katzman R: Normal pressure hydrocephalus, in Wells CE (ed): Dementia, ed 2. Philadelphia, Davis, 1977
17. Katzman R: The prevalence and malignancy of Alzheimer's disease. Arch Neurol 33:217-218, 1976
18. Katzman R: Vascular dementia. Presented at the Mini-White House Conference on Aging, Bethesda, Maryland, January 15, 1981
19. Katzman R, Karasu TB: The differential diagnosis of dementia, in Fields WS (ed): Neurological and Sensory Disorders in the Elderly. New York, Grune & Stratton, 1975, pp 103-134
20. Kiloh LG: Pseudo-dementia. Acta Psychiat Scand 37:336-351, 1961
21. Lipowski ZJ: A new look at organic brain syndromes. Am J Psychiatry 137:674-678, 1980
22. Lipowski ZJ: Organic brain syndrome: Overview and classification, in Benson DF, Blumer D (eds): Psychiatric Aspects of Neurologic Disease. New York, Grune & Stratton, 1975, pp 11-35
23. Marsden CD, Harrison MJG: Outcome of investigation of patients with presenile dementia. Br Med J 2:249-252, 1972
24. McHugh PR, Folstein MF: Psychiatric syndromes of Huntington's chorea, in Benson DF, Blumer D (eds): Psychiatric Aspects of Neurologic Disease. New York, Grune & Stratton, 1975, pp 267-286
25. Naeser MA: New methods in the CT scan diagnosis of dementia. Presented at the 2nd Conference of the International Study Group on the Pharmacology of Memory Disorders Associated with Aging, Zurich, Switzerland, April 3-5, 1981
26. Naeser MA, Gebhardt C, Levine HL: Decreased computerized tomography numbers in patients with presenile dementia. Arch Neurol 37:401-409, 1980
27. Noyes AP: Modern Clinical Psychiatry. Philadelphia, Saunders, 1953
28. Plum F: Dementia: An approaching epidemic. Nature 279:372-373, 1979
29. Post F: Dementia, depression and pseudodementia, in Benson DF, Blumer, D (eds): Psychiatric Aspects of Neurologic Disease. New York, Grune & Stratton, 1975, pp 99-120

30. Roth M, Tomlinson BE, Blessed G: Correlation between scores for dementia and counts of "senile plaques" in cerebral gray matter of elderly subjects. Nature 209:109–110, 1966
31. Schoenberg B: Epidemiology of dementia. Presented at the Mini-White House Conference on Aging, Bethesda, Maryland, January 15, 1981
32. Stengel E: Psychopathology of dementia. Proc Royal Soc Med 57:911–914, 1964
33. Taveras JM, Wood LH: Diagnostic Radiology. Baltimore, Williams & Wilkins, 1976
34. Tomlinson BE: The pathology of dementia, in Wells CE (ed): Dementia, ed 2. Philadelphia, Davis, 1977
35. Tomlinson BE, Blessed G, Roth M: Observations on the brains of demented old people. J Neurol Sci 11:205–242, 1970
36. Williams RS, Hauser, SL, Purpura DP, et al.: Autism and mental retardation. Arch Neurol 37:749–753, 1980

Commentary

Not everyone would agree with the vast enlargement of the concept of subcortical dementia presented in Chapter 6. Many current authorities would also dispute the downplay of the role cortical degeneration plays in many forms of dementia, most particularly the mental deterioration seen with advancing age. The broad picture expressed in Chapter 6 goes well beyond the ability of current data to support its suggestion that most dementia is treatable. Nonetheless, as adequate data is gathered it will almost unquestionably reveal that many treatable (even reversible) causes of dementia are currently misdiagnosed as Alzheimer's disease. It appears probable that a clearer picture will be forthcoming because of improved clinical and laboratory efforts and that many individuals with currently treatable dementia will be helped.

Among the many controversial problems that complicate the study of mental deterioration is the status of alcohol in the production of dementia. Strong opinions, both pro and con, dispute the influence of alcohol on mental functioning; whether alcoholic dementia exists as an etiologically specific entity has long been debated. With all learned disagreement aside, however, the fact remains that serious mental limitations are present in many individuals with a long history of alcohol abuse. In the following chapter, Dr. Cutting provides an updated, critical look at this problem and he also outlines a useful approach to the mental disorders commonly seen in chronic alcoholics.

John Cutting, M.D., M.R.C.P., M.R.C. Psych.

7
Alcoholic Dementia

Alcohol is one of the most potent and common causes of psychiatric morbidity. It is a risk factor in the genesis of all forms of psychiatric disorder—acute and chronic organic reactions, schizophrenia, affective psychosis, neurosis, and abnormal behavior. Alcohol may act as a disruptive agent in the psychosocial sphere or exert a direct effect on cerebral function. In the second case, its influence may be manifest acutely in nondependent subjects, during withdrawal in dependent alcoholics, or insidiously over the course of a heavy drinker's life. Alcoholic dementia is the term given to this last effect—a chronic organic reaction produced by a direct insidious effect of alcohol on cerebral function.

The term is misleading in some respects because it implies a severe, clinically obvious disease with gloomy outcome. Because the condition may be mild, clinically undetected, and with prospects of recovery, some writers have recommended the term psychologic deterioration. An even better but more cumbersome label, to emphasize the organic aetiology, would be neuropsychologic deterioration. The term dementia, however, will be retained in this chapter to mean a chronic organic reaction with extensive impairment of mental functions irrespective of severity or outcome.

To understand the nature of alcoholic dementia one must appreciate the range of other neuropsychiatric complications of alcohol. These may be mistaken for alcoholic dementia or may accompany it in the same patient. The bulk of the chapter will be devoted to clinical, pathologic, radiologic, and psychologic descriptions of alcoholic dementia. This will be followed by a discussion of the neuropsychiatric context in which it may arise.

Clinical Findings

Clinical descriptions of the condition go back to Magnus Huss, a Swedish physician, and Lawson, a British psychiatrist, in the last half of the 19th century. These descriptions were generally accepted by the German psychiatrists who founded modern psychiatry at the turn of the century. Bowman and Jellinek, American fathers into research of alcoholism and its complications, referred to the condition as chronic alcoholic deterioration.[7] Lewis, the most eminent British psychiatrist, gave the following description in 1952: "The patients exhibit deficiencies of memory and judgement, laziness, indifference, facile euphoria, and lability of mood, with failure to observe responsibilities, mendacity, gross lack of self-control, and general demoralisation."[26]

The discovery in the 1940s, and its general acceptance in the 1950s, of a vitamin deficiency as a cause of Korsakoff's syndrome resulted in a widespread belief that this and not alcoholic dementia was the most common chronic organic reaction in alcoholics. In the 1970s it became clear that alcoholic dementia had been unjustifiably neglected. Horvath could condemn the practice of "labelling any demented alcoholic as suffering from Korsakoff's psychosis" when he found that of 100 alcoholics with a chronic organic reaction, only 20 "showed its clear clinical features."[24] The remainder had deficits in areas of mental function other than memory, i.e., aphasia, apraxia and perseveration.

The tendency to overdiagnose Korsakoff's syndrome has been confirmed.[15] Between 1969 and 1975, 50 inpatients in the Maudsley Hospital in England were diagnosed as Korsakoff's syndrome and only 13 as alcoholic dementia. When the case notes of these were scrutinized, 17 patients diagnosed as Korsakoff's syndrome had an insidious onset to their cognitive impairment and had a global decline in intelligence. They resembled, almost exactly, the 13 diagnosed as alcoholic dementia. The clinical picture of alcoholic dementia can be extracted from Table 7-1 where the total of 30 patients with alcoholic dementia are compared with the remaining Korsakoff patients (preserved intelligence, acute onset) on whom there was sufficient information. A typical patient was a woman in her late 50s or early 60s, with failing intellect for about a year, a drinking history of over 10 years, marked mood change and cognitive impairment on mental state examination, an abnormal EEG and, surprisingly, a relatively favorable outcome if abstinence or reduced drinking was achieved.

Psychologic Findings

The clinical picture described above represents only a fraction of the true morbidity. The remainder is identified only by psychologic impairment, which may remain latent until discovered on psychologic testing

Table 7-1
Clinical Picture of Alcoholic Dementia and Korsakoff's Syndrome

	Alcoholic Dementia	Korsakoff's Syndrome
Number of patients	30	25
Age (mean)	61	52
Sex (% female)	60	36
Duration of illness (mo.)	13	0.7
Length of drinking history (years of drinking more than 150 ml/day abs alcohol)	19	15
Ophthalmoplegia on physical examination (%)	27	61
Mental state (%)		
Mood change	73	76
Delusions	24	44
Hallucinations	14	14
Investigations		
EEG abnormal (%)	69	0
Psychological status		
IQ (mean)	87	101
Outcome		
improved at followup (%)	66	14

or which may exert a subtle effect on personality and interfere with treatment.

Evidence for impairment in alcoholics without the classic clinical features described above was convincingly documented in many studies during the 1970s. Impairment on standardized tests for identifying brain damage such as the Halstead-Reitan battery, verbal-performance discrepancies on intelligence tests such as the Wechsler Adult Intelligence Scale (WAIS), and memory deficits on the Wechsler Memory Scale leave little doubt of this.

Although personality changes have been less reliably demonstrated, they conform to the pattern seen in dementia of other causes. Lack of drive, low vitality, emotional lability, denial and minimization of disability, and loss of social skills have been noticed.[6]

A disturbing feature for those involved in treatment is the finding that cognitive impairment is the best predictor of poor outcome[21]; it is more reliable than any other variable studied, including social status, age, length of drinking history, duration of abstinence, or previous compliance with treatment regimes.

The several psychologic formulations of the nature of alcoholic dementia offered fall into two classes. The first proposes that the psychologic impairment has a specific pattern which affects some functions more than others. The second regards all functions as equally vulnerable and attributes any apparent pattern to artefact, differential sensitivity of tests, or individual variations in performance. Proponents of the idea that alcohol has a differential effect on mental functions are further divided into those who believe that frontal lobe functions are selectively impaired and those who believe that alcohol has a predilection for the right hemisphere.

Those who implicate the frontal lobe, point to the similarity between the clinical picture in alcoholic dementia and that in patients with a frontal lobe tumor. Emotional lability, impaired judgement, poor appreciation of social cues, and lack of drive are common to both. Further, recognized tests of frontal lobe function—Wisconsin card sorting, verbal fluency, and manipulation of abstract concepts—have consistently discriminated well between alcoholics and controls. Tarter mustered such evidence to produce a convincing case for predominant frontolimbic dysfunction.[32]

One can produce an equally strong argument for right hemisphere dysfunction. Performance on visuo-perceptual tasks, when included in a battery of tests, has usually been worse than performance on verbal tasks. Pattern recognition memory was significantly worse in alcoholics than controls, whereas verbal memory was not significantly different[16]; 59 percent of 92 alcoholics were impaired on the Benton visual retention task compared with only 30 percent on the Walton-Black verbal learning[22]; block design and tactual localization with the left hand were the only significant associates with cerebral atrophy out of more than 20 psychologic measures.[3] Chandler and Parsons asked normals to carry out a visual search task after placebo and after a quantity of alcohol sufficient to raise their blood alcohol to 100 mg%.[12] Subjects were slower at searching for nonverbal items and items in the left visual field when intoxicated. A cerebral blood flow study by Berglund et al. showed a greater reduction in flow in the right hemishpere than in the left during the first week of abstinence.[2]

The strength of each of these cases is diminished by the failure to replicate the critical psychologic findings in some of the larger and better controlled studies.[30] At present, one must admit that the case for a specific neuropsychologic deficit is unproved.

Some of the critics who advocate a global decline in mental functions provide an attractive theory of their own. They cite the fact that age is the most consistent association with psychologic impairment and propose that alcohol induces a premature aging of the brain.[5] This explanation, however, has its detractors. Ron et al. found that alcoholics who started drinking late in their life developed cerebral atrophy at a faster rate than those who started drinking earlier.[30] This suggests that the association with age may reflect a greater susceptibility of older persons rather than premature aging itself.

Pathologic Findings

Pathologic evidence of the nature of alcoholic dementia comes from autopsy, air encepahlographic (AEG), and computerized tomographic (CT) studies. The most comprehensive postmortem study is that of Courville.[14] He found widespread cortical atrophy. Microscopically, there was evidence of cell loss, architectural disruption of cortical lamini, pigmentary degeneration, and glial proliferation. The frontal lobes were the site of the most extensive damage, followed by the parietal and temporal lobes. There was no consistent hemispheric predilection.

The frequent occurrence of cerebral atrophy was later confirmed by AEG studies.[8] Since the advent of CT scanning there have been 10 reported studies in alcoholics and all have found a substantial incidence of cerebral atrophy, despite different selection procedures, control groups, and indices of abnormality. Neither hemispheric bias nor frontal lobe involvement have been prominent. Most studies have shown abnormalities in all indices examined—width of cortical and interhemispheric sulci, width of Sylvian fissure, and ventricular size (planimetric ventricular-brain ratio or Evans' ratio). Some investigators claim that two distinct pathological lesions exist. Bergman et al. argued that alcoholics with cortical atrophy ran a different course than those with enlargement of the third ventricle.[3] They tentatively attributed the latter to an alcohol-induced communicating hydrocephalus. Wilkinson and Carlen distinguished a group with marked cortical atrophy from one with only moderate changes.[35]

Conclusion

Alcoholic dementia, whether recognised clinically, detected on psychologic testing, or identified radiologically or at postmortem, is a well-documented condition. The severe form has a characteristic clinical picture. Most instances are detected only by psychologic testing; here, the profile is variable, but most mental functions are affected to a greater or lesser extent. Radiologic investigations confirm an underlying atrophic process.

PREVALENCE

The prevalence of clinically obvious alcoholic dementia is not easily established. In the 1930s, before the diagnosis fell into disrepute, it was recorded in 3 percent of alcoholic psychiatric inpatients in the United States and accounted for 6 percent of acute or chronic organic reactions in such patients.[29] It accounted for 7 percent of all alcoholic psychoses, acute or chronic, in an English psychiatric hospital in the 1950s and 1960s.[15] Alcoholic dementia was diagnosed less often than Korsakoff's syndrome, but, as mentioned earlier, diagnostic criteria for the latter condition have been lax. In a study of 74 acute organic reactions referred to psychiatrists from the medical and surgical wards of a general hospital, an exacerbation of alcoholic dementia was the primary diagnosis in 4 percent of all cases and 21 percent of the alcoholics.[19] The proportion of cases of presenile dementia of all types in which alcohol is the major cause is a useful figure to know. It was incriminated in 7 percent of 100 cases admitted to a neurologic unit for investigation[27]; it was the fourth commonest cause, after Alzheimer's, multi-infarct and tumor.

Psychologic impairment has a much higher prevalence. Using the deterioration index of the WAIS, 50 percent of 108 inpatient alcoholics were impaired.[31] The same figure of 50 percent was found by Wilkinson and Carlen using the impairment index of the Halstead-Reitan battery.[35] The prevalence of moderate or severe CT scan abnormalities in inpatients is even higher. The mean for the 10 reported studies is 66 percent.

Reports of substantial morbidity among heavy drinkers in the community are particularly worrisome. Parker and Noble contacted 400 normal people, asked them to fill in a drinking questionnaire, and then gave them psychologic tests.[28] They classified 36 percent as heavy drinkers, with a daily consumption of 50 ml absolute alcohol (three doubles). This group had significant psychologic impairment relative to the lighter drinkers. Bergman et al. identified 18 heavy drinkers, defined in the same way, among a random sample of 200 men.[4] Forty percent of them had abnormal CT scans.

In conclusion, it is clear that the prevalence of alcoholic dementia is considerable. Radiologic screening is more sensitive than psychologic testing, and both identify considerably more than is clinically apparent. Morbidity is not confined to inpatient alcoholics but is present in some of those who regard themselves as social drinkers.

CAUSE OF ALCOHOLIC DEMENTIA

Although the condition is associated with an abnormal alcohol consumption by definition, the mechanism remains uncertain.

Alcoholic Dementia

Drinking History

There are various ways of measuring the quantity and pattern of alcohol consumption. Excess is usually defined as a daily intake of at least 150 ml or 120 gm of absolute alcohol. This is equivalent to two bottles of wine, seven pints of beer, half a bottle of spirits, or one bottle of sherry. The two most widely used measures are the number of years at which consumption was regularly at this level and the total lifetime consumption in litres of absolute alcohol. The pattern of drinking is expressed in terms of the balance between abstinence and drinking periods, usually in the last year. The length of abstinence immediately before testing is a potentially critical measure.

Neither lifetime consumption nor years of excess drinking have shown a consistent relationship with either psychologic or radiologic abnormalities. This is particularly true when the effect of age, the most consistent correlate of alcoholic dementia, has been partialled out statistically. Even when more individual estimates of heavy drinking have been used—i.e., years drinking at a typically heavy level, years over which there have been withdrawal episodes indicating dependence—the results have been disappointing. In some of the earlier studies, critical figures of between 10 and 15 years of excess drinking were quoted. This may still be a useful guide as the larger, better controlled studies have added a degree of complexity by indicating a number of factors which confound the issue. Chief among these are age, pattern of drinking, and length of abstinence before testing. For example, Ron et al. found that although both young and old alcoholics showed cerebral atrophy, different factors were active in each group. They noted that older alcoholics developed dementia after a shorter period of heavy drinking than younger alcoholics did; older alcoholics were slower to recover following abstinence; and both age groups were more vulnerable to continuous drinking and showed less impairment if they had a history of frequent withdrawal states.[30] Bergman et al. proposed a more complex interaction between age, drinking history, psychometric pattern, and pathologic findings.[3] Younger alcoholics at an early stage in their drinking history, they noted, developed deficits in abstracting ability related to cortical atrophy; older subjects, in contrast, showed memory impairment in proportion to the years of heavy drinking and this could be related to ventricular enlargement.

Other Potential Influences

Apart from age and drinking history, the only other consistent influence is the sex of the subject. Most psychologic and radiologic studies have excluded female alcoholics. Clinical studies, however, show an excess of women relative to the sex ratio in other types of alcoholic psychoses and in uncomplicated alcoholism.[15,29] These studies also suggest that women develop the clinical picture after a shorter period and lower consumption.

A history of other alcohol-related disabilities has, with one exception, little influence on the risk of developing alcoholic dementia. The exception is a history of frequent withdrawal phenomena—alcoholic psychoses in general[1] and delirium tremens in particular.[30] This pattern, indicative of interrupted drinking, confers a relative protection against alcoholic dementia. Other disabilities studied—dependence itself, memory blackouts,[33] liver disease,[25] and social decline (based on employment, marital, and forensic problems) have no independent influence. Guthrie and Elliott claimed that a history of poor nutrition was correlated with psychologic impairment, but this factor is notoriously difficult to measure.[22]

Conclusion

The cause of alcoholic dementia should be viewed as a complex interaction between age, sex, and certain critical aspects of a subject's drinking pattern. If one is asked for advice on what constitutes safe and what constitutes harmful drinking in this context, one needs some guidelines. A rough answer would be that harmful drinking is a daily consumption in excess of 150 ml of absolute alcohol for 10 years, expressed in terms of the preferred drink of an individual. Some might regard this as too generous an estimate. However, if one reduces this by a fifth for every additional risk category that an individual falls into—age over 50, female, and preference for regular as opposed to periodic drinking—then it becomes a flexible guide.

NATURAL HISTORY AND OUTCOME

The surprising and encouraging feature of alcoholic dementia is its tendency to remit during abstinence. This reversibility is evident in clinical, psychologic, and even radiologic measures. Of 30 patients with clinical evidence of alcoholic dementia, 66 percent of the 23 on whom there was adequate follow-up had improved.[15] Improvement was regarded as living an independent existence outside a hospital or sheltered accommodation for most of the follow-up period. The course of these patients was punctuated by relapses triggered by drinking bouts.

Many studies attest to psychologic improvement with abstinence. There is general agreement on three points. First, the rate of improvement is maximal during the first week of abstinence. Second, significant improvement continues for a further 4–8 weeks, but beyond this it is difficult to establish significant changes in test performance. Third, despite continuing abstinence or a substantial reduction in drinking for up to a year, psychologic functioning remains below what it would have been if the person had never drunk heavily. More detailed claims, i.e., that some functions improve more than others, are less soundly based.

Reversibility of the actual pathologic process, as demonstrated on CT scans, has been reported. Carlen et al. carried out repeat scans on eight alcoholics.[10] Of six abstinent subjects, four showed improvement in ventricular and sulcal indices; the two who continued drinking showed no improvement. Two subsequent reports, in which 23 alcoholics in both cases were scanned at intervals of between 2 to 9 and 12 months, respectively, showed an insignificant trend towards improvement in ventricular and cortical measures in abstinent subjects and no trend in those who continued drinking.[11,30] Carlen and his colleagues suggested that there might be regrowth of neurons, particularly their dendritic processes, along with the supporting glial and vascular tissues. Any permanent atrophy would represent disappearance of this nervous and supporting tissue.

In summary, alcoholic dementia has a favorable prognosis if abstinence or a marked reduction in drinking is maintained. Clinical remission and psychologic improvement will ensue and, although not so well-documented at present, pathologic reversibility is possible. This optimistic account should encourage physicians and psychiatrists to be alert to the condition as a potentially treatable form of dementia. It must be admitted, however, that the management of alcoholism is compromised by the advent of dementia. Such patients show less compliance with treatment regimes than alcoholics with other disabilities. Nevertheless, the improvement is so striking after even short periods of abstinence that a general reduction in consumption is worth striving for even if abstinence is not a realistic goal.

RELATED ALCOHOLIC NEUROPSYCHIATRIC DISORDERS

The range of disorders which may mimic or complicate alcoholic dementia are best appreciated by relating them to the effect of alcohol on cerebral function (Table 7-2) and to the stage of the alcoholic process when they appear (Fig. 7-1).

Table 7-2
Classification of Alcoholic Neuropsychiatric Disorders

Intoxication phenomena
  Pathologic intoxication
  Memory blackouts

Withdrawal phenomena
  Simple withdrawal state
  Delirium tremens
  Convulsion and pastictal state
  Atypical alcoholic psychosis

Associated "functional" psychiatric disorders
  Schizophrenia
  Depression
  Mania
  (Alcoholic hallucinosis)
  Behavior disorders, i.e., morbid jealousy

Chronic and nutritional conditions
  Alcoholic dementia
  Wernicke's encephalopathy
  Korsakoff's syndrome

Intoxication Phenomena

These phenomena comprise *pathologic intoxication* and *memory blackouts*. Pathologic intoxication refers to an episode of uncharacteristic behavior during a drinking bout. This usually involves violence that is out of keeping with the person's behavior when sober. The condition is well reviewed by Coid.[13] Memory blackouts (blankouts, palimpsests) are periods of several hours, during which a person was drinking, for which there is no subsequent recollection. Such amnesic spells have been extensively documented by Goodwin.[20]

In each of these conditions, doubt exists as to whether high blood alcohol is the only precipitating factor. In the case of pathologic intoxication, some predisposition—a latent personality trait or epileptic tendency—has been proposed. In the case of blackouts, additional considerations are the effect of the dependence process itself and alcoholic dementia.

A review of the literature indicates that the overriding factor in both phenomena is a high blood alcohol level which can arise in any individual regardless of whether he is dependent or not. Personality factors or unrecognized cerebral dysfunction may increase the likelihood of an unaccustomed burst of violence. Considerable tolerance of the intoxicating effect

Alcoholic Dementia

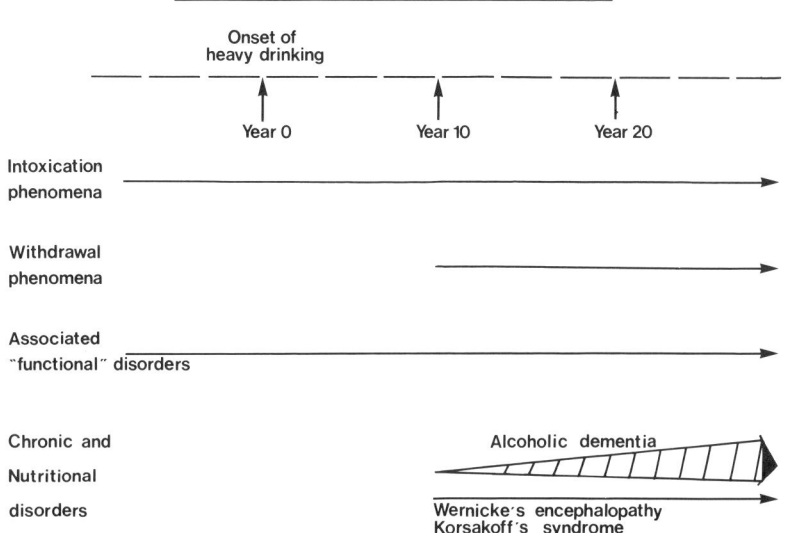

Fig. 7-1. Risk periods for neuropsychiatric disorders

of alcohol is required to drink sufficient amounts in the course of an evening to induce blackouts; such tolerance is more common in dependent persons but may occur in social drinkers.

Both conditions may be mistaken for or compounded by alcoholic dementia, which may be marked by unprovoked outbursts of irritability and aggression and by fluctuating disturbances of memory.

Withdrawal Phenomena

These comprise the *simple withdrawal state, delirium tremens, convulsions* and their neuropsychiatric sequelae, and *atypical forms of alcoholic psychoses*. They share in common an appearance during absolute or relative withdrawal from alcohol in an alcohol-dependent person.

The simple withdrawal state is made up of two symptom clusters.[23] The physical cluster is comprised of the well-known "shakes" and nausea. Less well-known but equally common is an affective cluster in which the patient feels awful, guilty, panicky, and dreads the day ahead. Transient abnormal visual and auditory experiences are uncommon and there is no clouding of consciousness. By definition, these appear in some degree in all alcohol dependent individuals within 12 hours of the last drink.

Delirium tremens (DTs) is qualitatively different from simple withdrawal. It develops in less than half of prolonged withdrawal phases and its onset is delayed by up to 72 hours from the time of the last drink. Clouding of consciousness, vivid visual and auditory hallucinations, terror, and cardiovascular changes mark the picture. The factors that determine which subjects will develop DTs are not certain, but the presence of alcoholic dementia does not constitute a risk factor.

A convulsion may supervene and a postictal confusional state may complicate the picture.

The form of the psychiatric disorder may differ from any of these and may include such extensive psychopathology that it is taken for a depressive, manic, or schizophrenic psychosis. One can describe it in terms of the functional disorder that it most resembles or label it an atypical alcoholic psychosis.

These conditions are all transient and begin to punctuate the mental life of an alcoholic at the same time as alcoholic dementia supervenes. The affective component of the simple withdrawal state and the cognitive impairment of delirium tremens may be mistaken for the more persistent changes of alcoholic dementia. One not infrequently encounters a delirious illness whose resolution is prolonged beyond the usual 3–5 days typical of delirium tremens. It is probable that such instances are due not to delirium tremens, but to either Wernicke's encephalopathy where the ophthalmophegia has resolved or been missed, or to an acute exacerbation of alcoholic dementia which takes weeks rather than days to return to baseline.

Associated "Functional" Psychiatric Disorders

The conditions discussed so far are acute or chronic organic reactions whose development is due almost entirely to the effect of alcohol on cerebral function. The distinction between organic and functional disorders, however, is merely a convenient divvision into those where cerebral dysfunction is the overriding etiologic consideration and those where it plays a subsidiary or as yet unknown role. Heavy alcohol consumption increases the risk of *schizophrenia, depression,* and *mania.* The clinical picture in such cases is indistinguishable from that seen without cerebral dysfunction. The condition of *alcoholic hallucinosis* was once regarded as distinct from both delirium tremens of schizophrenia. This distinction relies on diagnostic criteria for the latter conditions. These diagnostic criteria have become broader in the past 10 years, and cases that were previously regarded as alcoholic hallucinosis must be reassigned to delirium tremens, schizophrenia, and even affective psychosis.

The extent of drinking required to increase the risk of these conditions is not known, but it is assumed that as alcohol is only one of several factors (i.e., genetic, psychosocial), the risk period begins at the onset of heavy drinking. Because mood change is common, the affective disorders may enter the differential diagnosis of alcoholic dementia.

Chronic and Nutritional Disorders

This category includes alcoholic dementia itself, *Wernicke's encephalopathy,* and *Korsakoff's syndrome.* The latter two, sometimes grouped together as the Wernicke-Korsakoff syndrome, have a controversial relationship with alcoholic dementia.

Wernicke's encephalopathy is an acute organic reaction with transient ophthalmoplegia and ataxia. It is caused by thiamine deficiency, which, in developed countries, is nearly always a consequence of prolonged, heavy alcohol consumption. The critical pathology is in the midbrain, particularly the dorsomedial nucleus of the thalamus and the mamillary bodies. The condition resolves completely within two months with prompt and adequate thiamine replacement.

Korsakoff's syndrome is a chronic organic reaction in which a disorder of memory predominates over other mental impairment. The cause and pathology are identical to that of Wernicke's encephalopathy, and it is generally believed that Korsakoff's syndrome is the sequel to undiagnosed, inadequately treated, or refractory Wernicke's encephalopathy. The outcome is gloomy for the established disorder, despite zealous treatment.

Some authors still believe that alcoholic dementia and Korsakoff's syndrome are merely mild and severe versions, respectively, of the same disorder. They point out the similarity in clinical presentation, the prominent memory impairment which they share, and the demonstration of cortical atrophy in otherwise typical cases of Korsakoff's syndrome.[34] Such similarities are only superficial. The weight of evidence accumulated in the past decade lends much greater support to their status as distinct clinicopathologic entities. In practice, however, the distinction is compounded by the presence of alcoholic dementia in virtually all cases of Korsakoff's syndrome, as the latter requires for its development a drinking history sufficient to induce an invariable degree of alcoholic dementia.

Clinically, however, Korsakoff's syndrome can be distinguished from alcoholic dementia in a number of ways. It appears a decade earlier, is relatively more common in men, has an acute onset, a shorter drinking history, and ophthalmoplegia can usually be detected at its outset. It has a poor outcome once established.

The pattern of psychologic deficit is also distinctive, although methodologic problems have made this a more controversial issue. The central distinction is the preservation of intelligence in Korsakoff's syndrome and its decline in alcoholic dementia. Most investigators, however, have been forced to define the former empirically as a chronic organic reaction in alcoholics where the memory quotient of the Wechsler Memory Scale is substantially lower (15 points) than the intelligence quotient on the WAIS. Psychologic distinctions must therefore be argued on the basis of more specific differences in test performance. Further, few studies of Korsakoff's syndrome have included both alcoholic and nonalcoholic controls, and it is unclear in most studies whether a deficit is a feature of Korsakoff's syndrome or alcoholic dementia. The studies that have taken this into account suggest that Korsakoff patients have a deficit in verbal memory superimposed on the more general intellectual impairment, which is seen in the majority of prolonged, heavy drinkers.[9,18,35]

The best evidence for a pathologic distinction comes from two sources. The postmortem study of the Wernicke-Korsakoff syndrome of Victor et al. revealed an invariable association between amnesia and damage to the dorsomedial nucleus of the thalamus; cortical atrophy was present in only 27 percent of cases.[34] Wilkinson and Carlen defined Korsakoff's syndrome as the presence of either a 15-point discrepancy between memory and intelligence quotients or ophthalmoplegia.[35] There was no relationship between age, memory quotient, and CT changes in their study, suggesting that amnesia was an effect of subcortical lesions not shown on the scan; other alcoholics showed the usual relationship between age, generalized neuropsychologic deficits, and CT changes.

In summary, the nature of alcoholic dementia can only be understood with reference to other neuropsychiatric disorders with which alcohol is associated. The wide range and florid presentation of some of these have probably been responsible for the widespread neglect accorded to alcoholic dementia, whose influence on the life of the alcoholic, although more subtle, is no less pernicious.

REFERENCES

1. Berglund M, Leijonquist H: Prediction of cerebral dysfunction in alcoholics; a study of health insurance records. J Stud Alcohol 39:1968–1974, 1978
2. Berglund M, Bliding G, Bliding A, Risberg J: Reversibility of cerebral dysfunction in alcoholics during the first seven weeks of abstinence—a regional cerebral blood flow study. Acta Psychiatr Scand [Suppl] 286:119–127, 1980
3. Bergman H, Borg S, Hindmarsh T, et al.: Computed tomography of the brain and neuropsychological assessment of male alcoholic patients and a random sample from the general male population. Acta Psychiatr Scand [Suppl] 286:77–88, 1980a
4. Bergman H, Borg S, Hindmarsh T, et al.: Computed tomography of the brain, clinical examination and neuropsychological assessment of a random

sample of men from the general population. Acta Psychiatr Scand [Suppl] 286:47-56, 1980b
5. Blusewicz MJ, Dustman RE, Schenkenberg T, Beck EC: Neuropsychological correlates of chronic alcoholism and aging. J Nerv Ment Dis 165:348-355, 1977
6. Boeke PE: Some remarks about alcohol-dementia in clinically-treated alcoholics. Br J Addict 65:173-180, 1970
7. Bowman KM, Jellinek EM: Alcoholic mental disorders. J Stud Alcohol 2:312-390, 1941
8. Brewer C, Perrett L: Brain damage due to alcoholism. Br J Addict 66:170-182, 1971
9. Butters N, Cermak LS: Neuropsychological studies of alcoholic Korsakoff patients, in Goldstein G, Neuringer C (eds): Empirical Studies of Alcoholism. Cambridge, Mass, Ballinger, 1976, pp 153-193
10. Carlen PL, Wortzman G, Holgate RC, et al.: Reversible cerebral atrophy in recently abstinent chronic alcoholics measured by computed tomography scans. Science, 200:1076-1078, 1978
11. Carlen PL, Wilkinson DA: Alcoholic brain damage and reversible deficits. Acta Psychiatr Scand [Suppl] 286:103-118, 1980
12. Chandler BC, Parsons OA: Altered hemispheric functioning under alcohol. J Stud Alcohol 38:381-391, 1977
13. Coid J: Mania a potu: A critical review of pathological intoxication. Psychol Med 9:709-719, 1979
14. Courville CB: Effects of Alcohol on the Nervous System of Man. Los Angeles, San Lucas Press, 1955
15. Cutting J: The relationship between Korsakov's syndrome and alcoholic dementia. Br J Psychiatry 132:240-251, 1978a
16. Cutting J: Specific psychological deficits in alcoholism. Br J Psychiatry 133:119-122, 1978b
17. Cutting J: A reappraisal of alcoholic psychoses. Psychol Med 8:285-295, 1978c
18. Cutting J: Differential impairment of memory in Korsakoff's syndrome. Cortex 15:501-506, 1979
19. Cutting J: Physical illness and psychosis. Br J Psychiatry 136:109-119, 1980
20. Goodwin DW: Blackouts and alcohol-induced memory dysfunction, in Mello NK, Mendelson JH (eds): Recent Advances in Alcoholism. National Institute of Mental Health, Bethesda, Maryland, 1971, pp 508-536
21. Gregson RAM, Taylor GM: Prediction of relapse in men alcoholics. J Stud Alcohol 38:1749-1760, 1977
22. Guthrie A, Elliott WA: The nature and reversibility of cerebral impairment in alcoholism. J Stud Alcohol 41:147-155, 1980
23. Hershon HI: Alcohol withdrawal symptoms and drinking behavior. J Stud Alcohol 38:953-971, 1977
24. Horvath TB: Clinical spectrum and epidemiological features of alcoholic dementia, in Rankin JG (ed): Alcohol, Drugs and Brain Damage. Toronto, Addiction Research Foundation of Ontario, 1975
25. Lee K, Moller L, Hardt F, et al.: Alcohol-induced brain damage and liver damage in young males. Lancet 2:759-761, 1979

26. Lewis A: Alcoholic psychoses, in Horder L (ed): British Encyclopaedia of Medical Practice, 2nd Ed, vol 10. London, Butterworth, 1952, pp 394–402
27. Marsden CD, Harrison MJG: Outcome of investigation of patients with presenile dementia. Br Med J 2:249–252, 1972
28. Parker ES, Noble EP: Alcohol consumption and cognitive functioning in social drinkers. J Stud Alcohol 38:1224–1232, 1977
29. Pollock HM: Use and effect of alcohol in relation to mental disease before, during and after prohibition. Ment Hygiene 24:112–124, 1940
30. Ron MA, Acker W, Lishman WA: Morphological abnormalities in the brains of chronic alcoholics. Acta Psychiatr Scand [Suppl] 286:41–46, 1980
31. Soulariac A, Chavannes N, Maisoneve G: Perspectives psychometriques d'une etude de la deterioration mentale chez les alcooliques chroniques. Ann Med Psychol (Paris) 128:1–14, 1970
32. Tarter RE: Psychological deficit in chronic alcoholics: A review. Int J Addict 10:327–368, 1975
33. Tarter RE, Schneider DU: Blackouts: Relationship with memory capacity and alcoholism history. Arch Gen Psychiatry 33:1492–1496, 1976
34. Victor M, Adams RD, Collins GH: The Wernicke-Korsakoff Syndrome, in Contemporary Neurology Series vol 7. Philadelphia, Davis, 1971
35. Wilkinson DA, Carlen PL: Relationship of neuropsychological test performance to brain morphology in amnesic and non-amnesic chronic alcoholics. Acta Psychiatr Scand [Suppl] 286:89–101, 1980

Commentary

Dr. Cutting has presented a body of evidence suggesting that a specific mental deterioration can result from prolonged alcoholic abuse, therefore an alcoholic dementia. He has also emphasized the frequency with which this problem is associated with other alcohol related neurobehavior disorders. The latter problems both disguise and complicate the clinical picture of alcoholic dementia and make it almost impossible to define a consistent syndrome. Nonetheless, the portion of a chronic alcoholic's psychiatric status which is due to the mental deterioration associated with alcohol abuse deserves recognition as Dr. Cutting has clearly demonstrated that a considerable reversibility of the mental deterioration is possible if proper health measures (abstinence, good nutrition) are carried out. Not only has Chapter 7 offered a method for diagnosing alcoholic dementia but it has also provided a sharp reinforcement for the well-accepted need for abstinence in this problem.

One troublesome diagnostic problem that is increasingly recognized by practitioners of both neurology and psychiatry is pseudodementia, which encompasses an apparent dementia associated with recognized psychiatric problems. Pseudodementia can be a complicating factor in several disorders (schizophrenia, hysterical reaction) but the term usually refers to the dementia picture that can accompany severe depression. The incidence of both depression and dementia increase sharply with advancing age and they account for the largest segment of neurobehavior problems in the older age group. That two such common disorders would coexist in a number of patients seems probable; that one may mask the other also appears perfectly reasonable. Unfortunately, the two disorders respond quite differently to pharmacologic agents; incorrect medication based on incorrect diagnosis can produce a deterioration in either. Depression, dementia, and pseudodementia are easily cross-diagnosed[1] and appropriate therapy demands an ability to separate them. In the following chapter, Dr. Wells faces this challenging problem and helps clarify our approach to these two common disorders.

REFERENCES

1. Post F: Dementia, depression, and pseudodementia, in Benson DF, Blumer D (eds): Psychiatric Aspects of Neurologic Disease. New York, Grune & Stratton, 1975, pp 99–120

Charles E. Wells, M.D.

8
Pseudodementia and the Recognition of Organicity

Dementia is a diagnosis that has generally been regarded as self-evident. Indeed, the syndrome is usually recognized with ease by the lay public, and demented patients are most often brought to physicians for care only after the diagnosis has already been made, and correctly too for the most part, by family members. The putative accuracy of these diagnoses did not come into serious question until after it was recognized that some cases of dementia resulted from treatable disorders. Then, as patients thought to have dementia began routinely to come under serious diagnostic scrutiny, it became evident that not all who appeared on initial evaluation to be demented were actually so. In virtually every series of patients with "dementia," examples have been found of patients suffering primarily from functional psychiatric disorders mistakenly thought to be dementia.[19] In the last such series reported, 20 percent of the patients were diagnosed as having primary functional psychiatric disorders instead of dementia, the largest percentage yet recorded.[7]

Studies of another sort have lent support to the premise that the diagnosis of dementia is not always straightforward. Nott and Fleminger reported that of 35 patients initially diagnosed as having presenile dementia, 20 (57 percent) failed over a 5- to 23-year follow-up (mean, 10 years) to have the progressive mental deterioration that would confirm the original diagnosis.[11] It was their impression that this group mistakenly diagnosed as demented "consisted mainly of people with marked personality difficulties and neurotic symptoms or affective disorder." In a similar study, Ron et al. found that the original diagnosis of presenile dementia was supported in only 35 of 51 patients (69 percent) who were followed up for 5-15 years (mean, 9 years).[14] Both of these studies emanated from major teaching hospitals in Great Britain.

Such evidence of diagnostic fallibility has led to the study of pseudodementia—"the syndrome in which dementia is mimicked or caricatured by functional psychiatric disorders."[18] Several studies of the clinical features of this syndrome have now been published. [8,12,18] Rather than restate their findings, in this essay I shall seek to examine some of the conceptual sets and biases that give rise to this diagnostic confusion with the hope that by focusing on the clinical features of dementia and pseudodementia in a different perspective, diagnostic problems may be lessened.

ORGANIC VERSUS FUNCTIONAL DISORDERS

Psychiatrists and physicians in general, usually divide disorders manifested by abnormalities of affect, behavior, and/or cognition into two groups—the organic disorders and the functional disorders. These terms are derided by some, and in certain groups their use predictably leads to expressions of outrage, for does not the term "functional" in this context imply nonorganic and must not all disorders have an organic basis? Such devotion to semantic purity is regarded by some as commendable, and by others as precious, but in any event, it is not very helpful either conceptually or practically. As clinicians we need a label for those disorders of affect, behavior, and/or cognition that result from demonstrable chemical, physical, or pathologic alterations of brain tissue; similarly, we need a label for those disorders in which no such alterations can be demonstrated. Convenience and communication are both served by referring to the first group as organic disorders and the latter as functional disorders. Much of the progress in 20th Century psychiatry can be charted by the reassignment of disorders from the functional to the organic group as medical science uncovered more and more specific biologic aberrations in the causation of psychiatric illness.

The distinction between functional and organic disorders is important, because diagnostic and therapeutic approaches differ for the two groups, at least in theory if not always in practice. The recognition that a disorder is functional leads in due course to the diagnosis of a specific functional disorder. By its very definition, however, the assignment of a specific functional diagnosis does not carry with it information about specific underlying biologic defects in brain function. Thus, no matter how much one may learn observationally about the functional disorders, medical (primarily pharmacologic) treatment remains largely symptomatic because the underlying cerebral pathophysiologic alterations remain unknown. This symptomatic approach to treatment is reflected in the classification of the drugs most often used in their treatment—antipsychotics, antidepressants, anxiolytics.

The recognition that a disorder is organic, on the other hand, usually leads to the diagnosis of a specific underlying medical disease, one for which there is often, but certainly not always, some knowledge of the chemical and pathologic defects responsible. It is through an appreciation of these biologic defects that disease-specific therapy is developed. This is not to say that symptomatic treatment is unimportant in the organic disorders, but it does imply that therapy becomes increasingly targeted toward specific pathophysiologic processes as the basic organic substratum of a disorder unfolds. The distinction, therefore, between functional and organic disorders is, at our present level of knowledge, of prime clinical importance in determining the course of medical investigation and medical therapy. Functional and organic disorders may, of course, coexist, but even so, the distinctive aspects of each must be recognized.

There is no intent in the above statements to deny or to minimize the importance of psychotherapy as a treatment modality for both the functional and the organic disorders. A consideration of psychotherapeutic techniques as symptomatic or disease-specific is, however, beyond the purview of this discussion.

Because the distinction between functional and organic disease is important, and because it is often difficult to make on clinical grounds alone, physicians have often tried to rely on ancillary diagnostic procedures to make the distinction for them. Neuropsychologic testing has been used extensively to help with this differentiation, but problems abound if the clinician tries to rely on these procedures alone.[3] Help has also been sought and, to varying degrees, found from skull radiography, electroencephalography, computed cranial tomography, cerebrospinal fluid examination, and many other procedures. All of these diagnostic procedures have their limitations, however, and at present "no single test, nor any combination of tests, reliably differentiates between functional and organic disease . . . ."[20] The physician must then, in the last analysis, rely on clinical acumen to make this basic diagnostic distinction.

THE FOCUS ON COGNITION

Why is the distinction between functional and organic disorders often so clinically perplexing? I would suggest that in large measure this is because changes in cognition alone are too often used as the basis for the differentiation. Abnormalities in cognition are considered, correctly enough, to be the hallmark of the organic disorders, but abnormalities in cognition not only may be present, but indeed may be prominent in some if not in most functional disorders. To equate cognitive loss with organicity then is to fall into a serious clinical error.

Cognitive Changes in Functional Disorders

Lipowski defines cognition as "all the processes involving symbolic operations, namely perceiving, remembering, creating imagery, and thinking."[9] Cognition is evaluated clinically by careful attention to the complexities of the psychiatric interview, by the mental state examination, and by neuropsychologic testing.

Cognitive changes have probably been studied more extensively in schizophrenia than in any of the other functional disorders, but it is the cognitive changes associated with depression that seem to have resulted most often in diagnostic problems between dementia and pseudodementia. There is general agreement that both complaints of cognitive loss and evidence of cognitive dysfunction are common in depressive disorders, and especially so in older patients. Such observations led Folstein and McHugh[5] to suggest that there is actually a dementia syndrome of depression, one that usually improves significantly when the depressive disorder is treated successfully. These investigators documented in elderly patients both the impairment of cognitive functions during an episode of depression and improvement with resolution. Others have noted that dementia appears to worsen markedly if a depressive disorder is superimposed and that patients return to the baseline if the depression is treated successfully.[15,16]

Cognitive changes in mania are less clearly established, but there is ample anecdotal evidence that attests to cognitive impairment in manic psychoses also. In general, however, cognitive impairment in affective disorders is less global and less severe than in the primary organic disorders, and it is rare for cognitive impairment to dominate the clinical picture in affective disorders. When it does so, it is usually designated as a depressive pseudodementia.

Cognitive impairment is also a frequent finding in schizophrenia, but that is not to say that the pattern of cognitive loss is exactly the same in most cases of schizophrenia as in dementia. Nevertheless, disorientation, impairment of memory, reduced intellectual capacity, and poor ability to concentrate are observations frequently made in schizophrenia.[17] Similar abnormalities in performance may be observed on some neuropsychologic tests in both schizophrenic and demented subjects. On the Gorham Proverbs Test, for example, schizophrenic and organic patients demonstrate similar limitations in their capacity for abstract conceptualization.[4] As is true for the affective disturbances, cognitive impairment in schizophrenia is usually less severe and less pervasive than in the organic syndromes, and it seldom dominates the clinical picture. The evidence for cognitive impairment is less clear in the personality disorders, but examples of pseudodementia (as reflected by impaired cognition) in personality disturbances are well described in the medical literature.[14,18]

Cognitive losses are thus a feature of both functional and organic disorders. So long as cognitive abnormalities per se are interpreted as prima facie evidence for organicity, mistakes in diagnosis between these two groups will continue and, moreover, will be frequent. It would appear that psychiatrists, psychologists, and neurologists, by centering their attention on impaired cognition in the organic disorders, have unwittingly created a situation in which cognitive dysfunction is often regarded as diagnostic of organicity, whereas cognitive dysfunction should for the most part be considered merely the sine qua non for the diagnosis of organicity.

THE IMPORTANCE OF BEHAVIORAL AND AFFECTIVE CHANGES IN THE DIAGNOSIS OF ORGANIC DISORDERS

Clinicians should not only recognize but should also attend to the fact that the organic disorders produce changes in both behavior and affect in addition to the well-known changes in cognition. The diagnosis of organicity should, therefore, be based on changes observed in all three of these key clinical manifestations of brain function. Unless changes are evident in behavior and affect as well as in cognition, and unless these changes are congruent with each other (that is, unless they are in keeping with one another so far as severity is concerned), the dysfunction should not, without serious questioning, be attributed primarily or entirely to an organic disease process.

Behavioral and Affective Changes with Organicity

With rare exceptions, changes in these three key manifestations of brain function (cognition, behavior, and affect) move in tandem in the organic brain disorders.

Changes in Cognition

Cognitive functions have been studied extensively and described at length in the literature on organic brain disorders. With focal brain disease, changes may be confined to only one or two specific cognitive functions; e.g., abnormalities may be limited to language function alone in lesions involving only the dominant frontotemporal region, or memory may be preferentially impaired in lesions of the hypothalamic or third ventricular region. In practice, such cases are seldom seen primarily by psychiatrists unless the aphasic or amnesic defect is misperceived as a global dementing process.

With disease processes that involve the cerebral hemispheres diffusely, several or many of the individual cognitive functions are usually impaired. Whether these individual functions are measured by the mental state examination or by specific neuropsychologic tests, one expects impairment to be demonstrable in a variety of functions. With diffuse disease, the accuracy of performance may vary between different cognitive spheres (e.g., language functions may be more or less severely impaired than functions dependent on visuo-spatial perceptions), reflecting differences in the severity of the pathologic process from one area of the brain to another. The level of impairment should, however, be roughly the same on different tests designed to evaluate the same specific cognitive function. With organic disease, for example, it would be surprising to find significant impairment of short-term memory on one test and near perfect performance on another. When an organic process has been the prime diagnostic consideration, the surprise should be sufficient to suggest the possibility of a functional disorder.

Changes in Behavior

Evidence for behavioral change is derived from two sources: history and direct behavioral observation.

The history is, of course, the primary feature that points to the possibility of an organic process. So far as the recognition of dementia is concerned, however, the history is often an unreliable indicator, in at least two ways. First, a history that suggests dementia may be lacking even in fairly far advanced disease if the patient leads a sedentary, passive, and constricted life without exposure to new or different situations calling for innovative responses. This is especially likely if the patient's daily needs are largely met by an overly protective spouse. In these cases, observation outside the routine and habitual environment or a significant alteration in that environment may bring the dementia to light.

On the other hand, the patient's cognitive and behavioral aberrations may be exaggerated by the patient or the family providing the history. This is especially likely in the patient with a pseudodementia who complains of severe cognitive impairment and who is cared for by someone willing to compensate for this severe impairment. Curiously enough, the families of patients with dementia often believe them to be more capable of caring for themselves than they actually are, whereas the families of patients with

Pseudodementia and Organicity

pseudodementia often do not expect of them as much as they are capable of doing.

The patient's behavior may be observed in four settings: psychologic testing, psychiatric interview, an unfamiliar environments, and the familiar environment.

Psychologic testing is often regarded as a precise ancillary diagnostic procedure for measuring the brain's cognitive function, and in many ways it is. At the same time, one should not forget that it is also a standardized method for measuring *motivated* behavior. The psychologist who only scores test performance and fails to observe how the patient addresses various tasks and the strategies used for solving them is missing a great deal of valuable data. A low score on a test of intellectual function, for example, has an entirely different meaning if the patient erred by offering "near miss" answers than if the patient offered largely "don't know" responses.

Surprisingly, behavior during the psychiatric interview (as contrasted with the specific verbal material produced) is an often neglected source of behavioral data. Here the examiner specifically looks for the correlation or lack of correlation between interview performance and the history provided by the patient or caretaker, between the fullness and exactness of responses provided to specific questions and that provided in spontaneous communications. Does the patient who complains of impaired concentration appear to focus sustained attention on topics raised during the interview, especially on those topics raised spontaneously by the patient? Does the patient with complaints of poor memory organize large amounts of historic data accurately in unstructured portions of the interview, only to respond inadequately when asked for specific bits of information? Does the patient attend to each nuance of cognitive dysfunction and immediately call it to the attention of the examiner? Is the patient more aware of cognitive slippage during the psychiatric interview than the examiner is? Inconsistencies such as those suggested by the questions above should always be noted and attempts made to explain them.

Study of patients' behavior in an unfamiliar environment is a surprisingly powerful diagnostic tool which is also frequently overlooked. The hospital, the usual setting for this, is especially valuable, first, because it is an unfamiliar situation which requires adjustment to a new and different set of demands and second, because the patient can be observed in various situations without being aware of the scrutiny. Dementia may become more evident, as manifested by the patient who becomes lost on the unit, cannot find the toilet, fails to recognize staff or learn their names, or has difficulty dressing. In the same setting, close observation may reveal inconsistencies in behavior that suggest pseudodementia—i.e., the patient who is disoriented about time upon questioning but appears promptly for each meal without being called, or the patient who complains of poor memory but consistently calls a staff member by the same incorrect name, or the person who recalls no more than three or four digits on mental state examination but manages to look up telephone numbers in the directory and to recall them for dialing.

One suspects that much would be learned if patients could be observed in their usual environments, but this technique is seldom employed in medical evaluations. Home visits by nurses or social workers have been reported to be valuable, sometimes revealing neglect of nutritional and hygienic needs in demented patients which might not otherwise have been suspected.

Behavioral assessment is perhaps the most essential clinical element in the separation of functional from organic psychiatric disorders, in the separation of pseudodementia from dementia. Behavior is, however, perhaps the most difficult clinical element to measure, collate, and codify. The assessment of behavior as summarized in the preceding paragraphs still relies on the meticulous study and description of many individual events in a patient's life. Is there any wonder that psychiatrists and psychologists have sought simpler methods by which such diagnostic distinctions might be made?

Affective Changes

Affective change was listed in DSM-11 as a prime manifestation of the organic brain syndromes, as they were then called.[1] In DSM-III, it is not included among the diagnostic criteria for dementia,[2] yet affective changes are common in the organic mental disorders, and they should be explored routinely in patients in whom organicity is suspected.

Depression is said to occur frequently early in the course of dementing illnesses. Reifler et al. reported that 33 percent of mildly demented geriatric patients were depressed.[13] Liston found that symptoms of depression were present in over 50 percent of patients with presenile dementia; more importantly, a depressive spectrum disorder had been the initial diagnosis in over a quarter of them.[10]

As one reads about these patients though, one is uncertain about the nature of the "depression." Are these feelings truly those of depression, or are they better described as ill-defined dysphorias? One notes too that many of the usual criteria for the diagnosis of depression (sleep difficulty, loss of energy, agitation or retardation, loss of interest in usual activities, slow thinking) are manifestations of dementia as well. Thus the specificity of affective changes early in the course of dementia remains in doubt.

With more advanced dementia, however, affective changes are common and often prominent. These are described in DSM-II as a lability and shallowness of affect, yet this does not really throw much light on the situation. As Hollender noted some years ago: "These [affective changes associated with organic brain disease] are difficult to assess and to measure, and comparatively little has been written about them."[6]

Shallowness is perhaps not the best description for the affective changes that accompany dementia. They might better be described as inappropriate affective responses, whether in response to the patient's personal condition or to situations arising in the environment. This inappropriateness may be manifested either qualitatively or quantitively.

Demented patients generally experience less dysphoria and depression than might be expected of persons with so much impairment. They usually seem to be unaware of the gravity of their condition and thus do not appear to suffer commensurately. This inappropriateness of affect sometimes reaches the level of euphoria. At the same time that these patients appear unconcerned about events that others would regard as devastating, they may worry unaccountably about trivial matters, as though the radii of their concern had narrowed to include only the mundane.

Affective responses are usually distorted quantitively as well. Minor disappointments or failures may give rise to sadness and tears; trivial obstacles or frustrations, to rage. Though intense, such feelings are for the most part short-lived and tightly stimulus bound, being justifiably described as labile. If intense depression or euphoria is sustained in the demented patient, the physician should suspect a superimposed affective disorder and not accept the affective changes as simply a manifestation of the organic brain dysfunction itself. Such a patient should be treated appropriately and specifically for the affective disorder itself. This does not deny the rare occurrence of organic affective syndromes precipitated by structural or metabolic changes, in which affective abnormalities are evident in the absence of significant cognitive loss. These organic affective syndromes are unusual, however, and should not distract us from the major focus of this essay.

CONCLUSIONS

In summary, it is my thesis that functional psychiatric disorders are often mistaken for organic mental syndromes because too much importance is accorded in the diagnostic process to the mere presence of cognitive impairment. At the same time, too little attention is granted to the behavioral and affective changes which are characteristic and integral features of organic brain dysfunction.

We have been mesmerized by our search for *the* test of cognition (or *the* combination of tests) which will unfailingly differentiate the functional from the organic. Some of our neuropsychologic measures are better than others, and some indeed have a fair degree of validity, but none approaches infallibility, and none will. The cognitive losses seen in functional disorders resemble those in organic syndromes too closely to allow much optimism that a perfectly differentiating neuropsychologic test will ever be devised.

At the same time, study of the behavioral and affective changes that occur in organic disease has been neglected. We lack sophisticated instruments to measure behavioral changes in organic disease (unless neuropsychologic testing be regarded largely as a measure of behavior), and we also lack tests specifically designed to evaluate the affective changes that accompany organicity. Perhaps even more important, we are completely without instruments that assess the congruence or lack of congruence between changes in these three key indicators of brain function.

Until such instruments are developed and validated, we are left to a large degree dependent upon our clinical acumen for the differentiation between pseudodementia and dementia, between primarily functional and primarily organic disease. The clinician must therefore appreciate that in the presence of cognitive impairment, accurate diagnosis may ultimately rest upon the accurate assessment of behavior and affect. When changes in these three features (cognition, behavior, and affect) are qualitatively characteristic of organicity and are quantitively congruent with one another, the diagnosis of organic brain disease is extremely likely, if not certain. Lacking these, however, the clinician should at least suspect the presence of a functional disorder, whether primary or superimposed upon an underlying organic process.

REFERENCES

1. American Psychiatric Association: Diagnostic and Statistical Manual of Mental Disorders, ed 2. Washington, American Psychiatric Association, 1968
2. American Psychiatric Association: Diagnostic and Statistical Manual of Mental Disorders, ed 3. Washington, American Psychiatric Association, 1980
3. Crockett D, Clark C, Klonoff H: Introduction—an overview of neuropsychology, in Filskov SB, Boll TJ (eds): Handbook of Clinical Neuropsychology. New York, Wiley, 1981, pp 1–37
4. Elmore CM, Gorham DR: Measuring the impairment of the abstracting function with the Proverbs Test. J Clin Psychol 13:263–266, 1957
5. Folstein MF, McHugh PR: Dementia syndrome of depression, in Katzman R, Terry RD, Bick KL (eds): Alzheimer's Disease: Senile Dementia and Related Disorders (Aging, vol 7). New York, Raven Press, 1978, pp 87–93

6. Hollender MH: Early psychologic reactions associated with organic brain disease in the aged. NY State J Med 59:802–809, 1959
7. Hutton JT: Dementia reconsidered (letter-to-editor). JAMA 245:1025–1026, 1981
8. Kiloh LG: Pseudo-dementia. Acta Psychiat Scand 37:336–351, 1981
9. Lipowski ZJ: Delirium. Acute Brain Failure in Man. Springfield, Illinois, Thomas, 1980, p 60
10. Liston EH Jr: Occult presenile dementia. J Nerv Ment Dis 164:263–267, 1977
11. Nott PN, Fleminger JJ: Presenile dementia: The difficulties of early diagnosis. Acta Psychiat Scand. 51:210–217, 1975
12. Post F: Dementia, depression, and pseudodementia, in Benson DF, Blumer D (eds): Psychiatric Aspects of Neurologic Disease. New York, Grune & Stratton, 1975, pp 99–120
13. Reifler B. Larson E, Hanley R: Coexistence of dementia and depression in geriatric outpatients. Am J Psychiatry 139:623–626, 1982
14. Ron MA, Toone BK, Garralda ME, et al.: Diagnostic accuracy in presenile dementia. Br J Psychiatry 134:161–168, 1979
15. Shraberg D: The myth of pseudodementia. Am J Psychiatry 135:601–603, 1978
16. Snow SS, Wells CE: Case studies in neuropsychiatry: IV. Diagnosis and treatment of coexistent dementia and depression. J Clin Psychiat 43(11): 439–441, 1981
17. Wells CE: Dementia, pseudodementia, and dementia praecox, in Fann WE, Karacan I, Pokorny AD et al. (eds): Phenomenology and Treatment of Schizophrenia. New York, Spectrum, 1978, pp 39–48
18. Wells CE: Pseudodementia. Am J Psychiatry 136:895–900, 1979
19. Wells CE: Diagnosis of dementia. Psychosomatics 20:517–522, 1979
20. Wells CE: The differential diagnosis of psychiatric disorders in the elderly, in Cole JO, Barrett JE (eds): Psychopathology in the Aged. New York, Raven Press, 1980, pp 19–31

Commentary

Dr. Wells has provided considerable insight to the similarities and differences between dementia and depression that will help resolve the troublesome pseudodementia problem. There was little reason for separation in the past as dementia was considered untreatable and therapy for depression was limited to individual psychotherapy, a harmless exercise for the dement. The situation has changed dramatically in the past few years. There are now a number of effective treatments for depression and, as stressed in Chapter 6, many treatments are available for dementia. The treatments to be used for the two disorders are radically different, however, and a correct diagnosis is of paramount importance if proper treatment is to be given. Incorrect therapy based on misdiagnosis may prove harmful. Not only is it unwise to give electroshock therapy to a demented individual but, even more serious, the anticholinergic properties of many of the antidepressant drugs adversely affect the abnormal cholinergie system of patients with Alzheimer's disease, producing a psychosis. On the other hand, relegation of a patient with a depressive pseudodementia to an untreatable status (Alzheimer's disease) is a cruel waste. Diagnostic errors in either direction are potentially disastrous for the patient. Dementia and depression are extremely common and, in some instances, produce sufficiently similar phenomena that they can be cross-diagnosed. Although it is anticipated that the next decade will see increasing numbers of specific and effective therapies for both disorders, the value of treatment will depend directly on the accuracy of diagnosis, at present a narrowly practiced and difficult art.

Among the most disturbing problem patients from the borderland between neurology and psychiatry are those tortured creatures who suffer chronic pain. Pain, and its management, is within the province of all medical practitioners and, in most instances, specific, pathology-correcting treatment effectively controls the pain. The patient who fails to respond to such management, however, may undergo multiple investigations and treatments including traumatizing x-ray examinations, addictive pharmacologic management, and destructive surgical procedures. If the symptoms are not controlled, the pain patient is often referred to a neurologist or psychiatrist, usually with a poorly veiled suggestion that it is the patient's fault that correct and well-executed treatment has failed to control the pain. Thus, physically, metabolically, and pschologically traumatized and maintaining a well-developed disdain for the medical profession, the individual with chronic pain has always proved inordinately difficult to manage. In Chapter 9 Dr. Blumer proposes an explanation of the chronic pain problem, provides data to support his theory and, most important, suggests treatment that has proved successful for a number of pain-prone individuals.

Dietrich Blumer, M.D.

9
Chronic Pain as a Psychobiologic Phenomenon: The Pain-Prone Disorder

CHRONIC PAIN: NEUROLOGIC OR PSYCHOLOGIC PHENOMENON?

The sizeable group of patients with chronic and disabling pain of obscure origin appears to present a complex neurologic and psychiatric problem. In most cases, however, repeated and thorough examinations fail to reveal plausible somatic causes of the distress. The persistent desire of these patients to obtain a physical explanation for their suffering, and their rigid bias against any psychiatric inquiry are typical. Psychiatrists challenged to make an evaluation frequently lack experience with this type of patient and cannot see a cause of the pain beyond a somatic lesion. The patient, who claims to have no emotional or interpersonal problems other than those caused by the pain, may then return to his physician with a clear bill of good mental health and continue to be treated as a patient with a physical disorder. The agony of chronic pain evokes much compassion and specialists tend to respond with additional investigations and procedures indigenous to their specialty. The patients are often mistreated as a result and subjected to excessive investigations, procedures, and operations. Because the pain is chronic, they tend to be maintained on analgesics, and because the pain has no clear neurologic cause, muscle relaxants or antianxiety drugs are often prescribed.

The number of clinics specializing in chronic pain has grown rapidly. Admission to a pain clinic usually involves still another series of costly diagnostic procedures. Pain clinics may use a variety of nonspecific treatment approaches in a shotgun manner. Transcutaneous electrical nerve stimulation, nerve blocks, acupuncture, relaxation training, hypnosis, group therapy, and behavior-modification procedures are among the treatments employed. Fordyce has pioneered a systematic behavioral treatment approach for chronic pain and has emphasized that treatment for chronic pain cannot be effective unless it is directed away from the peripheral focus of the complaint.[15,16] In this approach, the pain complaint is steadfastly ignored and increased activity is systematically encouraged; thus a degree of rehabilitation and unlearning of the sick-role is achieved.

When confronted with a patient who insists he suffers from a bodily pain, the physician must be particularly aware of the strict, well-proved criteria for the neurologic nature of the pain complaint. Abnormalities that frequently occur in individuals who never experience a significant pain problem must not be unquestioningly accepted as explanations for the pain.[14,22] Likewise, if a patient has undergone surgery for his pain, it does not follow that he now has a vaguely defined "peripheral pain-generator."[43] Indeed, a majority of the problem patients with chronic pain experience pain in more than one part of their body, and the site of the pain may undergo peculiar shifts. Moreover, a large majority of these patients develop their pain without trauma or following a trivial injury.

In an effort to explain the persistent phantom body pain of paraplegics after complete transection of the spinal cord, Melzack and Loeser set forth the concept of "pattern generating mechanisms" consisting of abnormally active neuron pools above the cord section, a state they observed in a single patient.[31] The relationship of this abnormal neuronal activity to pain appears highly uncertain, and such a concept does not seem to apply to most patients with chronic pain of obscure origin, whose distress has never shown any neurologic pattern. Melzack and Loeser do recognize the importance of central mechanisms in the perception and perpetuation of chronic pain. The nature of central mechanisms in chronic pain needs to be understood. Current notions of psychogenic pain, as defined in the American Psychiatric Society's Diagnostic and Statistical Manual III, are vague and nonspecific.

The physician's persistence in searching for a peripheral source of the chronic pain is based on his training to view pain as a somatosensory phenomenon and the patient's insistence that something must be wrong right where it hurts. If nothing can be detected there, the pain must then be either contrived or imaginary. The idea that a psychic phenomenon can be experienced as bodily pain appears strange and abhorrent. Yet evidence for this phenomenon is abundant.

PAIN AND DEPRESSION

There is a large and well-identified group of patients with a high incidence of bodily pains that are clearly related to their mental state. It is commonplace to hear depressed individuals complain about aches and pains. Sixty to 100 per cent of depressed patients complain of bodily pain.[49,51] When a patient complains of pain for which no organic basis can be found, the clinician is well-advised to suspect the presence of an underlying depression.[18] Indeed, chronic pain has been viewed as a sign of masked depression by a number of authors.[17,23,28,29]

Most authors who have experience with chronic pain agree that most chronic pain patients are depressed.[1,11,15,21,34,43,44,50] Increased somatic preoccupation, sleep disturbances, fewer interests, weakened relationships, decreased libido, appetite changes, and irritability are cited as typical symptoms of depression among chronic pain patients. Psychologic testing of these patients tends to show that they are depressed, although the depression may be masked by the absorption in the somatic symptom.[43] Effective treatment efforts for chronic pain are identical to those for chronic depressive states and include antidepressants alone or in combination with neuroleptics,[10,20,24,27,33,36,45,48,51] electric convulsive treatment (ECT),[9,10,30,39] or, for extreme and otherwise intractable cases, psychosurgery.[46,47] Relief from pain and depression tend to be concomitant.[10,33,45,48,51]

The chronic pain patient typically blames his depressed state and all his misfortunes on the pain. It seems natural to assume that depression would be a consequence of chronic pain. If one keeps in mind that the pain far exceeds any established somatic cause, however, and that a primary mental state of agony is commonly associated with bodily experienced pain, a parsimonious explanation can be intimated. The chronic pain is the principal manifestation of a muted state of agony, i.e., a depressive symptom. Pain comes from pain.

The concept of chronic pain as masked depression is not completely satisfactory, however. Our experience over the past 18 years has led us to view chronic pain rather as a specific variant of depressive disease with characteristic clinical, premorbid, psychologic, and genetic aspects. It has been possible, since our earliest report 16 years ago, to describe a large number of chronic pain patients as a homogeneous clinical group.[3,4,5] Over the last few years, we have been able to further document the biologic aspects of this disorder, which we view as a psychobiologic entity.[6] A number of authors have confirmed certain psychologic characteristics of chronic pain patients that set this group apart from overtly depressed patients.[13,19,32,37,38] Following George Engel's original description of the pain-prone patient,[13] we have termed this psychobiologic disorder the pain-prone disorder.[5]

CHRONIC PAIN AS A VARIANT OF DEPRESSIVE DISEASE: THE PAIN-PRONE DISORDER

Our identification of the pain-prone disorder is based on the evaluation of over 900 patients with chronic pain who had no significant related somatic disorder. The majority of the patients were seen in psychiatric consultation and about one third of the group was also treated at the Henry Ford Hospital Pain Clinic in Detroit, Michigan. Patients were evaluated by a special questionnaire, interview, and by psychologic testing.[2,3,5,6]

Demographic Data

Women were more affected, the female to male ratio being 1.7:1 (569:331 patients). Onset of the chronic pain ranged as early as infancy and as late as age 80, with the mean onset at 39 years. Thus, the disorder begins most frequently in mid-life. The patients were evaluated after their pain persisted over an average of 6.5 years. The average education was 12th grade. The entire spectrum of socioeconomic classes was affected, but the disorder was found most prevalent (67 percent) in the lower-middle class, among blue-collar workers.

Clinical Presentation

The characteristics of the pain-prone disorder are listed in Table 9-1. Over 90 percent of patients present with a *continuous* chronic pain of obscure origin. They wake up with the pain and go to sleep with it. The pain seems mechanical to the patient since it intensifies with activity, although it does not fully stop with rest. In spite of recurrent negative examinations, they persist in their pronounced *somatic preoccupation* with the painful parts of their body. An insistent *desire for a surgical solution* is marked in many. The group averaged over one surgical procedure for pain per patient. Pain-prone patients focus all their misery on their pain and demand to have it removed.

Even after years of disabling pain and dependence on others (next-of-kin and the helping profession), most patients maintain a "solid citizen" image of themselves; they strongly *deny difficulties in their interpersonal*

Table 9-1
Pain-Prone Disorder

Clinical Traits
   Continuous Pain   } Somatic presentation
   Somatic Preoccupation
   Denial of conflicts   } "Solid citizen"
   Idealization of self and
     family relations

Premorbid Traits
   Relentless activity   } Ergomania
   Overachievement
   Courting of failures   } Masochism
   Masochistic bonds
   Intolerance of success

Depressive traits
  Anergia
  Anhedonia
  Insomnia
  Depressive mood
    and despair

Family History
  Unipolar depression
  Alcoholism
  Chronic pain
  Crippled relative

Psychodynamics
  Alexithymia

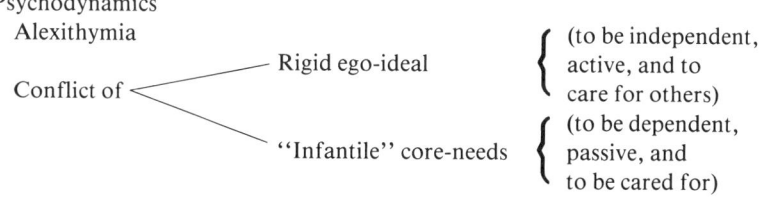

Conflict of — Rigid ego-ideal { (to be independent, active, and to care for others)
           "Infantile" core-needs { (to be dependent, passive, and to be cared for)

Biological markers
  Short REM latency
  Nonsuppression on Dexamethasone Suppression Test

relationships, often *idealize their family relationships,* and view themselves as independent. They have a strong aversion to any scrutiny of their personal life.

Premorbid Traits

The history before the onset of the pain shows an excessive work performance, often since childhood or early adolescence, and a relentless activity with little ability to enjoy leisure time. The original industriousness and overactivity of these patients is highly characteristic, and we have chosen the term *"ergomania"* for these premorbid traits because it is broader and less vernacular than the popular term "workaholism." In addition to the habit of working like slaves in service to the family, patients often have a history, not only of submissiveness, but of overt *masochism.* This is found in about a quarter of the patients. Their tendency to choose a spouse who is brutal, alcoholic, promiscuous, or otherwise abusive brings on prolonged suffering, with pain paradoxically beginning when there is relief from the abuse. These patients tend to be intolerant of success.

Depressive Traits

Following onset of pain, the patients completely lose their initiative and zeal for work. The contrast between their frantic premorbid activity and the morbid fatigue and helplessness is striking. This *anergia* becomes associated with *anhedonia*—an increasing inability to enjoy social life, leisure time, and sexual relations. While the appetite is frequently well maintained, *insomnia* often develops. Anergia, anhedonia, and sleep disorders are characteristic traits of depressive disorders; patients, however, almost invariably attribute these to the pain. This is the prime reason why the depression remains masked. The suffering is experienced physically more than mentally, and when questioned about a *depressed mood,* about one third of the patients deny it strongly, although they may admit to being in despair, over the pain.

Family History

About half of the patients report a *next-of-kin who is crippled* or deformed. Less fortunate, penalized, and in need of special consideration, such a relative may perhaps serve as the object of unconscious identification. A slightly smaller number of patients report a relative with *chronic pain.*

Alcoholism or overt *unipolar depression* that requires psychiatric treatment and hospitalization, not only in several of the patients themselves, but very frequently among their relatives, is an important finding. This finding places the pain-prone disorder in Winokur's depression-spectrum disease.[52] Winokur defines the depression-spectrum disease as an illness manifesting itself by the coexistence of unipolar depression (in the female) and alcoholism (in the male) within the same family.

Psychodynamic Factors

The psychodynamic factors behind the anxiously maintained image of the "solid citizen" can be detected by sensitive psychologic tests, by the study of the few patients who lend themselves to intensive psychotherapy, or by scrutinizing the clinical findings. Such a finding would be the change from a prematurely responsible, overly active, and industrious individual to a passive-dependent suffering invalid.

The patients clearly tend to show all the features of alexithymia. This inability to recognize and verbalize one's feelings is common in patients with psychosomatic and addictive disorders.[6,25,42] Patients display little emotionality unless depressive affect is openly manifesting itself. They cite tragic life events in a detached manner, while focusing all concern on the body parts in pain. Beneath the stoic and detached attitude there is a different set of concealed core issues. The need to be accepted and to depend on others is very strong; marked needs to receive affection and to be cared for are also present. These basic "infantile" needs have never been acknowledged by the patients. Their passive-submissive trends to the extreme of masochism, and their eagerness to be accepted by others were formerly manifested in their subservient industriousness for the sake of the family. Anything socially unacceptable is guilt-provoking and is anxiously concealed and controlled, including the need to be dependent, to remain passive, to receive affection, and, particularly, any hostile-aggressive trends. By relentless activity and work performance, their inner insecurity and guilt may be soothed and a certain acceptance gained until the dilemma eventually becomes too painful. After a significant loss or disappointment, with or without the advent of a painful injury or ailment, a shift occurs which is drastic in its outward effect. It transforms the "solid citizen" into an invalid and heightens the same painful dilemma. The need to be dependent, to be passive, and to be catered to which has asserted itself is still unacceptable, and the urge to be viewed as a strong and independent individual persists. This explains the enormous need to maintain a physical problem as the culprit. With the failure of the "solid citizen," however, the suffering becomes overt. The lack of a secure inner core, the need to be accepted by a "dominant other," as well as the conflict of guilt and concealed rage and aggression, are indeed indicative of depressive disorders.

It is obvious that the need for material security is a dominant motive in the ergomanic phase. Although a need for financial compensation after injury undoubtedly heightens anxiety and worsens disability in many patients, it is not a decisive factor. In a series of 234 patients with long-standing chronic pain evaluated at Massachusetts General Hospital, none had been admitted if a compensation issue was still pending.[5] Pain generally persists after completion of litigation.

Biologic Markers for Depression in Chronic Pain

Patients with chronic "psychogenic" pain appear to suffer from a specific depressive type of disease, with somatized pain as the prime expression of a concealed mental agony (pain-prone disorder). This view is supported by clinical, premorbid, and psychodynamic findings, as well as by the presence of biologic factors (i.e., response to antidepressants and a family history of affective disorders).

The family histories of these patients that are positive for unipolar depression and alcoholism suggest a *psychobiologic disorder*. The study of well-recognized biologic markers for depressive disease has further confirmed this notion.[8]

Biologic markers of depression include shortened rapid eye movement (REM) latency in sleep[26] and nonsuppression in the Dexamethasone Suppression Test (DST).[12] The study of both markers in 20 consecutive pain-prone patients with insomnia clearly showed abnormal REM latency and/or DST nonsuppression in half of the clinically and psychologically homogeneous group. The average REM latency of the entire group was measured at 60 minutes. There was a highly significant correlation between DST cortisol level and REM latency, and both biologic markers tended to predict response to antidepressants. These findings confirm that the pain-prone disorder can be viewed as a variant of depressive disease.

GUIDELINES FOR TREATMENT

Recognition of the pain-prone individuals is of paramount importance for all physicians. They are the many patients who desire endless and costly physical studies and interventions but who do not get well. They must be examined because they may suffer from a somatic disorder, even if it is only from a condition incidental to the pain. But once the disorder is recognized and the origin of the pain is understood, physical investigations must be reasonably curbed and useless surgical procedures avoided. The patient must then be oriented to the nature and treatment of his condition. The condition can be explained in the following terms. Pain can and commonly does occur (or persist) in the absence of a mechanical factor. Although there are no hidden, undiscovered ailments, this type of pain is nevertheless very real and is related more to a condition of the nervous system than to an injury. A depressive tension state plays a role, and the condition can be treated.

Analgesics and antianxiety agents are contraindicated. They provide no sustained relief, are habituating, and tend to exacerbate the depression and pain. Antidepressants, on the other hand, are not habituating. They should be administered patiently and systematically in sufficient doses (150-300 mg/day for the major tricyclic antidepressants) and with careful monitoring of side effects.[7,41] While insomnia may improve promptly, pain and the other depressive traits tend to improve about 10-30 days after institution of an appropriate antidepressant regimen. Activity and continuation of work need to be encouraged. The physician may have to repeatedly insist to the patient that the proper treatment for the pain has been chosen. A concerted, supportive, but rather forceful intervention needs to be carried out and the next-of-kin must be involved. Referral to a psychiatrist is necessary when depression becomes severe, when there is a significant suicidal risk, or when other serious psychiatric complications occur. The effective behavioral modification practiced by some pain clinics, with persistent de-emphasis of the pain and gradual reactivation, generally needs to be carried out, at least initially, on a well-staffed inpatient unit.

Chronic pain is the single predominant problem in the rehabilitation of disabled workers.[40] Settling for compensation payments and finally for a disability pension may be unavoidable in many cases, but is obviously an undesirable solution for individuals without significant physical impairment who are in the midst of their best earning years and whose working capacity has been their very strength. Joint efforts of physician, rehabilitation specialist, and employer may be required, and time is an important factor. Like the soldier with battle-fatigue who has been removed too far from action for too long and will not be able to return to the front line, the previously overachieving worker with the pain complaint will find it very difficult to function at work again if he has been away from his job for a long time. In the meantime, his position in the family as the respected breadwinner may crumble and much discontent if not open strife set in. Diminished activities and social life can result in a monotony which further increases the depression. The individual may become a permanent victim of work-fatigue. The customary extended and futile physical investigations and procedures are undoubtedly well-intended, but they may have a crippling effect. Physicians must learn to promptly recognize and treat the pain-prone disorder. Pain-prone patients can be maintained at work if they are promptly and properly treated.

The relentless work habits and submissive-masochistic attitude are typical of the premorbid phase of the pain-prone disorder and represent obvious warning signals. Efforts toward a more balanced lifestyle and toward self-assertion would appear to be of preventive value. It is equally important to foster an appreciation of feelings and an ability to deal with close relationships.

EPILOGUE

A significant group of patients with chronic pain of obscure somatic origin present a coherent psychopathologic syndrome, with characteristic clinical, premorbid, genetic, and psychodynamic traits. We have termed this syndrome the pain-prone disorder. It requires specific treatment. Its recognition permits a more effective early intervention and suggests specific preventive measures for pain-prone individuals. Chronic pain disguises a basic depressive type of disorder and ceases to be a puzzle as soon as the pain is understood as the expression of muted depression—an anguish and agony which is bodily experienced—rather than a somatic phenomenon. Further, the pain-prone disorder must be viewed not simply as masked depression, but rather as a specific variant of depressive disease. Pain-prone patients have demonstrated a high incidence of shortened REM latency and of nonsuppression on the Dexamethasone Suppression Test—well-recognized biologic markers for depressive disease.[8]

About 20 years ago, George Engel provided a lucid analysis of "psychogenic" pain and the pain-prone patient.[13] However, to this date the disorder has remained ill-defined. The many sufferers of chronic pain typically deny that there is anything wrong with them psychologically and seek out physicians trained to focus on somatic conditions. Consequently, their condition generally has escaped proper study and analysis. A review of the work of a prominent neurologist with the gift of astute psychiatric observation, nevertheless, documents that the pain-prone disorder is not merely a disorder of modern times.

In his monograph *The Traumatic Neuroses (Die Traumatischen Neurosen)* published in 1892, Hermann Oppenheim, a prominent contemporary of Charcot, presented the observations he collected at the Nervenklinik of the Charité in Berlin in the years from 1883 to 1891. He dealt with those disorders of the nervous system that had not occurred through direct damage of the nervous system but "by way of a shock in the broadest sense of the word."[35]

Oppenheim criticized the preoccupation of many of his colleagues with the phenomenon of the *railway spine*. He opposed both the popular diagnosis of "myelitis," as well as the customary alternative diagnosis of malingering, for the victims of railroad or other accidents who had developed a disabling condition in the absence of a definable neurologic lesion. He stated that there was nothing specific to railway accidents, that the injuries were very variable and often rather trivial. He emphasized that the spinal theory for these conditions had to be rejected, that a cerebral site of the disorder must be recognized, and that the disorder was of the nature of a neurosis. While emphasizing the functional nature of the disorder, he maintained that his patients with traumatic neurosis were different from the hysterics described by Charcot. He maintained that the former were characterized by a basic and persistent melancholic dysphoria and that their condition had to be differentiated from the hysterics whose manifestations were highly variable. Pain was the leading symptom in his patients, and the psychic alteration was characterized foremost by "hypochondriacal-melancholic dysphoria, anxiety states, and abnormal irritability," with the anomaly of mood representing the core of the emotional disorder. The patients' avoidance of social life, diminished interest in their own family, and manifestations of apathy and indifference showed a close relationship to melancholia in its pure form. Their single, central concern was the accident they suffered and its consequences. The patients easily became tearful, and the intensity of the dysphoria was sometimes heightened to the point of preoccupation with suicide. Sexual desire was frequently diminished or abolished. Loss of appetite was a rare finding, while insomnia was one of the most commonly associated symptoms.

In an effort to explore the predisposition for traumatic neurosis, Oppenheim reviewed the personnel files of the railway employees and discovered that they had been steady workers before their illness. He listed alcoholism as a predisposing factor in some. He also described how the neurosis developed over the period of several months to a more full-blown picture. There appeared to be no increased mortality, but a complete cure was judged to be the rare exception among the severe cases of the disorder. Complete cure could be observed in some mild cases while more severe cases, at best, showed a significant improvement. He pointed out that with the termination of litigation the disorder tended to continue unchanged.

The therapeutic measures he recommended included the avoidance of emotional excitement, prompt dispatch of litigation, and rehabilitation at work by assignment of an easier job void of emotional stress. Oppenheim expressed little enthusiasm for the various popular treatments of his time (e.g., immobilization, massages, and electrical stimulations). He emphasized that therapy had to be directed particularly towards the emotional life. Rest in the country was felt to be particularly helpful. He stressed the calming role of the physician and importance of assuring the patient that the condition was treatable and not dangerous to his life. Ignoring the complaints or meeting them with incredulity would lead to a loss of trust on the part of the patient, worsen his condition, and render treatment ineffective.

Oppenheim's treatise on the victims of traumatic neurosis presents a familiar picture. His patients of nearly a century ago had been steady workers, though some depended on alcohol. Following a trauma, which may have been trivial, they began to suffer from pain and a variety of less frequent somatic complaints, became totally preoccupied with the injury, inactive, and unable to return to work. They developed insomnia, withdrew from social life and sexual relations. They did not suffer from an obscure disorder of the spine or of the peripheral nerves. Their principal disorder was rather of a psychic nature. They were neither hysterics nor malingerers, and their disorder was not for the benefit of litigation. The symptoms of melancholia were predominant, and theirs was a chronic condition akin to depression.

REFERENCES

1. Black RG: The chronic pain syndrome. Surg Clin North Am 55:999-1011, 1975
2. Blumer D: Psychiatric aspects of chronic pain: Nature, identification and treatment of the pain-prone disorder, in Rothman RH, Simeone FA (eds): The Spine, ed 2. Philadelphia, Saunders, in press.
3. Blumer D: Psychiatric considerations in pain, in Rothman RH, Simeone FA (eds): The Spine, vol 2. Philadelphia, Saunders, 1975, pp 871-906
4. Blumer D: A study of patients with "psychogenic" pain. Paper presented at the American Psychosomatic Society, Philadelphia, 1965
5. Blumer D, Heilbronn M: The pain-prone disorder: A clinical and psychological profile. Psychomatics 22:395-402, 1981
6. Blumer D, Heilbronn M: Chronic pain as a variant of depressive disease: The pain-prone disorder. J Nerv Ment Dis, in press.
7. Blumer D, Heilbronn M, Pedraza E, Pope G: Systematic treatment of chronic pain with antidepressants. Henry Ford Hos Med J 28(1):15-21, 1980
8. Blumer D, Zorick F, Heilbronn M, Roth T: Biological markers for depression in chronic pain. J Nerv Ment Dis, in press.

9. Bornstein B: Sur le phénomène du membre fantôme. Encéphale 38:32–46, 1949
10. Bradley JJ: Severe localized pain associated with the depressive syndrome. Br J Psychiatry 109:741–745, 1963
11. Brena SF: Chronic pain: America's Hidden Epidemic. New York, Atheneum/SMI, 1978
12. Carroll BJ, Feinberg M, Greden JF, et al.: A specific laboratory test for the diagnosis of melancholia. Standardization, validation, and clinical utility. Arch Gen Psychiatry 38(1):15–22, 1980
13. Engel G: "Psychogenic" pain and the pain-prone patient. Am J Med 26:899–918, 1959
14. Finneson BE: Clinical portrait of a patient with industry-related chronic low back pain, in LeRoy PL (ed): Current Concepts in the Management of Chronic Pain. Miami, Symposium Specialist, 1977, pp 37–43
15. Fordyce WE: Learning processes in pain, in Sternbach RA (ed): The Psychology of Pain. New York, Raven, 1978, pp 49–72
16. Fordyce WE: Behavioral Methods for Chronic Pain and Illness. St Louis, Mosby, 1976
17. Forrest AJ, Wolkind SN: Masked depression in men with low back pain. Rheumatol Rehabil 13:148–153, 1974
18. Freedman DX, Smith RJ, Lehmann H, et al.: Depression today, part one, recognizing and diagnosing depression. Thirty-first Winter Scientific Meeting of AMA, December 1977, New York, CME Communications, 1978
19. Gentry WD, Shows WD, Thomas M: Chronic low back pain: A psychological profile. Psychosomatics 15:174–177, 1974
20. Hatangi VS, Boas RA, Richards EG: Post-herpetic neuralgia: Management with antiepileptic and tricyclic drugs, in Bonica JJ, Albe-Fessard D (eds): Advances in Pain Research and Therapy, Vol 1. New York, Raven, 1976, pp 583–587
21. Hendler NH, Fenton JA: Coping with Chronic Pain. New York, Clarkson Potter, 1979
22. Hitselberger WE, Witten RM: Abnormal myelograms in asymptomatic patients. J Neurosurg 28:204–206, 1968
23. Kielholz P: Masked Depression. Bern, Hans Huber, 1973
24. Kocher R: Die Behandlung chronischer Schmerzen mit Psychopharmaka. Schweiz Med Wochenschr 108:686–691, 1978
25. Krystal H: Alexithymia and psychotherapy. Am J Psychother 33(1):17–31, 1979
26. Kupfer DJ, Spiker DG, Coble PA, et al.: Sleep and treatment prediction in endogenous depression. Am J Psychiatry 138(4):429–434, 1981
27. Lascelles RG: Atypical facial pain and depression. Br J Psychiatry 112:651–659, 1966
28. Lesse S: The multivariant masks of depression. Am J Psychiatry 124 (Suppl):35–40, 1968
29. Lopez-Ibor JJ: Masked depression. Br J Psychiatry 120:245–258, 1972
30. Mandel MR: Electroconvulsive therapy for chronic pain associated with depression. Am J Psychiatry 132:632–636, 1975

31. Melzack R, Loeser JD: Phantom body pain in paraplegics: Evidence for a central "pattern generating mechanism" for pain. Pain 4:195-210, 1978
32. Merskey H: Pain and personality, in Sternbach RA (ed): The Psychology of Pain. New York, Raven, 1978, pp 111-128
33. Merskey H, Hester RA: The treatment of chronic pain with psychotropic drugs. Postgrad Med J 48:594-598, 1972
34. Merskey H, Spear FG: Pain: Psychological and Psychiatric Aspects. London, Baillière, Tindall and Cassell, 1967
35. Oppenheim H: Die Traumatischen Neurosen, ed 2. Berlin, August Hirschwald, 1892
36. Paoli F, Darcourt G, Cossa P: Sur l'action de l'imipramine dans les états douloureux. Rev Neurologique 102:503-504, 1960
37. Parkes CM: Factors determining the persistence of phantom pain in the amputee. J Psychosom Res 17:97-108, 1973
38. Pilowsky I, Spence ND: Illness behavior syndromes associated with intractable pain. Pain 2:61-71, 1976
39. Pisetsky JE: Disappearance of painful phantom limbs after electric shock treatment. Am J Psychiatry 102:599-601, 1946
40. Rowe ML: Low back pain in industry. Journal of Occup Med 2:161-169, 1969
41. Schatzberg A: Drug management of treatment resistant depression. McLean Hosp J 1:89-101, 1976
42. Sifneos PE: Clinical observations on some patients suffering from a variety of psychosomatic diseases. Proceedings of the Seventh European Conference on Psychosomatic Research, Basel, Karger, 1967
43. Sternbach RA (ed): The Psychology of Pain. New York, Raven, 1978
44. Sternbach RA (ed): Pain and depression, in Kiev A (ed): Somatic Manifestations of Depressive Disorders. Amsterdam, Excerpta Medica, 1974, pp. 107-119
45. Sternbach RA: Pain: A Psychophysiological Analysis. New York, Academic, 1968
46. Sweet WH: Central mechanisms of chronic pain (neuralgias and certain other neurogenic pain), in Bonica JJ (ed): Pain. New York, Raven, 1980, pp 287-303
47. Sweet WH, Obrador S, Martin-Rodriguez JG: Neurosurgical Treatment in Psychiatry. Baltimore, University Park Press, 1977
48. Turkington RW: Depression masquerading as diabetic neuropathy. JAMA 243(11):1147-1150, 1980
49. VonKnorring L: The experience of pain in depressed patients. Neuropsychobiology 1:155-165, 1975
50. Walters A: Psychogenic regional pain alias hysterical pain. Brain 84:1-18, 1961
51. Ward NG, Bloom VL, Friedel RO: The effectiveness of tricyclic antidepressants in the treatment of coexisting pain and depression. Pain 7:331-341, 1979
52. Winokur G, Behar D, VanValkenburg MD, et al.: Is a familial definition of depression both feasible and valid? J Nerv Ment Dis 166:764-768, 1978

The Pain-Prone Disorder

Commentary

Pain is a broad, ubiquitous, and challenging problem; it responds to many treatments but evades any single explanation. Dr. Blumer isolated a group of chronic pain patients who present a comparatively consistent clinical picture—a specific premorbid personality and a characteristic family history. The term pain-prone patient was suggested. It was noted that a similar constellation of findings was demonstrated late in the last century by Oppenheim, a well-known German neurologist. At that time, Oppenheim was strongly attacked by many of his contemporaries who viewed the traumatic neuroses as manifestations of either spinal lesions, hysteria, or malingering. The present concept of the pain-prone disorder will undoubtedly also give rise to considerable controversy.

Dr. Blumer clearly outlined the kinship between the clinical presentation and the personal background of the pain-prone patient to that seen in depression. In addition, the presence of positive Dexamethasone Suppression Tests and shortened REM latencies in sleep EEG recordings—both considered biologic markers for depression—and the response to antidepressant medication in many patients indicate that the pain-prone disorder is related to the affective disorders. If the pain-prone disorder can be considered to be a form of chronic depression, one needs to investigate to what degree the same underlying biologic disorder can be established. Thus, the chronic pain patients that fit the criteria of the pain-prone disorder, may have the same basic neurotransmitter defects that are seen in depressed patients. When patients with the pain-prone disorder cannot only be identified as a group but indeed respond to specific treatment, a major step in the process of managing chronic pain will have been reached.

In the field of iatrogenically generated disorders, one of the most prevalent and troublesome conditions facing today's psychiatrist is a neurologic complication—the movement disorder that has come to be called tardive dyskinesia. Between the actual occurrence of the disturbance and the potential of its happening, tardive dyskinesia has produced a severe limitation on the medical management of many psychiatric disorders, particularly the psychotic diseases. While tardive dyskinesia provides another complication to an already difficult treatment problem, it appears inevitable that the pharmacologically produced movement disorders will lead to significant advances as more is learned of their nature. In this sense, tardive dyskinesia represents one of the more obvious borderline problems; it is a neurologic dysfunction which produces significant limitations to psychiatric treatment but holds promise of insights into cerebral metabolic abnormalities causing or accompanying the major psychoses. In the following chapter, Drs. Goetz and Klawans provide a practical and clinically oriented discussion of tardive dyskinesia including parameters for proper diagnosis, currently held theories as to the pathophysiology of the dysfunction, and, based on the latter, suggestions for management. From the mountains of material on tardive dyskinesia continuously appearing in the current literature and from their own experience, the authors have distilled an understandable approach to this serious problem.

Christopher G. Goetz, M.D.
Harold L. Klawans, M.D.

10

Tardive Dyskinesia

In the psychiatric literature, the term extrapyramidal syndrome (EPS) has traditionally comprised a wide variety of drug-induced movement disorders.[3,8,35] It has recently become increasingly clear that the natural history, pathophysiology, and pharmacology of individual movement disorders are distinct, so that this unifying term is obsolete and may in fact be a source of therapeutic confusion.

Specific diagnostic entities traditionally considered under EPS have included acute dystonias, akinesia, parkinsonism, rabbit syndrome, akathisia, and tardive dyskinesia.

This latter term, tardive dyskinesia, represents a specific example of extrapyramidal dysfunction. Tardive dyskinesia is a disorder with a clinical spectrum, natural history, prognosis, and pharmacology distinct from other extrapyramidal syndromes seen in psychiatric patients or in patients receiving psychotrophic agents. This discussion focuses on the current understanding of tardive dyskinesia, on the pathogenesis and pathophysiology, as well as on recent concepts of therapeutic interventions for managing the iatrogenic disorder. A brief overview discussion of the extrapyramidal system and its anatomy and pharmacology precede the discussion of tardive dyskinesia.

THE EXTRAPYRAMIDAL SYSTEM

The extrapyramidal system involves the nuclei and pathways of the central nervous system that relate to motor activity, but are not directly part of the classic descending pyramidal tracts. Three major characteristics help to contrast this system with the pyramidal system. First, the extrapyramidal system is multisynaptic; second, it does not have its own descending spiral cord tract; and third, lesions in the extrapyramidal system are characterized by poor integration of motor activity but not weakness.[14,16]

The pyramidal system most simplistically viewed is a two-cell system. To understand the basic anatomy, it is best to use an example and trace the pathway for volitional movement of the right foot. The first cell body is located in the left motor cortex and its axon travels through the left internal capsule, left descending pyramidal tracts of the brain stem, and crosses in the medullary pyramidal decussation continuing in the right lateral cortical spinal tract to the right anterior horn cell. The second cell body is located in the right anterior horn cell and its axon travels out of the spinal cord to the muscles of the right foot. Damage to the pyramidal system anywhere along this pathway will result in right foot weakness. The presence of spasticity or flacidity, increased or decreased reflexes, atrophy and fasiculations will help in differentiating which cell of the two-part system is damaged.

In contrast, the extrapyramidal system involves inputs from multiple brain stem and deep cortical nuclei that modulate this pyramidal function. Such nuclei include the substantia nigra in the midbrain, and the basal ganglia—a collective term for the striatum (caudate nucleus and putamen), globus pallidus, and subthalamic nucleus. The nuclei send ascending information primarily to the motor cortex via the thalamus for modulation of the pyramidal system. Since there is no extrapyramidal spinal cord pathway, information from extrapyramidal nuclei must be first integrated and then descend in the final pathway of the lateral cortical spinal tract. When the extrapyramidal nuclei and integrating axons are damaged, there is abnormal motor function, but since the two-cell pyramidal system is uninvolved, there is no weakness. Instead, poor control or integration of movement, either hypokinetic (pathologically slow) or hyperkinetic (pathologically overactive) movements are seen. Hence, although the term extrapyramidal indicates that this is a motor system that is nonpyramidal, it should not suggest that extrapyramidal function is independent of or in conflict with pyramidal activity. The two systems are closely integrated both anatomically and functionally so that strength and coordination are effected simultaneously in the normal situation.

Pharmacologic studies of extrapyramidal function have focused primarily on the striatum, where there are high concentrations of two major putative neurotransmitters that act antagonistically to one another, dopamine and acetylcholine.[6] Striatal dysfunction in the form of structural disease or biochemical imbalance of dopaminergic-cholinergic activities has been linked to a number of abnormal involuntary movement disorders. These movement disorders, while all extrapyramidal, have distinctly different pharmacologic bases, so that considering them all as a single entity (EPS) is confusing and therapeutically hazardous. For example, parkinsonism is felt to relate to a diminished activity of dopamine at selected striatal dopamine receptor sites.[60] In Parkinson's disease, cells whose axons project to the striatum die, leaving the striatum depleted of dopamine. Parkinsonism due to primary striatal degeneration is also seen, and drugs that block striatal dopamine receptors will induce the same parkinsonian effect.[73] Although parkinsonism is a disorder of the dopaminergic system, changes in striatal cholinergic function will influence parkinsonian features. Acetylcholine antagonizes striatal dopaminergic function, so that in parkinsonism where there is an absolute underactivity of dopamine, there is a relative overactivity of acetylcholine. Hence, there are two potential arms of therapy for parkinsonism—amplification of dopaminergic function or antagonism of cholinergic activity.[60]

In contrast to parkinsonism, the various forms of chorea are felt to relate to overactivity of dopamine at selected dopamine receptors in the striatum.[61] These receptors are most likely distinct from the dopaminergic receptors related to the pathophysiology of parkinsonism. Similarly to parkinsonism however, the same antagonism between dopamine and acetylcholine can be demonstrated. While chorea is aggravated by dopaminergic precursors or agonists and ameliorated by dopamine-receptor blockade or dopamine depletion, cholinergic alterations will also modify the abnormal movement. Absolute overactivity of dopaminergic function can be viewed as a relative underactivity of cholinergic function and hence reasonable treatment for chorea would include cholinergic amplification. This treatment has been shown to be effective with the use of short-acting cholinergic agents, and reports of putative cholinergic precursors have been favorable in many cases.[5,32,63] Other neurotransmitters may also play a role in the pathophysiology of chorea and parkinsonism, but these have not been proved.

TARDIVE DYSKINESIA—CLINICAL SPECTRUM

Lingual-facial-buccal dyskinesias are abnormal involuntary, persistent, movements of the tongue, lips, and facial muscles,[91] initially described as an integral part of the hyperkinesias of Huntington's chorea and other choreatic states. Following the introduction of neuroleptics into the practice of psychiatry in France in 1952, reports began to appear in the late 1950s of an extrapyramidal disorder characterized by persistent dyskinesias often of a lingual-facial-buccal nature which were associated with the long-term administration of neuroleptics. The late appearance led Uhrbrand and Faurbye in 1960 to apply the term "tardive dyskinesia" (TD).[96] By definition this term implies an iatrogenic disease due to chronic neuroleptic therapy.

The early description of this syndrome stressed abnormal motor movements affecting the face, the so-called bucco-lingual masticating syndrome. This consisted of involuntary mouthing, chewing, sucking, and licking movements of the tongue. Later, the syndrome description was broadened to include a variety of abnormal muscular manifestations, including choreoathetoid-type movements of the fingers, hands, arms, and feet, and ballistic-type movements particularly of the arms, as well as axial hyperkinesias and diaphragmatic movement resulting in grunting and difficult breathing. As the condition was studied more, the mouthing movements were further refined to include puckering, panting, smacking, and tongue movements inside the mouth. The clinical picture closely resembles L-dopa-induced dyskinesias and other choreatic disorders, both in the character of the movement abnormality and in the diversity of the individual symptoms.

As indicated, TD is by definition an iatrogenic disorder related specifically to chronic neuroleptic administration. Phrases such as spontaneous tardive syskinesia are hence self-contradictions and should be discarded. Spontaneous lingual-facial-buccal dyskinesias (i.e., chorea) may be a manifestation of Huntington's disease, senile chorea, and other degenerative neurologic syndromes, but are not TD.

EPIDEMIOLOGY

A number of population studies have been conducted to establish the frequence of TD and the significance of such factors as sex, age, and type of underlying psychiatric disease. The prevalence of TD has been estimated to range from 0.5 to 56 percent of patients treated with long-term neuroleptic agents.[2,12,25,99] This wide variance may be partly explained by the patient selection process and the diagnostic methods used to define TD. Those studies where patients were chronically institutionalized and older tended to report the highest incident of TD while studies that focused on middle-aged and younger patients reported lower incidences.[9,10,56] Smith et al. used the Abnormal Involuntary Movement Scores (AIMS) to assess the prevelance of TD and demonstrated that abnormal movement scores tend to be more severe with increasing age in both men and women up to age 70.[93] In patients over 70, the mean AIMS decreased in the male population sampled, and continued to increase in females. Hence, the often quoted 2:1 female to male prevalence ratio of TD was true only for patients over 70; otherwise no sex difference was seen.[93]

Other factors besides age and sex that have been studied in relation to the epidemiology of TD include length of hospitalization, history of neuroleptic-induced extrapyramidal syndromes, and type of schizophrenia. No established patterns have emerged to clarify these epidemiologic issues, and it appears that these factors are not significant to the development of TD.[53] Jus et al. reported a higher prevalence of TD in those schizophrenics with an insidious rather than acute onset of their psychiatric disease. They felt, however, that this may be an epiphenomenon since the insidious clinical presentation was more characteristic for the older patient population as a whole.[53] Furthermore, they concluded that the prevalence of TD was significantly higher if the mean age was higher at the beginning of medication therapy, again a possible reflection of age alone.

The fact that neuroleptic drugs are associated with the development of TD might suggest that the greater the total amount of neuroleptic a patient has received, the higher the risk of severity of TD. Two studies suggested an association between total amount of neuroleptic received and TD, although a third study using higher neuroleptic doses indicated no relation.[26,28,85]

Smith et al. reviewed drug history and TD in over 100 patients and concluded that total neuroleptic received over many years was not the main variable related to the development of TD. Instead, they found a positive correlation between the maximal amount of neuroleptic administered in any one year and the TD score. These results suggest that the temporal schedule and daily amount of neuroleptic administered may be epidemiologically more important than the total amount of medicine a patient receives.[93] No increased prevalence of TD in patients chronically treated with antiparkinsonian drugs has been definitely established.[1,39,54] In fact, one study reported a lower prevalence of TD in patients receiving concurrent neuroleptic and antiparkinsonian drugs than in patients receiving neuroleptics alone.[2]

NEUROPATHOLOGY

The observation that TD frequently remains permanent even after discontinuation of the antipsychotic drugs[24,87,96] has led investigators to search for a permanent structural alteration in the brains of TD patients. Neuropathologic studies following acute or chronic administration of antipsychotic drugs in laboratory animals have not demonstrated specific or localized neuropathologic changes in the brain beyond those secondarily produced by the diverse systemic effects of these drugs.[51,88] Although there is a single report of reduced neuronal cell count in the basal ganglia of rats chronically receiving phenothiazines,[80] this is of uncertain significance since degenerative changes or gliosis were not observed. Postmortem neuropathologic changes in man following chronic phenothiazine treatment in patients without extrapyramidal complications have usually consisted of scattered areas of neuronal degeneration and gliosis without convincing localization.[88] Individual patients with drug-induced parkinsonism or TD have been reported to have postmortem changes in the globus pallidus and putamen,[83] caudate nucleus and substantia nigra,[45] and in the inferior olive, where other investigators have reported no significant neuropathologic abnormality in patients with TD.[49]

Christensen has reported the presence of neuronal degeneration and gliosis of the substantia nigra in 27 of 28 brains from patients with chronic oral dyskinesias, 21 cases of which were attributed to antipsychotic drugs, while only 7 of 28 matched control brains, showed similar changes.[17] Although the reported nigral degeneration and gliosis may represent a toxic effect of the drug, their occurrence in some elderly individuals without TD raises the possibility that they may be accompanying events of aging and not directly related to the appearance of TD. The fact that no obvious anatomic alterations are associated with the development of TD has led investigators away from microscopic studies and initiated a more thorough evaluation of receptor-site dynamics, neurochemistry, and pharmacology of the disorder.

PATHOGENESIS AND PATHOPHYSIOLOGY

Although the pathologic sequence of changes underlying the development of TD remains unknown, the similarity of the abnormal movements to other forms of chorea suggests a common biochemical basis. A number of clinical and pharmacologic observations have helped to clarify the pathophysiology of the movements seen in TD and suggest etiologic as well as therapeutic implications. In summary, there is substantial evidence that the pathogenesis of TD relates to chronic dopamine-receptor site blockade, while the pathophysiology of the disorder relates to the resultant receptor site hypersensitivity.

The first clues concerning the pathophysiology of TD came from the observation that the neuroleptics, those agents associated with the development of TD, are the same agents known to cause drug-induced parkinsonism. Parkinsonism is felt to result from deficient dopaminergic activity in the striatum.[61] The fact that the neuroleptics can induce a parkinsonian syndrome suggests that these agents may alter central dopaminergic balance and thereby chemically simulate the structural abnormality seen in Parkinson disease. Biochemical studies have corroborated these hypotheses and have shown that the neuroleptics act by blocking dopamine receptor sites in the limbic system and the striatum.[50]

This blockade of dopamine receptors in the striatum is felt to underlie the neuroleptic-induced parkinsonism so often seen within the first weeks or months after neuroleptic induction. These studies show that neuroleptics affect the dopaminergic system and that at least initially, this effect is one of functional underactivity of dopamine at dopamine receptor sites of the striatum.

This blockade may be thought of as a form of chemical denervation or functional inactivation of dopamine receptors in the striatum. If the blockade is complete at any receptor site, then this receptor is prevented from receiving its normal neurotransmitter influence. This does not imply that the blockade is complete for all dopaminergic receptors throughout the striatum. This is an important concept, for it implies that not all receptors are blocked to the same extent by a single agent. If the latter were true, then chemical denervation could only occur following complete blockage of all dopamine receptors, which would necessarily be accompanied by a severe form of drug-induced parkinsonism.

A second clue concerning the pathophysiology of TD comes from the observation that these dyskinesias are remarkably similar and often indistinguishable from the abnormal movements seen in Huntington's disease and levodopa-induced dyskinesias. These latter two movement disorders are felt to relate to a heightened response of the dopamine receptor sites in the striatum. The similarity of TD to movement disorders whose pathophysiology is better understood suggests that TD may also relate to altered sensitivity of the striatal dopaminergic system.

Whereas parkinsonism results from underactivity of the dopaminergic system, these dyskinesias appear to result from overactivity. The neuroleptics would then appear to be associated with both dopaminergic syndromes, initially parkinsonism, implicating dopamine underactivity, and eventually TD implicating dopamine overactivity. The explanation behind this apparent dichotomy relates to the fact that after chronic blockade, receptor function is altered. There is a large body of evidence demonstrating that after prolonged denervation, a receptor site becomes hypersensitive to ambient amounts of neurotransmitter exposure. This results in an enhanced response of the postsynaptic cell to neurotransmitter concentrations that previously led to only low rates of baseline firing. This phenomenon of denervation hypersensitivity has been extensively studied in the peripheral receptor site system and has been shown to apply to the dopaminergic striatal system as well. Ohye and his associates showed that after prolonged denervation, the postsynaptic striatal cells fire with enhanced frequency to ambient dopamine that previously caused only low, baseline firing rates.[78] A similar behavioral hypersensitivity can be seen in animals after chronic neuroleptic administration.[46] The ultrastructural basis for this chronic hypersensitivity has been studied in detail and it appears that hypersensitivity relates pathophysiologically to alterations in dopaminergic-receptor site populations. After chronic neuroleptic administration to animals, there is an increase in the number of striatal dopamine receptors that clearly parellels the behavioral changes.[15,46] Analogous alterations may underlie the pathophysiology of TD in humans.

Dopamine turnover studies are consistent with the gradual development of denervation hypersensitivity. Cerebrospinal fluid levels of homovanillic acid, the major metabolite of dopamine, tend to increase acutely following the administration of neuroleptics.[11] Within the first few weeks of treatment, this elevation tends to decrease so that after chronic treatment there is generally decreased turnover of dopamine.[42,82,89]

The question of which dopamine receptor sites are sensitized is of central importance to an understanding of the pathogenesis and pathophysiology of TD. If TD results from prolonged blockade of the same dopaminergic receptors whose less chronic blockade leads to parkinsonism, then some degree of parkinsonism would be a prerequisite for the subsequent occurrence of drug-induced TD. Furthermore, these dyskinesias should occur in the same muscles supplied by the same receptors which were involved in the parkinsonian manifestations. This is clearly not the case, as TD often occurs in patients who have had no past history or evidence on physical examination of drug-induced parkinsonism.[61] Additionally, although patients with TD tend to have fewer hypokinetic parkinsonian symptoms than neuroleptic-treated patients without TD, case reports demonstrate that patients may suffer simultaneously from both TD and drug-induced parkinsonism.[19,33,38]

These observations suggest the possibility of more than one dopamine-receptor site in the striatum. There is, in fact, evidence from cellular recordings that at least two different dopamine-receptor populations exist in the striatum. Dopamine receptors of the striatum have been demonstrated to respond to dopamine with facilitation or inhibition. Since the response of a receptor to a transmitter is a property of the receptor site and not the transmitter, two different responses suggest two different receptors. When dopamine activates one type of receptor, the neuron is hyperpolarized or inhibited. These receptors could be called dopamine-inhibited receptors. The second receptor responds to dopamine stimulation with depolarization or facilitation, and could be called the dopamine-facilitated receptor. Parkinsonism is usually related to decreased activity of dopamine at the dopamine-inhibited receptors.

It is of interest that while the neuroleptics block both types of dopamine receptors, the degree of blockade is different for the two populations. The dopamine-facilitated neurons are blocked by levels of haloperidol or chlorpromazine that do not block the action of dopamine at dopamine-inhibited receptor sites. Only with larger doses of the neuroleptics are the dopamine-inhibited receptors also blocked.[23] This observation, together with the observation that TD can occur independently of drug-induced parkinsonism suggests that the two disorders both relate to dopamine, but to different receptor populations. One could visualize TD as an abnormal hyperactive response of dopamine-facilitated receptors to dopamine, while parkinsonism relates to a lack of response of the dopamine-inhibited receptors to dopamine.

No large studies measuring receptor-site populations in humans with TD have been performed, although receptor-site measurements from brains of schizophrenics have been investigated. Owen et al. demonstrated increased dopamine-receptor sensitivity both in receptor numbers and affinity as measured by spiroperidol binding in postmortem brains of schizophrenics.[79]

These biochemical changes were seen in patients who were receiving neuroleptic agents at the time of death, as well as patients who were not receiving medication. Those patients who were currently receiving medication, however, demonstrated a greater degree of receptor-site sensitivity. No information was reported on the incidence of TD in these patients so that these data cannot be applied directly to the pathophysiology of TD. Significantly, however, dopamine-receptor site sensitivity was increased in the caudate nucleus and putamen as well as the nucleus accumbens of the limbic system. The former two basal ganglia are felt to be related to movements and motor disorders, while the latter limbic dopaminergic nucleus has been suggested to relate to the pathophysiology of psychosis.

A similar study by Lee et al. reported increased haloperidol binding in the caudate nucleus, putamen, and nucleus accumbens of brains from patients with schizophrenia.[69] Again the prevalence of TD in these patients was not discussed. Since ^{3}H-apomorphine binding was not altered in these brains, it was suggested that neuroleptic-induced alteration in receptor-site binding in all three dopamine-rich areas were predominantly related to postsynaptic receptors.[75]

A number of investigators have attempted to demonstrate dopaminergic hypersensitivity in patients with TD by the use of various neuroendocrine tests. Neuroendocrine interest in relation to TD and dopamine stems from the observation that there is a readily accessible and well-defined hypothalamic dopaminergic pathway that involves prolactin and human growth hormone (HGH) control.[20,67,68,70,74] If TD represents or is associated with a diffuse hypersensitive response of dopaminergic systems, neuroendocrine hypersensitivity may be expected. If a selective striatal alteration underlies the pathophysiology of TD, however, necessary neuroendocrine changes in dopaminergic function would not be anticipated. Cohen et al. reported normal prolactin response after exposure to thyrotropin-releasing factor in four schizophrenic patients with TD, and could demonstrate no hypothalamic dopaminergic supersensitivity.[21] Similarly, the prolactin measurement in patients with TD challenged with apomorphine showed no enhanced or hypersensitive response when compared with normals.[37]

Growth hormone measurements after apomorphine challenge have suggested the same lack of hypothalamic hypersensitivity. One study failed to show evidence of any difference between normal controls and TD patients, while a second study, using the same apomorphine dose reported that chronic schizophrenics, both with and without TD, showed slight but not significantly lower growth hormone levels than controls.[37,81,95] Although growth hormone responses in acute schizophrenia appeared higher than controls, these responses cannot be viewed as relative to TD, since TD is seen by definition after prolonged neuroleptic therapy for chronic disease. Neuroendocrine studies have hence not revealed evidence of hypothalamic hypersensitivity in patients with TD. These data would suggest that if TD relates to dopaminergic hypersensitivity, it is a selective hypersensitivity of certain receptor populations. Because of the clinical similarity of TD to Huntington's chorea, the probable level of selective hypersensitivity would be the striatum. Studies of striatal receptor-site hypersensitivity in nonschizophrenic patients with TD have not yet been reported.

DIFFERENTIAL DIAGNOSIS

Tardive dyskinesia usually begins after 1–2 years of chronic neuroleptic treatment, and hence is temporally distinct from other extrapyramidal disorders such as drug-induced parkinsonism or dystonia. These latter conditions tend to occur earlier in the course of neuroleptic therapy. Drug-induced parkinsonism is felt to relate to dopaminergic receptor-site blockade in the striatum. The clinical features of parkinsonism which include bradykinesia, resting tremor, rigidity, and loss of postural reflexes appear to result whenever striatal receptor sites do not receive appropriate dopaminergic stimulation. Resting tremor is rarely misdiagnosed as TD, except in cases where there is tremor in the jaw region. Jaw tremor is also referred to in the psychiatric literature as "rabbit syndrome," since the patients have rhythmic and repetitive movements that resemble a rabbit's munching.[55,94,97] Since parkinsonism and TD are based on very distinct pharmacologic alterations that require very different management, the addition of another term, regardless of how colorful it may be, tends to obscure essential distinctions. Resting tremor, whether oral-facial or limb, tends to occur coincident with commencement or increase in neuroleptic medication and is associated with other parkinsonian features. It relates pathophysiologically to decreased activity of dopaminergic function at the striatal level and is therefore treated in the same manner as other parkinsonian features.

Neuroleptic-induced dystonias are seen early in the course of chronic neuroleptic therapy and are not confused with TD since a dystonia is a sustained abnormal and involuntary posture. The fine, irregular movements that characterize chorea are not seen. Dystonic manifestations can be quite diverse although the most common clinical signs involve the eyes and neck, leading to dramatic oculogyric crisis or severe torticollis spasms.

It is important to distinguish TD from other hyperkinetic syndromes, especially stereotypic mannerisms and agitation related to psychotic behavior and akathisia associated with early administration or recent elevation in dose of neuroleptics. A wide variety of mannerisms are seen in the psychotic population, and these peculiar behaviors may resemble oral-facial dyskinesias or limb chorea.[73] In the vast majority of cases, however, they are highly ritualistic in character and consistent in anatomic distribution, which distinguishes them from the unpredictable irregularity of choreiform movements. Furthermore, mannerisms are usually conscious and symbolically significant to the patient, whereas TD is often completely unrecognized or of little concern. The former movements also are seen as part of the early psychotic state and do not usually emerge after prolonged drug treatment.[34] A psychotic or mentally deranged patient with early-onset chorea or dystonia should raise the additional important diagnostic considerations of extrapyramidal disorders like Huntington's chorea, dystonia musculorum deformans, and Wilson's disease.

An initial glance at TD patients might suggest that they are agitated, since there is an abundance of movement often with shifting in the chair, irregular tapping of feet, or strange mouthing movements. While these behaviors might suggest an overly nervous person, TD does not resemble the hyperactivity seen in psychotic states like manic-depressive illness or involutional psychosis. In the latter cases, a generalized psychomotor activation is seen characterized by overactivity but well-coordinated movements and often exaggerated expressions of affect.

Finally, akathisia must be differentiated from TD. Akathisia is a state of motor restlessness that occurs following early administration or an augmentation of neuroleptic dose.[3,4,74] It is not clear, however, that this effect relates specifically to extrapyramidal dysfunction. Akathisia does not occur naturally—except in very rare occurrences of Parkinson's disease—in any extrapyramidal disorder.[90] While it does occur coincident with neuroleptic administration, there are no data to confirm that akathisia relates to neuroleptic effects on dopaminergic activity or the extrapyramidal system. While it can be mildly modified by the administration of anticholingeric agents, the effect of this drug class on akathisia is much less marked than in cases of drug-induced parkinsonism.[73] The hallmark of akathisia is the striking complaint of inner tension, a need to move about and resist inactivity. Usually, the patient feels forced to shuffle his feet restlessly and may feel unable to sit or lie down. Akathisia can be differentiated from TD in its natural history, since the former occurs coincident with medication induction or dosage increase and is not associated with fine involuntary movements so characteristic of TD. The patient interview also helps since the movements of akathesia are felt to be secondary to the internal restlessness, whereas TD is not necessarily associated with mental agitation of any sort. In fact, often the patient is unaware of his TD.

A recent report suggesting new diagnostic categories for late-onset drug-related dyskinesias included "withdrawal dyskinesia" and "covert dyskinesia.[41] The former was defined as self-limited TD, resolving within 12 weeks after drug withdrawal; covert dyskinesia was defined as dyskinesia seen with discontinuation or reduction of neuroleptic dose without spontaneous abatement. The distinctions, of theoretic interest, are not practical however, since in a patient who develops dyskinesia after medication withdrawal, the diagnosis would first be withdrawal dyskinesia for 12 weeks and, if there was no abatement, the diagnosis would be changed to covert dyskinesia. The change in diagnosis gives no insight into pharmacology and pathophysiology, and the time of 12 weeks is at best arbitrary. As the authors of the report admitted, these distinctions may confuse rather than clarify clinical thinking.

PHARMACOLOGIC THERAPY

With this pharmacologic background, one can consider therapeutic options in terms of the pathogenesis and pathophysiology of TD. If the pathogenesis of the disorder relates to chronic dopaminergic receptor-site blockade and the pathophysiology relates to the resultant denervation hypersensitivity, agents that interrupt this sequence would be of potential benefit. Reserpine acts by blocking the reuptake of dopamine, norepinephrine, and serotonin into the intraneuronal storage vesicles. In this way, reserpine depletes the brain of dopamine. Since it acts presynaptically, this drug would allow less endogeneous dopamine to be released onto the presumed hypersensitive dopamine receptor, thereby simulating a more normal dopaminergic homeostasis. Reserpine given in doses of 1–5 mg/day has been shown to reduce TD in a number of clinical trials.[36,44] The potential side effects of hypotension and psychologic depression must be monitored carefully. Reserpine-induced depression is infrequent in schizophrenics without a history of affective disorder.

Jus et al. have recently reported treating TD based on a concept of slow desensitization of dopamine receptor sites.[52] They hypothesized that since a long period of time was required to build up striatal hypersensitivity, a prolonged and slow decrease in neuroleptic blockade might resolve the problem. They treated 62 chronic schizophrenics with TD by a very slow (average period of 3.9 years) progressive stepwise diminution of neuroleptic and antiparkinsonian medication. At the same time, they administered slowly increasing doses of reserpine or, when clinically necessary to control psychosis, a more sedating neuroleptic rather than the long-acting phenothiazines. Their long-term results were disappearance of TD in 37 percent, improvement in 42 percent, and no effect in 21 percent of patients. No patients demonstrated progression of their abnormal movements. This long-term inpatient study has not yet been expanded to include outpatients.

Tetrabenazine, a synthetic benzoquinolone derivative which depletes monoamines by a mechanism similar to that of reserpine, is more rapid in onset, more selective for central nervous system activity, and has less hypotensive effects than reserpine. Given in doses 100–300 mg/day, tetrabenazine has reduced or abolished TD in several clinical trials—most of these cases, however, were acute or lasting less than 6 months.[13,57,59,72] Agents that deplete central dopaminergic stores serve as the mainstay of present therapy for TD.

Formerly, TD was often treated by increasing the dose of neuroleptics. This short-sited treatment generally abates the abnormal movements but clearly is contraindicated. This method of therapy treats the pathophysiology of TD but aggravates the pathogenesis by potential further denervation and subsequent hypersensitivity. Epidemiologic evidence shows a direct relationship between the incidence of TD and the duration of neuroleptic therapy. In the individual patient, abnormal movements show a gradual progression over time, beginning usually with mild, localized lingual-facial-buccal dyskinesias and later becoming more severe and generalized. As neuroleptic therapy becomes prolonged, there is both an increase in the severity of abnormal movements and an increase in the number of body areas involved. As discussed in the section of epidemiology, the issue of age relative to prevalence of TD can be difficult to separate from chronicity of medication. Nevertheless, it appears that the longer the pathogenesis persists the more frequently and severely the physiology will be disrupted.[24,61,73] For these reasons neuroleptics have no role in the routine treatment of TD.

An additional therapeutic option is the manipulation of other neurotransmitters. There is a well known and accepted balance between dopamine and acetylcholine in the striatum. While Parkinson disease relates primarily to dopamine alteration, the cholinergic system is known to modify the movements of the disease.[60] Presumably, since dopamine is already decreased, decreasing the cholinergic influence as well would re-establish the relative neurotransmitter balance and reinstitute the former homeostasis, but at a different absolute level. Under the same premise, if TD relates to an increase in dopaminergic effect, elevating the cholinergic effect would re-establish the former homeostasis, but again at a new neurotransmitter level. In fact this appears to be the case; anticholinergic agents appear to aggravate the abnormal movements of TD and cholinergic agents may ameliorate them. Klawans and Rubovits administered intraveneous physostigmine to patients with TD and demonstrated clear abatement of the abnormal movements.[64] Although this study demonstrates the importance of neurotransmitter balance to the pathophysiology of TD, since physostigmine cannot be given orally, this therapy has not been of practical benefit to patients. Orally available precursors of acetylcholine include choline chloride and phosphatidylcholine (lecithin). In short-term studies, both agents have been reported to be useful in the control of TD.[27,31] Long-term controlled studies have not yet been conducted and these drugs remain experimental. Dimethylaminoethanol (Deanol) was originally reported to be efficacious in the treatment of TD, but more extensive studies have not corroborated this finding.[13]

Using the same concept of dopaminergic-cholinergic antagonism relative to TD, but with a focus on early or presymptomatic detection, Chouinard et al. advocated the very short-term use of anticholingerics.[18] They acutely exposed patients on chronic neuroleptic therapy to small doses of anticholinergic drugs to see whether these doses uncover or precipitate choreatic movements. If subclinical dyskinesias could be transiently unmasked by this alteration of dopaminergic-cholinergic balance, this precipitation would theoretically warn the clinician that striatal hypersensitiviy is developing. Appropriate reduction of the neuroleptic or introduction of dopaminergic depleting agents could then be instituted as an

early intervention. The efficacy of such treatment is unproved, and the distinction between this short-term provocation course of anticholinergic therapy and the chronic exposure to anticholinergic drugs is essential. The latter course has been suggested, although not proved to be associated with an enhanced chance of developing TD.
Other agents have also been tried but remain unproved in the treatment of tardive dyskinesia.

1. Lithium: In two short-term studies mild improvement has been reported in TD with lithium therapy.[43,86] Other studies report no improvement or exacerbation.[29,92] Additionally, re-emergence of old TD quiescent for several years was seen in a patient when lithium therapy was introduced.[7] The interaction of lithium with the dopaminergic system is not understood although lithium accelerates synaptic reuptake of norepinephrine.[22]

2. Baclofen (in patients who have to be maintained on neuroleptics): As a presumed GABA-agonist, baclofen has been suggested to affect the dopaminergic system at the level of the striatum or substantia nigra.[65]

3. Levodopa: Following initial worsening there are reports of amelioration.[40]

4. Alpha-methyldopa: One report suggested amelioration while another indicated no change in TD after methyldopa therapy.[58,98]

5. Clonazepam: A benzodiazepam derivative, this drug is used in the treatment of seizure disorders. It has been reported to improve dyskinesia in 42 patients given 1-3 mg/day.[77]

6. Manganese: Small series have reported on the successful treatment of TD with manganese chelete 60 mg/day.[47,66,76]

7. Electroconvulsive therapy: Previously, it was suggested that ECT could increase the likelihood of the development of TD in patients receiving neuroleptic drugs.[24,30,96] These reports, however, lacked significant historic and drug treatment information so that direct association could only be conjectured. In fact, a recent report suggested that TD may be ameliorated after ECT.[84] The patient reported had had a stable degree of abnormal movement before ECT and showed a sudden dramatic and sustained improvement after the first three ECT treatments.

Again, these are all short-term studies in small groups of patients. None of these modalities can be definitely recommended at this time.

RECOMMENDATIONS

The following principles should help to decrease the incidence of TD.

1. Decrease the number of subjects at risk. Neuroleptics should only be used where clearly indicated and continued only when efficacy is clear.
2. Keep the daily dosage as low as possible.
3. Avoid chronic anticholinergics if possible. Since anticholinergic agents clearly exacerbate already present TD, it is possible that with chronic administration, these drugs may alter the striatal neurochemical balance and potentiate the development or abnormal movements de novo.[61]
4. Keep the duration of therapy as short as possible. Most schizophrenics are maintained on neuroleptics to control chronic symptoms or prevent exacerbation. In the latter group it is quite possible that neuroleptics can be withdrawn for at least some period of time without a severe exacerbation (drug holiday). It is possible that such drug holidays might decrease the overall incidence of TD. Data collected from animal studies suggest that drug-free periods should be at least 1 month long to be effective.[61] The decision to withdraw neuroleptics must be individualized for each patient, and the relative morbidity of the abnormal movements must be weighed against the danger of a psychotic exacerbation.
5. Early detection and drug withdrawal when possible.
6. In the event that neuroleptics are absolutely required, we tend to switch the medication to thioridazine. This decision is based on several considerations. First there appears to be some relationship between drug-induced parkinsonism and TD, and thioridazine has the lowest incidence of drug-induced parkinsonism of available neuroleptics. Evidence already sited from animal experiments also suggests that some agents may be less likely to induce receptor hypersensitivity than others. In animals, thioridazine is a much weaker blocker of striatal dopamine receptors than other neuroleptics. Furthermore, in our laboratory, we have been unable to produce receptor-site hypersensitivity measured either biochemically or behaviorally with chronic thioridazine but can easily produce this state with other phenothiazines and haloperidol in equivalent doses.[71] There is no human data to establish a lower incidence of TD with thioridazine but because of the above considerations, we feel that it is reasonable to substitute thioridazine in this situation. Clozapine, a neuroleptic not available in the

United States, has the lowest incidence of associated parkinsonism and appears to be a more specific dopamine-receptor blocker for the nucleus accumbens of the limbic system.[62]

It was common to attribute the low incidence of parkinsonism caused by thioridazine and clozapine to the ability of these agents to block central muscarinic receptors. The fact that these agents are both dopaminergic blockers and cholinergic blockers might suggest that they should have the highest likelihood of causing TD. This is certainly not the case. No reports of clozapine-induced TD have yet appeared. From a variety of animal behavior studies it is clear that clozapine and thioridazine are not equivalent to another neuroleptic (e.g. haloperidol) plus an anticholinergic agent.[71] The differences in incidence of parkinsonism may not be due solely to a neuroleptic's anticholinergic properties but may reflect a preferential ability to block specific striatal dopamine receptors.

With the exception of clozapine, the relative incidence of TD with different neuroleptics is not definitely known and although thioridazine can cause TD we tend to feel safer using this drug when neuroleptic treatment is necessary.

PROGNOSIS

Tardive dyskinesia may worsen initially following neuroleptic withdrawal, presumably because of better access of dopamine to striatal receptors. This exacerbation, however, is usually only a short-term effect. Tardive dyskinesias, in fact, are often reversible and may spontaneously remit following neuroleptic withdrawal. The earlier the symptoms are recognized and drugs withdrawn, the better the prognosis for recovery.[61] This is consistent with the view that TD is a progressive disorder. The chances that TD may become irreversible can be decreased by early detection and neuroleptic withdrawal, and patients should be carefully examined for dyskinesias at frequent intervals. In some cases, TD can disappear within 1-2 months after the discontinuation of neuroleptic therapy. Larger series with more prolonged follow-up after the withdrawal of antipsychotic drugs have shown that TD is more likely to remit completely.[2,92]

SUMMARY

The basic pathogenesis of TD appears to relate to chronic pharmacologic denervation of specific dopaminergic receptor sites in the striatum. The pathophysiology of the disorder relates to the resultant denervation hypersensitivity. The mainstay of treatment includes withdrawal of neuroleptics where feasible and the use of dopamine-depleting agents. Enhancement of the striatal cholinergic input offers potential ancillary benefit to the alleviation of abnormal movements. The benefit of manipulating other neurotransmitters remains experimental. Treatment of TD with neuroleptics themselves is clearly treatment with the presumed offending agent, and should be avoided. This short-sited therapy may temporarily abate the pathophysiology of the condition, but serves to aggrevate its pathogenesis.

REFERENCES

1. American College of Neuropsychopharmacology—Food and Drug Administration Task Force: Neurologic syndromes associated with antipsychotic drug use. N Engl J Med 289:20-23, 1973
2. Asnis FM, Leopold MA, Duvoisin RC, et al.: A survey of tardive dyskinesia in psychiatric outpatients. Am J Psychiatry 134:1367-1370, 1977
3. Ayd FJ: A survey of drug-induced extrapyramidal reactions. JAMA 175:1054-1060, 1961
4. Ayd FJ: Neuroleptics and extrapyramidal reactions in psychiatric patients. Rev Can Biol 20:451-459, 1961
5. Barbeau A: Phosphatidylcholine in neurologic disorders. Neurology 28:358,1978
6. Bartholini G, Stadler H, Lloyd KG: Cholinergic-dopaminergic interactions in the extrapyramidal system, in Calne DB (ed): Progress in the Treatment of Parkinsonism. New York, Raven, 1973, pp 233-241
7. Beitman BD: Tardive dyskinesia reinduced by lithium carbonate. Am J Psychiatry 135:1229-1230, 1978
8. Boston Collaborative Drug Surveillance Program: Drug induced extrapyramidal symptoms. JAMA 224:889, 1973
9. Bourgeois M, Boueilh P, Peyre C et al: Les dyskinesies tardives des neuroleptiques. Ann Med Psychol 135:660-679, 1977
10. Bourgeois M, Tignol J: Les dyskinesies tardives des neuroleptiques. La Nov Pres Med 6:3649-3650, 1977
11. Bowers MB Jr: 5-HIAA and HVA following probenecid in acutely psychotic patients treated with phenothiazines. Psychopharmacologia 28:309, 1973
12. Brandon S, McClelland HA, Prothero C: A study of facial dyskinesia in a mental hospital population. Br J Psychol 118:171-184, 1971
13. Brandrup E: Tetrabenazine treatment in persisting dyskinesias caused by psychopharmaca. Am J Psychiatry 118:551-552, 1961
14. Brodal A: Neurological Anatomy. New York, Oxford University Press, 1969, pp 151-254
15. Burt DR, Creese I, Snyder SH: Antischizophrenic drugs: Chronic treatment eleviates dopamine receptor binding in the brain. Science 196:326-328, 1977

16. Carpenter MD: Human Neuroanatomy. Baltimore, Williams and Wilkins, 1976, p 496-519
17. Christensen E, Moller JE, Faurbye A: Neuropathological investigation of 28 brains from patients with dyskinesias. Acta Psychiatr Scand 46:14-23, 1970
18. Chouinard G, de Moutigny C, Annable L: Tardive dyskinesia and antiparkinsonian medication. Am J Psychiatry 136:228-229, 1979
19. Chouinard G, Annable L, Ross-Chouinard A, et al.: Ethopropazine bentropine in neuroleptic induced parkinsonism. J Clin Psychiat 40:147-152, 1979
20. Clemens JA, Shaar CJ, Smalstig EB: Inhibition of prolactin secretion by ergolines. Endocrinology 94:1171-1176, 1974
21. Cohen KL, Cooper RA, Altshul S: Prolactin levels in tardive dyskinesia. N Engl J Med 46:294, 1979
22. Colburn RW, Goodwin FK, Bunney WE Jr, et al.: Effect of lithium on the uptake of nordrenaline by synaptomes. Nature 215:1395, 1967
23. Cools AR: Basic considerations on the role of dopaminergic, gabaergic, cholinergic and seratonergic mechanisms within the striatum, in Ellinwood EH, Kilbey MM (eds): Cocaine and Other Stimulants. New York, Plenum, 1977, p 210-216
24. Crane GE: Tardive dyskinesias in patients treated with neuroleptics: A review of the literature. Am J Psychiatry 124 (Feb Supp): 40-48, 1968
25. Crane GE: Persistant dyskinesia. Br J Psychol 122:395-397, 1973
26. Crane GE: Factors pre-disposing to drug-induced neurological side effects, in Forrest IS, Carr CJ, Usdin E (eds): Advances in Biochemical Psychopharmacology, vol 9. New York, Raven, 1974, pp 269-279
27. Crane GE: Deanol for tardive dyskinesia. N Eng J Med 292:926-928, 1975
28. Crane GE: Smeets RA: Tardive dyskinesia and drug therapy in geriatric patients. Arch Gen Psychiatry 30:341-343, 1974
29. Crews EL, Carpenter AE: Lithium-induced aggravation of tardive dyskinesia. Am J Psychiatry 134:933, 1977
30. Curran JP: Tardive dyskinesia—Side effect or not. Am J Psychiatry 130:406-410, 1973
31. Davis KL, Berger PA, Hollister LE: Choline for tardive dyskinesia. N Eng J Med 293:152, 1975
32. Davis KL, Hollister LE, Barchas JD, et al.: Choline in tardive dyskinesia and Huntington's disease. Life Sci 19:1507-1508, 1976
33. DeFraites EG Jr, Davis KL, Berger PA: Coexisting tardive dyskinesia and parkinsonism: A case report. Biol Psychiatry 12:267-272, 1977
34. Degwitz R, Binsack KF, Herkert H: Zur problem der persistierenden extrapyramidelen Hyperkinesen nach langfritiger anwendang von Neuroleptica. Nervenarzt 38:170-174
35. Detre TP, Jerecki HG: Modern Psychiatric Treatment. Philadelphia, Lippincott, 1971
36. Duvoisin RC: Reserpine for tardive dyskinesia. N Eng J Med 286:611, 1972
37. Ettigi P, Nair NPV, Lal S, et al.: Effect of apomorphine of growth hormone and prolactin in schizophrenic patients. J Neurol Neurosurg Psychiatry 39:870-876, 1976

38. Fann WE, Lake CR: On the coexistence of parkinsonism and tardive dyskinesia. Dis Nerv Syst 35:325-326, 1974
39. Fracchia J, Sheppard C, Merlis S: Combination medications in psychiatric treatment. J Am Geriatr Soc 19:301-307, 1971
40. Freidhoff AJ, Bounett K, Rosengarten H: Reversal of two manifestations of dopamine receptors supersensitivity by administration of L-dopa. Res Commun Chem Pathol Pharmacol 16(3): 1977, pp 411-423
41. Gardos G, Cole JO, Tarsy D: Withdrawal syndromes associated with antipsychotic drugs. Am J Psychiatry 135:1321-1324, 1978
42. Gerlach J, Thorsen K, Fog R: Extrapyramidal reactions and amine metabolites in CSF during haloperidol and clozapine treatment of schizophrenia. Psychopharmacologia 40:341, 1975
43. Gerlach J, Thorsen K, Munkvad I: Effect of lithium in neuroleptic induced tardive dyskinesia compared with placebo in a double-blind cross-over trial. Pharmakopsychiatr Neuropsychopharmakol 8:51-56, 1975
44. Goetz CG, Weiner WJ, Klawans HL: Treatment of the choreas, in Barbeau A (ed): Disorders of Movement. Philadelphia, Lippincott, 1981, p 29-41
45. Gross H, Kaltenbach E: Neuropathological findings in persistent dyskinesias after neuroleptic long term therapy, in Cerletti A, Bove FJ (eds): The Present Status of Psychotropic Drugs. Amsterdam, Excerpta Medica, 1968
46. Hitri A, Weiner WJ, Borison RL, et al.: Dopamine binding following prolonged haloperidol pretreatment. Ann Neurol 3:134-140, 1978
47. Hoffer A: Tardive dyskinesia treated with manganese. Can Med Assoc J 117:859, 1977
48. Hunter R, Earl CJ, Janz D: A syndrome of abnormal movements and dementia in leukotomized patients treated with phenothiazines. J Neurol Neurosurg Psychiatry 27:219-223, 1964
49. Hunter R, Blackwood W, Smith MC, Cummings JN: Neuropathological findings in 3 cases of persistent dyskinesias following phenothiazine medication. J Neurol Sci 7:763-773, 1968
50. Iversen IL: Dopamine receptors in the brain. Science 188:1084-1089, 1975
51. Julou L, Ducrot R, Ganter P, Maral R, et al.: Chronic toxicity, side effects and metabolism of neuroleptics of the phenothiazine group, in Proceedings of the European Society for Study of Drug Toxicity, vol 9: Toxicity and Side effects of Psychotropic Drugs, International Congress Series no. 145. Amsterdam, Excerpta Medica, 1968, pp 35-51
52. Jus A, Jus K, Fontaine P: Long-term treatment of tardive dyskinesia. J Clin Psychol 30:73-79, 1979
53. Jus A, Pineau R, Lachance R, et al.: Epidemiology of tardive dyskinesia. part I. Dis Nerv Syst 37:210-214, 1976
54. Jus A, Pineau R, Lachance R, et al.: Epidemiology of tardive dyskinesia. part II. Dis Nerv Syst 37:257-261, 1976
55. Jus K, Jus A, Gautier J, et al.: Studies on the action of certain pharmacological agents on tardive and on the rabbit syndrome. Int J Clin Pharmacol 9:138-145, 1974
56. Kazamatsuri H, Chien CP, Cole JO: Treatment of tardive dyskinesia. Arch Gen Psychiatry 27:103-106, 1972

57. Kazamatsuri H, Chien CP, Cole JO: Treatment of tardive dyskinesias. I. Clinical efficacy of dopamine depleting agent, tetrabenazine. Arch Gen Psychiatry 27:95-99, 1972
58. Kazamatsuri H, Chien CP, Cole JO: Treatment of tardive dyskinesia. III. Clinical efficacy of a dopamine competing agent, methyldopa. Arch Gen Psychiatry 27:824-827, 1972
59. Kazamatsuri H, Chien CP, Cole JO: Long-term treatment of tardive dyskinesia with haloperidol and tetrabenazine. Am J Psychiatry 130:479-483, 1973
60. Klawans HL: The pharmacology of parkinsonism. Dis Nerv Syst 29:805-816, 1968
61. Klawans HL: The Pharmacology of Extrapyramidal Movement Disorders. Barger, Basel, 1973
62. Klawans HL: Animal models of tardive dyskinesia. Third International Symposium on Phenothiazine. Zurich, Sept, 1979
63. Klawans HL, Rubovits R: Cholinergic-anticholingeric antagonism in Huntington's chorea. Neurology 22:107-112, 1972
64. Klawans HL, Rubovits R: Effect of cholinergic and anticholinergic agents on tardive dyskinesia. J Neurol Neurosurg Psychiatry 37:941-947, 1972
65. Korsgaard S: Baclofen in the treatment of neuroleptic induced tardive dyskinesia. Acta Psychiatr Scand 54:17-24, 1976
66. Kunin RA: Manganese and niacine in the treatment of drug-induced dyskinesia. J Ortho Psych 5:4, 1976
67. Lal S, de la Vega CE, Courkes TL, Friesen HG: Effect of apomorphine on growth hormone, prolactin, luteinizing hormone and follicle stimulating hormone levels in human serum. J Clin Endocrinol Metab 37:719-724, 1973
68. Lal S, Martin JB, de la Vega CE, Friesen HG: Comparison of the effect of apomorphine and L-dopa on serum growth hormone levels in normal men. Clin Endocrinol (OXF) 4:277-285, 1975
69. Lee T, Seeman P, Tourtellotte WW, et al.: Binding of ^{3}H-neuroleptics and ^{3}H-apomorphine in schizophrenic brains. Nature 274:897-898, 1978
70. Lemberger L, Crabtree R, Clemens J: Inhibitory effect of ergoline derivative on prolactin secretion in man. J Clin Endocrinol Metab 39:579-584, 1974
71. Ljungberg T, Ungerstedt U: Evidence that the different properties of haloperidol and clozapine are not explained by differences in anticholinergic potency, in Ljungberg T (ed): Dopaminergic Mechanism Investigated with a New Method of Measuring Specific Behavorial Patterns. Stockholm, Karolinska, 1978
72. MacCallum WAG: Tetrabenazine for extrapyramidal motor disorders. Br Med J 1:760, 1970
73. Marsden CD, Tarsy D, Baldessarini RJ: Spontaneous and drug-induced movement disorders in psychiatric patients, in Benson DF, Blumer D (eds): Psychiatric Aspects of Neurologic Disease. New York, Grune & Stratton, 1975
74. Martin JB, Lal S, Tolis G, Freisen HG: Inhibition by apomorphine of prolactin secretion in patients with elevated serum prolactin. J Clin Endocrinol Metab 39:180-182, 1974

75. Nagy JI, Lee T, Seeman P, et al.: Direct evidence of presynaptic and postsynaptic dopamine receptors in brain. Nature 274:278-281, 1978
76. Norris JP, Sams RE: More on the use of manganese in dyskinesias. Am J Psychiatry 134:1448, 1977
77. O'Flanagan PM: Clonazepam in the treatment of drug induced dyskinesia. Br Med J 1:269-270, 1975
78. Ohye C, Bouchard R, Boucher, R, et al.: Spontaneous activity of the putamen after chronic interruption of the dopaminergic pathway: Effect of L-dopa. J Pharmacol Exp Ther 175:700-708, 1970
79. Owen F, Crow TJ, Pouler M, et al.: Increased dopamine-receptor sensitivity in schizophrenia. Lancet 1:223-226, 1978
80. Pakkenberg H, Fog R, Nilakantan B: The long-term effect of perphenazine enanthate on the rat brain. Some metabolic and anatomical observations. Psychopharmacologia 29:329-336
81. Pandey GN, Garver DL, Tamminga C, et al.: Postsynaptic supersensivity in tardive dyskinesia. Arch Gen Psychiatry 134:518-522, 1977
82. Post RM, Goodwin FK: Time dependent effects of phenothiazines and dopamine turnover in psychiatric patients. Science 190:388, 1975
83. Poursines Y, Alliez J, Toga M: Syndrome Parkinsonien consecutif a' la prise prolongee de chlorpromazine avec ictus mortel intercurrent. Rev Neurol (Paris) 100:745-751, 1959
84. Price TRP, Levin R: Effects of electroconvulsive therapy on tardive dyskinesia. Am J Psychol 135:991, 1978
85. Pryce IG, Edwards H: Persistent oral dyskinesia in female mental hospital patients. Br J Psychiatry 112:983-987, 1966
86. Reda FA, Scanlon JM, Kemp K, et al.: Treatment of tardive dyskinesia with lithium carbonate. New Eng J Med 291:850, 1974
87. Rodova A, Nashunek R: Persistent dyskinesia after phenothiazines. Cesk Psychiatr 60:250-254, 1964
88. Roizin L, True C, Kuigut M: Structural effects of tranquilizers. Res Publ Assoc Res Nerv Ment Dis 37:285-324, 1959
89. Scatton B, Garrett C, Julou L: Acute and sub-acute effects of neuroleptics in dopamine systhesis and release in the rat striatum. Naunyn Schmiedebergs Arch Pharmacol 289:419-434, 1975
90. Selby G; Parkinson's disease, in Vinken B, Bruyn GW (eds): Handbook of Clnical Neurology, vol 6, Diseases of the Basal Ganglia. Amsterdam, Elsevier, 1968, pp 173-211
91. Sigwald J, Banthee D, Raymondeaud C, et al.: Quatre cas de dyskinesia, facio-bucco-linquo-masticatrice a l' evolution prolongee secondaire a un traitment par les neuroleptiphques. Rev Neurol (Paris) 100:751-755, 1959
92. Simpson GM, Branchez MH, Lee HJ, et al.: Lithium in tardive dyskinesia. Pharmakopsychiatr Neuropsychopharmakol 9:76-80, 1976
93. Smith HM, Oswald WT, Kucharski T, et al.: Tardive dyskinesia: Age and sex differences in hospitalized schizophrenics. Psychopharmacologia (Berlin) 58:207-211, 1978
94. Sovner R, Diamascio A: Effect of bentrophine in the rabbit syndrome and tardive dyskinesia. Am J Psych 134:1301-1302, 1977

95. Tamminga C, Smith RC, Pandey G: A neuroendocrine study of supersensitivity in tardive dyskinesia. Arch Gen Psychiatry 34:1199–1203, 1977
96. Uhrbrand L, Faurbye A: Reversible and irreversible dyskinesia after treatment with perphenazine, chorpromazine, reserpine, ECT therapy. Psychopharmacologia 1:408–418, 1960
97. Villeneuve A: Rabbit syndrome—A peculiar extrapyramidal reaction. Can Psychiatr Assoc J 17:69–72, 1972
98. Villeneuve A, Boszormeny Z: Treatment of drug induced dyskinesias. Lancet 1:353–354, 1970
99. Villeneuve A, Lavallee JC, Lemieux CH: Dyskinesie tardive postneuroleptique. Laval Medical 40:832–837, 1969

Commentary

The authors clearly separated tardive dyskinesia, the iatrogenic, drug-induced movement disorder, from other extrapyramidal syndromes that occur in both neurologic and psychiatric patients with and without psychotropic medication. They emphasize that quite different pharmacologic abnormalities underly the various movement disorders and, therefore, equally specific treatments are indicated. By utilizing the distinct clinical picture of tardive dyskinesia and linking this to a specific psychopharmacologic dysfunction, the actors were able to suggest a rational treatment plan. Not all tardive dyskinesia can be controlled totally but the suggestions offered in Chapter 10 provide considerable assistance to the physician faced with treating this disorder. Even more important was the authors' strong emphasis on the importance of prevention through limiting use of neuroleptics to those patients who clearly will benefit and, even in these patients, keeping the dosage to a minimal effective level. Drug-induced movement disorders are such a major problem in psychiatric therapy that it is imperative that radically different treatment plans of the type outlined be instituted.

In a totally different vein and related to the above problem only in that it represents a mixture of neurologic and psychiatric malfunctions, brain trauma is nonetheless a neurobehavoior problem that almost always occupies the borderland between disciplines. Successful neurologic and neurosurgical treatment often produces inadequate results, ostensibly based on psychiatric complications. Psychiatric management of these patients, on the other hand, frequently fails because of "organic" factors. It is the rare individual who doesn't manifest both psychiatric and neurologic symptomatology after significant brain injury. In addition, the almost limitless mix of the areas of the brain that can be affected by trauma produces innumerable, almost random, combinations of neurobehavioral abnormalities. No single finding or group of findings can be considered a key characteristic of brain injury. When the vast breadth of symptomatology caused by brain injury is coupled with the varieties of premorbid personality traits, each brain trauma patient must be recognized as a unique phenomenologic entity. It is no wonder that for years the unsophisticated, cop-out diagnosis of "compensationitis" was offered; the complexities of brain trauma were beyond the knowledge of the day.

Brain injury has long been recognized as a major challenge for medical management but, partially because of the complexity involved, has generated only limited research. Most investigations have centered on finite but inadequate facets such as posttraumatic epilepsy, the treatment of subdural hematoma, and alterations of psychosocial status after brain injury, etc. All investigators agree that psychiatric complications are common and often devastating in the brain injured individual but these problems and the behavioral matrix upon which they appear have proved too diffuse for reliable "scientific" investigation. While offering no simple panacea, Dr. Alexander has put these problems into a meaningful perspective from which better understanding, improved research, and more practical management can be anticipated.

Michael P. Alexander, M.D.

11
Traumatic Brain Injury

Closed head injury is the conventional term for nonpenetrating injury to the head that results in brain dysfunction. While scalp, skull, and facial injuries may be extensive and important, injury to the brain is the most disabling or disturbing consequence of closed head injury. To emphasize the clinical primacy of brain damage the term traumatic brain injury (TBI) will be utilized here. This chapter has several sections: a review of the epidemiology and the pathophysiology of TBI, discussion of the neurobehavioral consequences of minor TBI and the postconcussion syndrome (PCS), and last, a detailed assessment of the neurobehavioral, neuropsychologic, and psychiatric aspects of major injuries. The review of major TBI will consider the course of recovery, the idiosyncracies of behavior in the various stages of recovery, the useful forms of clinical and formal assessment for the various stages, and the prognosis for meaningful recovery.

EPIDEMIOLOGY

Exact data on TBI have been difficult to gather for many reasons: under-reporting of minor injuries, over-reporting of major injuries at large medical centers, deaths before reaching hospitals, etc. There are some surveys, however, that have attempted to document the size of the population which has suffered a TBI. In Scotland, TBI cases constitute almost 10 percent of all emergency room visits[18] with an annual rate of

Table 11-1
Estimated Incidence of Neurologic Disorders

	Incidence	Prevalence
Stroke	200/100,000	
Epilepsy	40/100,000	400–600/100,000
Multiple Sclerosis	2/100,000	30–60/100,000
Parkinson's Disease	18/100,000	170/100,000
Huntington's Disease	0.5/100,000	3–7/100,000
Motor Neuron Disease	1/100,000	5/100,000
Duchenne's Muscular dystrophy	14–28/100,000 (live births)	3/100,000†
Myasthenia Gravis	0.4/100,000	4/100,000
All TBI	200/100,000	439/100,000‡
Severe TBI	20/100,000	Unknown

*Powerful effects of geography
†Total population
‡Measured as hospital admission rates

All figures except TBI from Kurtze JF, Kurland LT. The epidemiology of neurologic disease, in Baker AB, Baker LH (eds): Clinical Neurology, vol 3. Hagerstown, N.Y., Harper & Row, 1973, Ch 48

1775 per 100,000 population. Approximately 50 percent of these emergency room visits occur after 5:00 P.M., and an average of 22 percent are associated with alcohol use. In both Britian[31] and the United States[32] hospital admissions for TBI occur at a rate of about 200 new cases per 100,000 population per year. In the United States, 10 percent of these admissions are for longer than 3 weeks and, if this figure is used as a rough estimate of severe TBI with survival, the incidence of new cases of significant TBI with survival is 20 per 100,000. Table 11-1 allows comparison with the estimated incidences of several well-known neurologic disorders. Overall, men are affected twice as often as women, but in the age group 15–24 years and in cases of motor vehicle accident, men are involved up to four times as often as women. The mortality of severe TBI is 50 percent[18] with most deaths occuring at the scene, in the emergency room, or within 48 hours of admission. TBI accounts for 15-20 percent of all deaths between the ages of 5 and 25 in Scotland.[31]

The total number of hospital admissions for TBI (old and new cases) in the United States in 1974 was 439 per 100,000 population.[32] This statistic emphasizes the total health burden of TBI and suggests that survival after TBI is not the only obstacle which these patients face. The most significant secondary obstacles are the profound effects of TBI upon cognition and behavior.

PATHOPHYSIOLOGY

The literature on the neuropathology of TBI primarily focuses on severe injuries for the obvious reason that few cases with minor head injury die acutely. A short review of the mechanics of brain damage in TBI, however, will provide a pathophysiologic foundation for understanding and anticipating the cognitive deficits to be described below for both minor and major injuries. The various factors which contribute to TBI are outlined in Table 11-2.

Ommaya and Gennarelli have summarized the mechanics of TBI.[48] Experimental evidence has demonstrated that the type of TBI that causes the greatest amount of brain damage is acceleration-deceleration; that is, the head suddenly stops moving usually by striking a solid object. Other types of closed head injury (crush injuries, a heavy item falling on the head, etc.) do not produce as much damage. Acceleration-deceleration movements produce two types of mechanical forces—contact and inertia. Contact events are those which deform the skull, cause skull fracture, and produce direct and contracoup cerebral injury. Inertial forces may be horizontal or rotational depending upon how the head is moving at the time of impact. Horizontal movements of the brain within the decelerating or stopped skull contribute to coup and contracoup lesions which are linearly related to the site and direction of impact. In summary, focal cortical lesions may be anywhere depending on the direction and site of head injury, but the gross rotatory and horizontal brain movements tend to produce cortical contusions in certain predictable sites. Both horizontal and rotary movements of the brain within a fixed skull may cause damage to cortical regions which are adjacent to rough bony surfaces such as the sphenoid wing (anterior temporal lobe) or orbital plate (orbitofrontal areas). Courville demonstrated the remarkably high frequency of brain

Table 11-2
Factors that Contribute to Pathologic Changes in TBI

Direct contact effects
　Contusion underlying the point of trauma (coup)
　Contusion linearly opposite the point of trauma (contracoup)
　Compression from overlying depressed skull fracture
　Compression from overlying hematoma

Inertia effects
　Diffuse impact damage
　　Widespread damage in cerebral white matter
　　Discrete lesions in corpus callosum
　　Discrete lesions in rostral brain stem
　Common cortical contusions independent of direction of impact
　　Orbitofrontal
　　Anterior temporal
　　Frontopolar

Secondary processes
　Secondary cerebral processes
　　Cerebral edema
　　Increased intracranial pressure with central herniation (Duret hemorrhages)
　　Increased intracranial pressure with uncal herniation and posterior cerebral artery entrapment (medial occipital infarction)
　　Multifocal ischemic changes

　Contributing secondary systemic processes
　　Shock (blood loss, ruptured viscera, sepsis, etc.) with hypotension
　　Pulmonary failure with anoxia
　　Long bone fracture with fat emboli

injury in the orbitofrontal, frontopolar, and anterior temporal regions in consecutively autopsied cases of TBI.[17] Ommaya and Genarelli confirmed the high frequency of contusions in those areas in experimental studies.[48] Computerized tomography (CT) scanning has also demonstrated the preponderance of frontal contusions. Clifton et al. demonstrated 64 contusions by CT scan in patients with severe TBI; 56 percent were anterior frontal in location.[16]

Rotational movements also generate gradients of stress within the brain substance. Some areas of brain are relatively free to move while others are not. Shearing forces are produced across the many small boundaries of moving and stationary brain. Widespread microscopic tissue disruption in the white matter results. Careful study of human brains after TBI has defined the areas of white matter most commonly affected.[12] Discrete lesions are seen in the dorsolateral brain stem tegmentum, usually bilaterally, and in the corpus callosum, just off the midline. When the lesions are large, there are grossly visible hemorrhages; most lesions, however, are microscopic. Lesions are also seen diffusely in the white matter; at times there are visible small hemorrhages although the lesions primarily are microscopic. Whether diffuse or focal, the microscopic changes are the same. Early lesions reveal only damaged axons with microhemorrhages; later the lesions show evidence of macrophage activity suggesting the removal of degenerating myelin and axonal structures. The final, stable phase reveals widespread white matter degeneration presumably secondary to diffuse axon disruption. This loss of white matter bulk can often result in marked secondary ventricular enlargement despite the fact that the basic neuropathologic event is a microscopic, albeit widespread, one.[57]

To summarize, the primary mechanics of TBI produce a fairly consistent pattern of brain injury. Cortical lesions may be anywhere but have a propensity for the frontopolar, orbitofrontal and anterior temporal regions. This observation has implications for the behavioral consequences of TBI (Table 11-3). Microscopic white matter lesions are scattered diffusely, but again there is a propensity for certain regions such as the corpus callosum and the brain stem tegmentum. This distribution of lesions also has implications for behavior (Table 11-3).

In addition to the primary contact and inertia forces, there are several secondary processes which may contribute to clinically significant brain injury. Increased intracranial pressure, which may follow contusions and subsequent edema, can cause shifts of the brain from one bony compartment to another. This shift compresses neurologic and vascular structures and produces additional damage. There are two common consequences. First, midline brain stem hemorrhages (Duret hemorrhages) are secondary to downward pressure on the midbrain during tentorial herniation.[1] As downward pressure proceeds, these secondary brain stem hemorrhages develop and produce progressively descending deterioration of brain stem function.[50] Second, compression of the posterior cerebral artery against the edge of the tentorium can produce ischemic injury to the medial occipital region. Unilateral or bilateral infarction in the posterior cerebral artery territories is a common result of sustained increased intracranial pressure with transtentorial herniation. In the autopsy series of Graham et al. 20 percent of cases had medial occipital infarction.[23] CT scanning of survivors also may reveal occipital infarction[33] secondary to tentorial herniation. Medial occipital infarctions may account for some neurologic deficits which would otherwise seem remote from the apparent focus of injury, in particular hemianopia, cerebral blindness, and alexia.

Table 11-3
Anticipated Deficits from Specific Lesions of TBI

Frontopolar contusions*
   Impaired judgment and insight
   Decreased problem solving and reasoning
   Apathy and diminished motivation

Orbitofrontal contusions*
   Impulsivity, excitability
   Impaired social judgment

Anterior temporal contusions
   Memory loss

Brain stem tegmentum lesions
   Loss of consciousness acutely, decreased attention chronically
   Vestibular dysfunction
   Various motor impairments (cerebellar outflow, pyramidal, extrapyramidal)

Diffuse white matter lesions
   Motor impairments?
   Poor cognitive endurance?
   Decreased concentration?

*Reprinted from Blumer D, Benson DF: Personality changes with frontal and temporal lobe lesions, in Benson DF, Blumer D (eds): Psychiatric Aspects of Neurologic Disease. New York, Grune & Stratton, 1975, pp 151–170

Finally, widespread microscopic ischemic lesions have been reported by Graham and co-workers.[23] These small areas of infarction are most prominent at the borderzones between arterial supplies especially the borderzone between anterior cerebral and middle cerebral arteries. Several pathophysiologic events combine to cause these widespread, small infarcts: (1) increased intracranial pressure which may decrease perfusion pressure in distal arterial beds, or (2) intracranial herniations with partial entrapment of blood vessels, combined with diminished systemic perfusion secondary to shock or blood loss, etc.

The above summary of the pathology of TBI is largely applicable to severe injuries, and many of the deficits seen in patients with severe TBI are in part predictable from the sites of damage (see below). Although evidence is sparse, there are data to suggest that the neuropathology of minor TBI also predicts and correlates with the clinical consequences. Oppenheimer[49] studied five patients with mild TBI who died because of various systemic reasons, typically fat emboli from long bone fractures.[49]

The postmortem examination of these patients was particularly helpful because it documented the presence of unequivocal microscopic changes following mild injury, i.e., axonal disruptions throughout the white matter with predilection for the midbrain tegmentum and the corpus callosum. The pathologic changes following mild TBI are qualitatively similar to those following severe TBI exept that cortical contusions are uncommon.

Review of the regions of brain with a high propensity for damage suggests some predictable behavioral consequences (Table 11-3). There are several important features about these observations. First, considerable variation exists between patients in the relative severity of the various components of the TBI. Some patients have extensive cortical contusions with brief loss of consciousness and apparently minor white matter injury; others have the opposite proportion. Each case must be assessed individually. Second, despite the emphasis on typical lesions, many patients have single idiosyncratic focal contusions because of the specific direction of impact in their injuries. Again, each case must be assessed individually. Third, despite the two caveats just listed, most patients with severe TBI do have very similar pathology, and the lesions and resulting behaviors are fairly predictable. Furthermore, these predictable behaviors will underlie whatever unique focal disturbances might also occur.

The last observation about the usual lesions of TBI and the typical behavioral consequences is sufficiently important that it stands alone. The areas of cortical damage following TBI represent the neocortical portions of the limbic system.[46] Traumatic brain injury is one of a very few diseases which routinely damages neocortical limbic areas in a symmetrical fashion while sparing, at least from gross injury, the remainder of the neocortex. There are two important corollaries of the unique limbic distribution of the lesions. First, patients recovering from TBI may have behavioral problems that are enormously out of proportion to other neurologic deficits--a normal neurologic examination does not reflect the degree of behavioral impairment caused by TBI. Second, the symmetrical, bilateral limbic damage may cause profound changes in behavior, affect, and emotion with less significant long-term cognitive impairments; standard neuropsychologic assessment may not reflect the depth of behavioral disorder.

MINOR HEAD INJURY

It is possible that no head injury is minor or totally free of TBI, but certain head injuries are conventionally regarded as minor. The term concussion has been used for these injuries, implying a brief loss or alteration of consciousness with rapid return to normal alertness and no evidence of neurologic dysfunction. Patients with such a clinical history abound. One careful study of all patients admitted to the hospital (the Royal Infirmary, Cardiff, U.K.) for TBI found that 73 percent of the patients who had the level of consciousness recorded were awake at the time of admission;[56] 85 percent of the admitted patients had a duration of unconsciousness less than 1 hour. With minor TBI, the duration of unconsciousness is less than 1 hour and usually less than 10 minutes. Upon awakening, the patient may vomit, have mild gait ataxia, and complain of unsteadiness. These immediate symptoms usually clear over a few hours and the patient returns to normal activities. Although it is clear that such patients can be identified clinically, it is less clear that they have no neurologic damage. As described in the previous section, Oppenheimer demonstrated neuropathologic changes in the brains of patients with concussion.[49]

Postconcussion Syndrome

The most troublesome behavioral sequela of minor TBI is the postconcussion syndrome (PCS), a characteristic cluster of symptoms that may present at the moment of injury or emerge days to weeks later. The symptoms of PCS are headache, dizziness (occasionally vertigo), impaired concentration, faulty memory, irritability, and lack of energy.[43] The elements of the PCS are surely related to the neuropathologic changes of concussion described by Oppenheimer[49] or to damage to peripheral neurologic organs such as the semicircular canals. All serious attempts to demonstrate physiologic dysfunction in patients with PCS have been successful. For instance, Harrison studied 108 patients with concussion; all complained of dizziness and 18 specifically complained of vertigo. Benign positional vertigo (i.e., vertigo induced by sudden changes in head position) was found in 17 patients, including 15 of the 18 patients with vertigo. All patients with vertigo had abnormal caloric testing, but in an unpredictable pattern. Patients with only dizziness recovered in an average of $2^{1}/_{2}$ months; patients with benign positional vertigo remained symptomatic for 1 year on average.[25] Dizziness may be due to damage to the inner ear structures—benign positional vertigo results and recovery may be very slow. There are no findings on examination which document this problem except nystagmus after sudden head movement. Dizziness may also be due to central damage to brain stem vestibular mechanisms—a less specific complaint results and the rate of recovery is unpredictable. White matter damage in the brain stem tegmentum is the presumptive cause of this second variety of dizziness. Rowe and Carlson evaluated 19 patients with minor TBI who had PCS. Electronystagmography (ENG) demonstrated unequivocal vestibular dysfunction in 11 (58 percent), and brain stem auditory evoked potentials (BAEP) were abnormal in 8 (42 percent). Only 21 percent of the patients had both normal BAEPs and ENG.[52] Thus, neurophysiologic methods document significant brain stem dysfunction which routine examination cannot detect.

The other major complaint in the PCS is impaired concentration. Clinical assessment of concentration is extremely primitive and subjective, but when the appropriate tools are used a deficit is readily demonstrated.[24] Using a special test of sustained attention, Gronwall and Wrightson could demonstrate that patients with PCS had a definite impairment in the rate at which a stream of information could be processed. Furthermore, the patient's subjective assessment of improvement paralleled the course of recovery of concentration and attention, as measured by their technique. When objective evidence of normal concentration and attention was obtained, the patient was ready to return to normal mental activities.[24] We believe that the irritability, lack of energy, and poor memory that patients with PCS complain of are secondary to the deficits in concentration. The specific neuropathologic substrate of impaired concentration is unknown, but damage to brain stem tegmentum reticular activating systems seems most probable.

There are individual variations in the PCS which are probably related to small differences in the exact distribution of brain injury.[59] These individual variations and the failure to demonstrate abnormalities with the usual clinical examination should not be construed as evidence that there is psychogenic exaggeration of symptoms. The PCS is a legitimate neurologic syndrome, as surely as torsion dystonia, idiopathic epilepsy, or other disorders in which the neuropathology is not glaring and physiologic measures may not be diagnostic. If the PCS is not complicated by additional psychologic factors, it should clear in 5-10 weeks.[24,25] Physicians may err by encouraging the patient to return to normal activities too soon. The patient may fail and feel anxious or guilty because he has been told that he is recovered. In the early PCS period, the patient should be continually reassured that his disability is understandable and self-limited. The patient should be told that complete recovery will take days to weeks, and he should be encouraged to return to work as he is able, without undue haste. If symptoms persist longer than 5 weeks, ENG and BAEPs should be performed to document continuing physiologic brain stem impairment. If the return to work is unduly delayed, additional psychologic stresses (job security, finances, etc.) may develop. Proper management requires carefully steering the patient's return to normal activities.

Accident Neurosis

The psychologic disturbances which accompany the basic PCS are a real problem. The most common psychologic disturbance has been dubbed accident neurosis.[45] Many of the original assumptions made about this disorder (measuring severity of TBI by presence of a skull fracture, presumed predisposing characteristics, etc.) were incorrect and have been criticized by Taylor.[60] The clinical phenomenon of accident neurosis, however, is certainly real. It is not limited to cases of head injury. Patients with back injury, neck injury, limb fractures, and chronic pain are also at risk for this disorder.[45] The exact frequency of accident neurosis is not known because it is inevitably reported in preselected groups. The symptoms of accident neurosis after head injury are a combination of exaggeration of the PCS and symptoms of depression and anxiety. Examination typically produces a highly dramatic elaboration of physical signs. Regardless of the original cause (head injury, chronic low-back pain, etc.), certain clinical features are common in accident neurosis. First, there is a higher incidence in men, in unskilled workers, and following industrial accidents. Second, there is a high frequency of compensation litigation. Third, there is a very low correlation between the severity of injury and the likelihood of subsequent litigation. In fact, there is a bimodal correlation between injury severity and frequency of claims; the highest incidence of litigation is in the cases with the most severe injuries and in the cases with the least severe injuries.

Long-term follow-up of cases with accident neurosis has been reported by Miller.[45] Most patients settle their claims out of court. The settlement took over 2 years to be reached (in 1960 in England) and was usually paltry given the long disability. Ninety percent of patients were back at work within 2 years after the settlement, and whatever else the settlement resolved, the patients usually stopped visiting physicians. We believe that this syndrome of accident neurosis is very real. It is not unique to minor TBI but, after concussion, probably evolves out of the PCS complaints. It has a psychogenic mechanism and its own clinical course.

Management of minor TBI depends upon the clear recognition of the two distinct disorders outlined above. Arguing that all symptoms after minor TBI are either PCS (the militant neurologic stance) or neurosis (the militant psychiatric stance) fails to recognize that there are two separate syndromes, that one of them is self-limited (PCS) and that the other is potentially preventable (accident neurosis).

Depression

Another important complication of minor TBI is depression. In a review of 200 cases of TBI referred specifically for medical-legal assessment, Miller found accident neurosis in 69 patients and depression in 9; the other patients had only neurologic dysfunction.[45] The depression improved with proper symptomatic treatment, including electroconvulsive therapy (ECT). In an evaluation of patients referred for psychiatric complaints after minor TBI, Merskey and Woodforde found a high frequency of depression (63 percent).[43] The patients complained of headache, dizziness, loss of memory, and loss of energy accompanied by mood depression and vegetative symptoms of depression. The patients in this study were selected on the basis of psychiatric complaints and the absence of any pending litigation. Depression following minor TBI may be a reaction to failure at normal activities in the absence of any obvious neurologic dysfunction. The symptoms may emerge out of and blend imperceptibly with those of PCS. Unlike accident neurosis, there is no dramatic overelaboration of symptoms or signs. The vegetative symptoms and depressed mood should suggest secondary depression. Recovery of depressed patients is usually not complicated by litigation obstacles, as it is in cases of accident neurosis. Recognition of depression and proper treatment (early reassurance and late antidepressants) should result in a favorable outcome.[43,45]

SEVERE TBI

Severe TBIs are defined and rated by either intake or outcome criteria. Intake criteria are the duration of unconsciousness and the duration of amnesia. Outcome criteria are motor and cognitive recovery and return to work or normal activities. The relevance of each of these facets to assessment of TBI deserves attention.

Intake Criteria

Loss of consciousness (coma) is the neurologic sign which identifies patients with TBI, but coma is not a unitary, uncomplicated phenomenon. There are many levels of unconsciousness. Many different neurophysiologic functions are independently altered during coma. Because the duration of coma is the most readily measured effect of TBI, it is essential that it be assessed and rated in a meaningful manner and that clear documentation of the termination of coma be made for every patient. Recognition of the importance of measuring changes in level of coma led Jennett to develop a simple assessment tool for depth of coma, the Glasgow Coma Scale (GCS).[30] This scale is a rating of the comatose patient's best response in three spheres: eye opening, gross motor activity, and verbalization. The scale score has several uses: indication of initial severity, moment-to-moment evaluation of status, determination that coma has cleared, and an evaluation of the return of vigilance, responsive movements, or attempted vocalization.

The period of amnesia (posttraumatic amnesia—PTA) is the time "between injury and the subsequent resumption of normal continuous memory."[65] By necessity this includes the duration of coma and subsequent confusion. The PTA is generally believed to be the single most useful assessment of TBI severity[65] but duration of the PTA is often hard to determine until it is over because the patient may go through a long period with normal responsiveness but impaired memory function.

Outcome Criteria

The outcome criteria of TBI are more difficult to define clearly. Neurologic recovery (hemiparesis, ataxia, cortical blindness, etc.) is straightforward, but less important than cognitive recovery as a determinate of quality of recovery.[7] Cognitive recovery has been defined many ways, including standard psychometric test instruments such as the Wechsler Adult Intelligence Scale (WAIS) and the Wechsler Memory Scale, neuropsychologic batteries, and idiosyncratic collections of cognitive tests. In the section on pathophysiology, the unique neuropathology of TBI was emphasized. Measures of cognition developed for normals (WAIS) or validated on patients with single focal-brain lesions may not provide adequate assessment of the exact nature of impairment of TBI.

Personality measures are also hard to evaluate. Various psychometric tools and psychiatric diagnostic scales have been utilized. Each contributes to our understanding of the problems of the TBI patient, but none describes the total behavioral problem. For that, careful clinical description is probably the most useful instrument.[38] Sociologic measures of severity of TBI have the advantage of being operationally simple—a patient returns home, to work, to normal leisure pursuits, to premorbid social contacts, etc. or he does not.

The Glasgow group have defined five broad categories of outcome—death, chronic vegetative state, severe disability (conscious but dependent in daily care), moderate disability (independent), and good recovery (at premorbid level of functioning).[30] The first two categories are distinct and narrow. The last three categories, however, contain many different levels of functional recovery, and attempts have been made to define more precisely the exact parameters of recovery.

For purposes of this chapter, severe TBI is defined as an injury that produces coma for at least an hour or PTA for at least 1 day. The following will review the stages of recovery from TBI from coma to stable recovery, describe the behavioral characteristics of each stage, and the bedside tests and supplementary evaluations which are appropriate and useful for each stage. An outline of the prognosis for long-term outcome after TBI will follow.

Stages of Recovery

Recovery from traumatic unconsciousness occurs in stages. Following prolonged unconsciousness, the rate of recovery is slow and the stages are easily identified. After brief unconsciousness, recovery may be

Table 11-4
Recovery From Severe TBI

Stage of Recovery	Step of Recovery
1. Coma	1. Restoration of gross wakefulness
2. Unresponsive vigilance	2. Development of purposeful wakefulness
3. Mute responsiveness	3. Recovery of speech
4. Confusional state	4. Resolution of period of PTA
5. Independent in daily selfcare; adequate social interaction	5. Cognitive improvement
6. Independent intellectually	6. Develop normal goal-directed behavior
7. Complete social recovery	

sufficiently prompt that none of the stages are clearly recognized although all probably occur. As outlined in Table 11-4, recovery progresses through the following stages—coma, unresponsive vigilance, mute responsiveness, diminishing confusion, independence in self care, intellectual independence, and full social recovery.[8,19]

Coma, Unresponsive Vigilance

The first two stages will be seen in the neurosurgical unit and although they have few behavioral issues relevant to this chapter, a few comments about evaluation, complications, and prognosis are warranted. As indicated above, the GCS was developed to monitor the course of coma and indicate deterioration that might escape superficial clinical assessment;[30] its clinical usefulness is in the intensive care unit. Even this primitive and early assessment will provide some prognostic information. In a survey of patients with severe TBI, the GCS score at 24 hours had the following correlation with a bad outcome of death or persistent vegetative state.[30] Patients in the highest category of responsiveness had a bad outcome of 6 percent; those in the lowest category had an 80 percent incidence of a bad outcome. Combining the GCS score with assessments of pupillary light response and of extraocular movements to vestibular stimula (calorics or oculocephalic reflexes) produced an overall accuracy of 98 percent in predicting a bad outcome. Neurologists or psychiatrists who first examine the patient at a much later time may still benefit from knowledge of these early measures.

The management issues during coma and unresponsive vigilance are neurosurgical and neurologic. There must be a conscientious search for factors that slow or complicate recovery to normal wakefulness. Examples of such factors are obstructive hydrocephalus,[37] which may be overlooked in a patient who has not recovered consciousness, and intracranial hematomas (epidural, subdural, and intracerebral) with mass effects or cerebral edema, etc. Assessment of coma requires CT scanning, spinal fluid analysis, and electroencephalography (EEG). In a comatose patient with no reversible structural brain lesions, the EEG may provide useful prognostic information. For instance, normal sleep activity (K-complexes, spindles, and slow-wave sleep) recorded during posttraumatic unconsciousness heralds a good recovery.[14]

Mute Responsiveness

When the patient moves into stage three, mute responsiveness, the change may not be immediately obvious. Nurses may report the first changes, i.e., the patient lifts his arm to be positioned, turns his head to avoid washing, grabs the bed rail on command, etc. Establishing this improvement is a challenge to the examiner. One must begin when the patient is rested as responsiveness may initially be fatigueable and intermittent. One should not request an act that might be performed by reflex action, such as squeezing the examiner's fingers. Because, by definition, the patient is not vocalizing at this stage and the level of responsiveness precludes writing, all requests should be for actions that have a high probability of being understood (in case there is an undetectable aphasia) and carried out (in case there is an unsuspected apraxia). Because patients are subject to both aphasia and apraxia,[21] the best tasks are eye movements (i.e., close your eyes, look up, etc.) which may be made more complex (i.e., close your eyes twice, look to the entrance, etc.). All response pathways—eye movements, mouth and face movements and limb movements—should be explored if there is any uncertainty. Typically several clinical parameters improve simultaneously from this point. The reliability and endurance of appropriate responses increase and the patient finally begins to vocalize. Although some patients with very severe TBI plateau at this stage, in our experience, most patients who reach this level, improve further. Bricolo et al. reported a similar experience in patients with very severe TBI (coma longer than 14 days.)[8]

At this stage of recovery, the primary clinical issues are again neurosurgical and the methods of investigation are the EEG and CT scan. The complicating process most difficult to detect at this stage is still obstructive hydrocephalus. In his review of 100 cases with severe TBI, Lewin specifically investigated for secondary hydrocephalus.[37] Twenty-six cases were identified and 12 benefited from surgical treatment. Nine of these cases were in clinical situations that suggested the diagnosis of unequivocal deterioration with increased intracranial pressure or delayed gradual deterioration. Three cases who improved after shunting would not have been suspected clinically. They had simply plateaued at an early stage of recovery. As described in the section on neuropathology, the late effect of diffuse white matter damage may be ventricular enlargment secondary to atrophy of brain structures. This secondary hydrocephalus ex vacuo and obstructive hydrocephalus may have similar CT appearances. Radionuclide cisternography will usually distinguish between the two processes.

The next step in recovery is the return of speech. The major clinical impact of this step is that a more detailed cognitive evaluation is made possible. When the patient is talking, the examiner is able to explore for problems in memory, language, and cognition. At this level of recovery, behavioral issues become the primary focus of management.

Confusional State

The earliest distinctive behavioral syndrome in recovery from severe TBI is the confusional state. Confusion is defined here as an inability to maintain a coherent stream of thought. The major features of the acute confusional state of TBI are listed in Table 11-5. The signs are not unique to trauma but have been described in several settings.[64]

Examination during the confusional state will reveal profoundly abnormal attention, and the staff caring for a confused patient should have a series of bedside tasks that provide easy day-to-day comparisons of attentional mechanisms. Such tasks should be simple yet require sustained attention, i.e., digit span forward and backward, serial subtractions or even merely counting backwards, reciting the months of the year backwards, reciting every third letter of the alphabet, and recognizing lengthy but common words spelled aloud (i.e., hospital), etc. Any member of the staff can give these tests on a regular basis, recording the number of errors and the time needed to complete the task. The results provide a simple clinical measure of diminishing confusion.

In all aspects of mental status testing, deficits in control of attention are prominent. There is difficulty establishing the patient's attention on new tasks, trouble maintaining attention against trivial competing stimuli (distractibility), and, paradoxically, trouble moving attention off of old

Table 11-5
The Early Behavioral Syndrome in Recovery From TBI

Severe attentional disturbance with confusion
Sleep/waking disturbance
Amnesia
Denial of illness
Confabulation
Perseveration

stimuli (perseveration). Abnormal at all times, attention often deteriorates with stress; the patient's confusion and all related signs such as confabulation may worsen as the day progresses or even as a single examination progresses. In our experience, patients with posttraumatic confusional state often have disordered sleep patterns; constant drowsiness and excessive sleeping, nocturnal wakefulness and daytime drowsiness, and constant wakefulness with only short, shallow sleep episodes are the three most common patterns.

During this period of confusion, new memories are not being formed normally; the patient is still in the PTA phase and remains disoriented. Associated disturbances are confabulation and denial of illness. Denial may be awesome; a patient with bilateral hemiparesis, a tracheostomy scar, double vision, a cast on one leg, multiple limb scars, and profound muscular wasting will blandly assert that he knows of no problems requiring hospitalization. The confabulation often has a particular flavor— occupational delirium. The patient will insist that he is in the hospital (or wherever he thinks that he is) to do his premorbid work and will propogate this confabulation wildly to account for the accoutrements of hospitalization.

CASE 1

JN is a 36-year-old radiology technician who suffered a severe TBI with prolonged coma (over 1 week). When examined 1 month later, he stated that he was in the hospital to perform ultrasound procedures on patients, denying that he had any injury. He became distressed that we were ruining his schedule by examining him; asserted that his hospital gown was an x-ray shield, and that it was customary for him to live in the hospital during busy periods.

Several studies have documented that the presence of confabulation and of denial, whatever the etiology, correlates with the severity of the confusion, not simply the presence of amnesia.[55,62]

Beyond attentional deficits and amnesia, the mental status examination may not be profoundly abnormal. Drawing and writing are commonly disturbed but in a manner very characteristic of confusional states,[15] with perseverations, repetitions, and failure to maintain a horizontal line. Reasoning and insight are impaired, as befits a patient who confabulates and denies self-evident infirmity. Within the limits of attention and possibly motor problems, language, praxis and visual discriminations are often intact.

Neuropsychologic testing is often not profitable during this period. Mandleberg has evaluated the effects of the early confusional state with standard psychometric tools (the WAIS).[40] Comparison of patients who were comparable in age but not in length of PTA revealed that, at equal

Traumatic Brain Injury

times after the TBI, patients still in the period of PTA did substantially worse on all WAIS tests than patients whose PTA had ended. This difference on the WAIS was particularly marked on the performance scale (nonverbal tasks). When the two groups were reassessed much later, no significant differences were found between the two groups. The confusional state has a profound impact on cognitive measures, particularly on performance tasks, but the poor performance while confused does not reflect eventual level of recovery.

Management of the confusional state of TBI requires that hospital protocol be adapted to deal with the attentional disturbance of the patient. A quiet room helps to prevent excessive stimulation. When agitation, in particular nocturnal agitation, becomes a problem for the ward, we treat with diphenhydramine HCl, 50–100 mg at bedtime. Standard hypnotics and tranquilizers often increase confusion, but, on occasion, antipsychotic medications are helpful in the management of agitation. One common error in the use of these medications is to use small doses throughout the night. No single dose is large enough to produce sedation, but the cumulative effect leaves the patient sleepy all the next day and even more awake the next night. An alternative dosage regimen is to use a small dose (1 mg of haloperidol, for example) at 6 and 9 PM and midnight. If the patient is not quiet by then, hold further treatment. The next night give 2 mg of haloperidol at 6 and 9 PM and midnight if needed, and so on, establishing the dose necessary to produce sedation at the required hour. It must be emphasized that antipsychotics often are ineffective, that they produce motor and behavioral side effects, and that they are treating a transient although difficult stage in recovery. If possible, behavioral manipulations should be used, i.e., a quiet room as mentioned, an aide or family member to stay with the patient during the night, and prevention of daytime napping, are all helpful measures.

Independent Self Care

As confusion abates, attention improves and sleep-wake cycles normalize, confabulations will diminish, memory will begin to improve, and the patient will achieve some insight into the reason for his hospitalization. During this process of recovery, patients typically become better able to care for their daily needs, often achieve continence of urine, and begin to interact more normally in structured situations. When coherent memories from one day to the next are demonstrated, the PTA is over, and it is reasonable to consider the patient in the next stage of recovery. The characteristics of this middle syndrome are listed in Table 11-6. The major process of the middle syndrome is improvement in cognition.

Table 11-6
The Middle Behavioral Syndrome in Recovery From TBI

Mild attentional disturbance
Improving amnesia
Unconcern about illness
Limited insight and reasoning

Examination early in this state will demonstrate persistently impaired attention with the attributes described previously but at a much milder level. Only the more difficult tasks of concentration will continue to be abnormal. The patient is often approximately oriented, knowing the hospital, the month and year, and some of what he has been told about his TBI, but he will continue to be uncertain about the duration of hospitalization and the interval since the accident. Further assessment of memory is one important part of the mental status examination. Demonstration that the retrograde amnesia (the amnestic gap for events immediately before the TBI) is becoming briefer, requires careful questioning about recent personal and historic events. If done properly, a shrinking retrograde gradient may be seen, i.e., the retrograde gap is progressively filled, beginning with remote memories and moving up to the time of the accident.[5] Whitty and Zangwill have reviewed the other routes which memory improvement may take.[64] The examiner must also be able to evaluate the patient's ability to form new memories. The easiest measures of ongoing memory recovery are taken at the bedside by asking the patient to identify his therapists or to remember a list of three to four words for 3 minutes.

The remainder of the mental status evaluation will reveal persistently poor stamina of cognitive functions; memory and attention may still deteriorate late in the day. Perseveration will be seen at these times. Writing and simple drawings will generally be normal. Reasoning, complex problem solving, and insight remain abnormal. At the bedside, explanation of idiomatic speech (what does it mean to say "warm-hearted," "feel blue," "give a cold shoulder," etc?), proverb interpretation, and multistep mental calculations may all reflect persistent impairment. While frank denial of illness is now uncommon, the patient may be unconcerned, minimize his deficits, and irritably insist on doing things which he cannot do (return to work for instance). Confabulation is uncommon and when it occurs, may have specific significance. As described previously, confabulation is usually seen in patients in confusional states. When this clears but confabulation persists, it is probable that the patient has suffered extensive bilateral anterior frontal lobe injury.[58] To re-emphasize, TBI is virtually unique because cortical lesions often involve limbic regions alone. Persistent extraordinary confabulation may be one unusual syndrome which requires such specific limbic lesions and is much more commonly seen in cases of TBI than any other etiology.

Formal neuropsychologic testing becomes a major tool of assessment at this stage, and much of the literature on TBI deals with the course of neuropsychologic deficits from this stage through total recovery. Much of the available data come from long-term studies in Scotland.[41,42] These investigators have given the WAIS to patients with TBI at intervals up to 2 1/2 years post injury and have compared cognitive outcome, as indicated by the WAIS scores, with an intake criteria of severity—length of coma or length of PTA. They found little correlation between cognitive outcome and PTA duration, although the rate of recovery of cognition was related to PTA duration. They found that the shorter PTA cases had more rapid recovery, but at 6 months post injury there was no effect of PTA on verbal IQ and by 12 months post injury there was no effect on performance IQ. Mandleberg tabulated some of the important cognitive changes that the WAIS scores might overlook[41]—slower rate of problem solving, loss of persistence or other changes in style, and alteration in strategy of problem solving. The long-term studies in Scotland have also included assessment of memory recovery using the Wechsler Memory Scale and various short-term memory tasks.[9-12] These studies found that memory function improves slowly and may continue to improve for well over 1 year after injury, that duration of PTA has a moderate correlation with the eventual outcome of memory function, and that long-term retention (1 hour) is proportionately more difficult for patients with TBI than normals.[11]

Additional neuropsychologic data are available from other sources which confirm and supplement the Scottish studies. Two studies have demonstrated a major disturbance in reaction time in patients with TBI.[44,61] Simple reaction time remains slow after severe TBI, perhaps a reflection of chronic hypoarousal following brain stem injury. Choice reaction time magnifies the impairment after TBI, and the difference from controls increases in proportion to the complexity of the choice to be made before reacting.[44] The choice reaction time correlates with the duration of PTA and with overall outcome at 1 year post injury.[61] These findings indicate that TBI slows decision making and reduces capacity for handling information. These deficits are reminiscent of the more subtle abnormalities found after minor TBI.[24] In a very thorough follow-up of patients with severe TBI, Levin et al. demonstrated that cognitive recovery, as reflected by WAIS scores (particularly the performance IQ), had some correlation with overall social outcome.[36] Likewise, memory function after a recovery period of at least 6 months correlated with overall outcome and remained abnormal in most cases. Finally, Lezak used a more difficult task of verbal memory and demonstrated persistent deficits up to 3 years after injury in 70 percent of cases with severe TBI.[39]

The course of cognitive recovery as reflected in neuropsychologic testing can be summarized as follows. The overlearned material of the verbal IQ scale of the WAIS recovers relatively quickly, and within 6 months the improvement in the verbal IQ begins to plateau. Eventual recovery of the verbal IQ shows no relationship to PTA. The performance IQ scale is more slow to recover and may have a closer correlation with the PTA.[36] Memory function improves even more slowly, and on tests of sufficient subtlety remains significantly impaired.[39] Information processing and decision making apparently never return to normal and probably are good indicators of the severity of injury.[44]

Neurologic and neurosurgical complications are uncommon in the later stages of recovery from TBI. Failure to improve or stalling at a premature plateau may be signs of an underlying reversible structural disorder in the early stages of recovery. When hydrocephalus or intracranial hemorrhages occur later in recovery, the course is more likely to be deterioration in neurologic or cognitive status. The signs of these structural lesions may not be those that are anticipated in "typical" cases with hydrocephalus or subdural hematomas in whom there is no underlying brain disease. For example, in a patient who already has cognitive changes, ataxic gait and incontinence because of the primary TBI—the typical triad-gait disorder, incontinence, and dementia—may not trigger consideration of the diagnosis of hydrocephalus. In the setting of TBI, we have seen hydrocephalus present as an increase in confabulation, sudden muteness, increased tone in the legs, and other unusual ways. Any deterioration in neurologic or cognitive status may signal development of a structural disturbance.

Management of this period of improving cognition does not usually require medication. The patient is better able to process multiple stimuli and may benefit from having a roommate, attending patient group meetings, and working on cognitive tasks. Judgment, reasoning, memory, concentration, and mental endurance are improving but not normal. The improvement in daily activities, when compared to the earlier confusional state, is so profound that many families and staff overestimate the patient's capacities at this middle stage. Hospital personnel and family members must attend to the patient's performance to prevent overstimulation. Also, performance failures secondary to fatigue might excite or discourage the patient. The patient is usually ready for discharge from the rehabilitation unit during this middle period of recovery. Patients who plateau within this phase of recovery will usually be independent in all daily tasks, will function well in structured situations, and will be safe at home alone. They are often not able to return to work.

Intellectual Independence

The next level of recovery from severe TBI is difficult to define exactly. The major issues are behavior, personality, and cognitive style. Recovery in these areas progresses simultaneously with cognitive improvement, but the residual disturbances in personality are long lasting, more difficult to objectively assess, and often most troubling to family members. The basic elements of the late behavioral syndrome are listed in Table 11-7.

The clinical mental status examination at this stage of recovery is often unremarkable. The tests of concentration listed previously will usually be normal. Memory assessment will demonstrate the amnestic gap (short retrograde amnesia and longer posttraumatic amnesia) and variable amounts of ongoing disturbance in forming new memories. The patients, however, often complain of being forgetful despite examination showing near normal mental status. More complex tasks of problem solving, strategy formation, and behavior modification are often still abnormal, but these tasks are usually not part of a bedside assessment. Motivation and interest in life seem blunted, and affect is often flat and unconcerned. The families often complain that the patient is unreasonable and irritable when pushed to perform daily activities.

Standard psychometric instruments show a plateau of improvement, but sufficiently sensitive tasks will still demonstrate unequivocal impairments. A carefully directed, clinically skilled neuropsychologic assessment at this point in recovery is one of the most useful interventions that can be made for the patient with TBI. Such an assessment will demonstrate subtle objective problems and outline the specific disturbances in higher level processes which impede the patient's final recovery.[63] Behavioral impairments are rarely seen in isolation after TBI; an adequate, detailed cognitive assessment will always reveal parallel intellectual deficits. For example, the "behavior" of apathy is paralleled by the cognitive impairment of failure to generate strategies to solve problems, disturbed concentration, and thus poor problem solving. These cognitive changes are not incompatible with an apparently normal IQ.

Table 11-7
The Late Behavorial Syndrome in Recovery From TBI

- Impaired concentration
- "Forgetfulness"
- Apathy
- Irritability
- Limited insight and reasoning
- Personality change

The personality changes of TBI are often profound. Lezak has described them as "characterologic" which is appropriate given the thorough alteration in behavior which they produce.[38] Lezak's tabulation of the elements of the personality change reflects our experience. Patients are unable to assess the impact of their illness upon others and thus seem to have no consideration for their families. They have reduced ability to monitor and control their behaviors and may then be impulsive and irritable. They have trouble analyzing and anticipating changes in their lives and thus seem to have decreased motivation, organizational and planning skills, and they become unnecessarily dependent upon others. They do not learn effectively from their own experience, and therefore these behaviors are often very persistent. Finally, emotional changes commonly accompany these personality changes; apathy, fatuousness, lability, and irritability are the most common.[38]

Attempts to quantify these behavioral changes have been made, but have generally not been very helpful. Levin and Grossman have studied 70 patients with a multiscale psychiatric rating instrument.[34] The resulting enumeration of psychiatric problems appears related to neurologic disturbances: conceptual disorganization, motor retardation, blunted affect, disorientation, etc. There was an increase in these kinds of disturbances with increasing severity of injury, but there was no certainty about the nature of the disturbance being measured. Analysis of a report by Levin et al. on patients with very severe TBI again demonstrated an increase in "psychiatric" deficits in the more severely injured cases, but the essence of the deficits was clearly cognitive.[36] For instance, signs of thought disorder were distractibility, tangentiality, and denial; signs of withdrawal behaviors were motor slowing and apathy. For the reasons outlined earlier, it is improbable that any instrument used to evaluate cases of TBI but validated on normals will provide useful insight into the abnormal brain mechanisms of TBI. Levin et al. clearly recognized that they were describing neurologically determined behaviors which characterize the patient with severe TBI, but these tests may be misleading to naive readers who really believe that a "psychiatric" disorder is being demonstrated.[36]

The characterologic behavior changes described above are similar to classic frontal lobe signs.[63] This resemblance may have an anatomic explanation, i.e., the very high frequency of frontal cortical contusions in TBI. It may also be that diffuse white matter damage causes these behavioral changes through mechanisms as yet undetermined. The proper management of the behavior problems described in this section is unknown. Whether the behaviors are attributed to frontal injury, diffuse injury, or a combination of both, little is known about prevention or management of personality change after severe TBI. In many patients, the behavioral changes slowly improve in a responsive setting of work and home, and

Traumatic Brain Injury

these patients, even if not exactly as they were before, can be considered to have made a complete recovery.

Post Traumatic Aphasia

There are three miscellaneous elements of recovery from severe TBI that should be briefly discussed before concluding—aphasia, epilepsy, and reactive depression. Patients with severe TBI often have abnormal language; usually the abnormality is limited to content (confusion, confabulation, perseveration, etc.) and not linguistic structure. Severe TBI, however, may produce a true language disturbance. When there is gross focal contusion or hemorrhage in the left hemisphere language zone, aphasia will result. In some patients there are language problems in the absence of any obvious focal lesion. Heilman et al. described 13 patients with TBI who had significant aphasia (out of 750 cases of TBI).[26] All 13 patients had fluent aphasia; 9 had anomic aphasia and 4 had Wernicke's aphasia, and several patients were alexic (see Benson[6] for a review of these syndromes). Analysis of the location of associated skull fractures suggested that either coup (left temporal fracture) or contracoup (right frontal fracture) injury to the left temporoparietal region produced the aphasia. Levin et al. approached the problem slightly differently. They methodically assessed language in 50 patients with TBI, none apparently clinically aphasic. The disturbance in language was related to the severity of the injury, not the site of injury. Traditional aphasic syndromes (Broca's and Wernicke's) were not seen. Impairment on the Token test was the most sensitive measure, and anomia was the most common disturbance.[35] Our experience supports these complementary observations. Patients with TBI often have word finding difficulties which are proportionate to their other cognitive deficits. Impairment on the Token test is probably in large measure due to posttraumatic confusion not to language disturbance. When a true aphasic syndrome occurs, it is almost always a fluent aphasia (anomic or Wernicke's) and many patients will have a left temporal contusion or hematoma on CT scan. Finally, we have seen three patients with severe TBI who have had pure alexia following prolonged coma.[6] CT scan demonstrated left occipital infarction secondary to left posterior cerebral artery entrapment during uncal herniation. Nonetheless, true aphasia is uncommon (1.7 percent of the cases of Heilman et al.[26]).

Posttraumatic Epilepsy

TBI may result in the development of epilepsy. There are two facets to posttraumatic epilepsy—early and late seizures. The exact incidence of both is uncertain, but data from the Mayo Clinic indicates that 2.1 percent of cases of TBI will have a seizure within the first week (early epilepsy) and that 1.9 percent will have a seizure at some point after the first week (late epilepsy).[3] Jennett has provided the best description of the characteristics of these two classes of seizures.[29] Early epilepsy is often focal (sensory or motor) and usually reflects the acute brain injury. About a quarter of these cases will also develop late seizures. Late epilepsy may take many forms, but complex partial seizures are common.[29] Patients with complex partial seizures may develop behavioral problems secondary to the seizure disorder,[4] and these problems complicate the posttraumatic behavioral disorder. The elements of the interictal behavioral syndrome of temporal lobe epilepsy are described elsewhere.[4] In brief, they are overinclusiveness (circumstantial speech, hypergraphia, and meticulousness), emotional intensity (hyperreligiosity, profound moralism, and aggressivity), and hyposexuality. The treatment of the interictal personality of temporal lobe epilepsy is not known. Anticonvulsants which control the seizures do not affect personality.

Reactive Depression

Patients with TBI are often young, often recover to a considerable extent, and most remember their past capabilities. Many are unconcerned about the change which has occured, but often as they improve, a reactive depression develops. The diagnosis of depression in the TBI population is difficult. Standard psychiatric rating tools are probably not adequate (see above). Some apathetic, unmotivated patients will admit to being depressed if asked directly, but do not complain spontaneously, have no vegetative signs, and are unable to formulate causes of their depression. Operationally, we accept a diagnosis of reactive depression in patients who spontaneously describe depressed mood, whose behavior reflects depression, and who demonstrate insight into the reasons for their depression. Patients with cognitive impairment whose alleged depression is only seen as a response to a direct stimulus are not considered depressed. We have had no success treating either category of patient with traditional antidepressants. Return to normal activities has been the best treatment.

Long-Term Outcome

The conclusion of this chapter should be a brief discussion of the eventual outcome of patients with severe TBI. Information about outcome depends on several factors, such as the severity of TBI included for study, the type of hospital at which the study is made (acute or rehabilitation), and the length of follow-up. Very few studies address exactly the same outcome question with the same parameters, and outcome conclusions require consolidation of data from several complementary sources.

There are four representative outcome studies of patients with severe TBI, selected on the basis of the duration of coma. The selection criterion varied from coma of at least 6 hours[30] to coma of at least 1 month.[37] All four studies began with the acute hospitalization. Several conclusions about outcome emerge from this wealth of data. First, mortality is high (35–50 percent), and most deaths occur early in hospitalization. Late deaths are usually secondary to complications such as pneumonia or sepsis.[8] A small percentage of patients remain in a persistent vegetative state. About 25–30 percent of survivors remain permanently severely disabled and dependent.[27,30] Of the remainder of the survivors about half have persistent moderate disability with dependence on others for some aspects of daily living or support, and the other half have essentially full recovery and return to premorbid activities.

Further delineation of the outcome of severe TBI comes from study of survivors only or from long-term follow-up of admissions to rehabilitation units. Two small but intensive follow-up studies of survivors of severe TBI reach similar conclusions.[20,44] Most patients eventually return to work and fairly normal activities—12 of 27 in one report with relatively brief follow-up;[44] and 19 or 23 in another with 6 years follow-up.[20] Cognitive deficits are common and provide the major obstacles to re-employment and the greatest distress to family members. Family strains and social withdrawal occur with high frequency. Oddy and Humphrey analyzed the effect of TBI on the social fabric with a 2-year follow-up of 54 patients selected by a criterion of PTA greater than 1 day.[47] Sixty-seven percent returned to work at 6 months and 82 percent by 12 months. Both physical and cognitive deficits influenced the return to work. Twenty-four percent of those patients working had problems with the work; these patients had demonstrably greater cognitive impairment. Social contacts were also decreased in patients with significant cognitive deficits. Family strains were often noted. Sibling conflicts were more common than child-parent conflicts. Family strains were more serious in the families with patients who had profound personality change. Patients with severe personality change after TBI are often displaced from the family and home. They gravitate to chronic psychiatric institutions where they may constitute a sizeable minority of patients with chronic "organic brain syndrome" (7 percent in a review at one such hospital[53]).

Gilchrist and Wilkinson reviewed their experience with severe TBI in a rehabilitation hospital.[22] Their patients were last evaluated from 1 to 15 years after discharge. Eighteen percent were institutionalized, 38 percent were home but inactive, 13 percent were home and working at a downgraded level, and 26 percent were engaged in fully normal activities.

From various portions of these three different types of studies (all acute hospitalizations, acute hospital survivors, and rehabilitation admissions), several generalizations can be made. Age at TBI is not a factor in survival of the primary brain injury itself, but increasing age increases mortality from secondary complications.[8] Age does not affect duration of coma,[13] but age has a powerful effect on recovery. There is a decreasing quality of survival with increasing age, particularly over age 60.[27] Duration of coma and of PTA also predict the final outcome, although not in an absolutely stratified manner.[36] Very few patients in coma for more than 1 month achieve full recovery.[37] Premorbid personality disorders adversely affect the quality and extent of recovery.[22,47]

The outcome in children with severe TBI is not greatly different than in adults. Cognitive deficits are the major factor that limit recovery, and the worst problems are persistent memory loss and behavior change.[28,51,54] About half of the survivors are able to return to school without adaptation. Overall level of recovery is roughly proportional to severity of injury as measured by PTA.

There are distressingly few concrete management suggestions that can be made for patients who have recovered to a stable plateau after TBI. The three major problems that remain after recovery are cognitive deficits, behavior change, and social disruption. No proved method of cognitive retraining exists, and research is desparately needed in this area. The behavior changes after severe TBI are poorly managed by standard psychiatric methods and medications. Social and vocational agencies established to deal with the problems of cerebral palsy, mental retardation, stroke, or physical disability fail to meet the specific needs of the patient with severe TBI. TBI remains a field where diagnosis and description far exceed management and rehabilitation.

SUMMARY

In this chapter, we have reviewed the epidemiology and pathophysiology of TBI. Many of the deficits which are seen following TBI are predictable from a knowledge of the characteristic pathology. We have reviewed the problems of the minor TBI; the PCS and secondary accident neurosis, both extremely common problems, are perhaps the most common neurologic disorders other than migraine headaches. We have reviewed the course, the evolution of typical recovery patterns, the range of outcomes, the clinical assessment and management of severe TBI, and the usual behavioral sequelae of TBI. Our emphasis has been on behavioral residua with little attention to the other neurologic problems which are well reviewed elsewhere.[31] Neurologists, neurosurgeons, psychologists, and psychiatrists will find that their interests meet over the problems of the patient with TBI, and all involved must have an organized approach to the behavioral problems unique to TBI.

REFERENCES

1. Adam JH: The neuropathology of head injuries, in Vinken PJ, Bruyn GW (eds): Handbook of Clinical Neurology, vol 23, part 1. Amsterdam, Elsevier, 1975, pp 35-65
2. Adams JH, Mitchell DE, Graham DI, Doyle D: Diffuse brain damage of immediate impact type. Brain 100:489-502, 1977
3. Annegers JF, Grabow JD, Groover RY, et al.: Seizures after head trauma: A population study. Neurology 30:683-689, 1980
4. Bear D, Fedio P: Quantitative analysis of interictal behavior in temporal lobe epilepsy. Arch Neurol 34:454-467, 1977
5. Benson DF, Geschwind N: Shrinking retrograde amnesia. J Neurol Neurosurg Psychiatry 30:539-544, 1967
6. Benson DF: Aphasia, Alexia, and Agraphia. New York, Churchill Livingstone, 1979
7. Bond MR: Assessment of psychosocial outcome after severe head injury, in Porter R, Fitzsimons DW (eds): Outcome of Severe Damage to the Central Nervous System (Ciba Foundation Symposium 34). Amsterdam, Elsevier, 1975, pp 141-157
8. Bricolo A, Turazzi S, Feriotti G: Prolonged post-traumatic unconsciousness. J Neurosurg 52:625-634, 1980
9. Brooks DN: Recognition memory and head injury. J Neurol Neurosurg Psychiatry 37:794-801, 1974
10. Brooks DN: Long- and short-term memory in head injured patients. Cortex 11:329-340, 1975
11. Brooks DN: Wechsler Memory Scale performance and its relationship to brain damage after severe head injury. J Neurol Neurosurg Psychiatry 39:593-601, 1976
12. Brooks DN, Aughton ME, Bond MR, et al.: Cognitive sequelae in relationship to early indices of severity of brain damage after severe blunt head injury. J Neurol Neurosurg Psychiatry 43:529-534, 1980
13. Carlsson CA, von Essen C, Loegren J: Factors affecting the clinical course of patients with severe head injuries. J Neurosurg 29:242-251, 1968
14. Chatrian GE, White LE, Daly D: Electroencephalographic patterns resembling those of sleep in certain comatose states after injuries to the head. Electroencephalogr Clin Neurophysiol 15:272-280, 1963
15. Chedru F, Geschwind N: Writing disturbances in acute confusional state. Neuropsychologia 10:343-353, 1972
16. Clifton GL, Grossman RG, Makela ME, et al.: Neurological course and correlated computerized tomography findings after severe closed head injury. J Neurosurg 52:611-624, 1980

17. Courville CB: Pathology of the Central Nervous System. Mountain View, California, Pacific, 1937, part 4
18. Editorial: Head injuries—from Accident Department to Necropsy Room. Lancet 1:589-591, 1978
19. Eson ME, Yen JK, Bourke RS: Assessment of recovery from serious head injury. J Neurol Neurosurg Psychiatry 41:1036-1042, 1978
20. Fahy TJ, Irving MH, Millac P: Severe head injuries. Lancet 3:475-479, 1967
21. Geschwind N: The apraxias: Neural mechanisms of disorders of learned movements. Am Sci 63:188-195, 1975
22. Gilchrist E, Wilkinson M: Some factors determining prognosis in young people with severe head injuries. Arch Neurol 36:355-359, 1979
23. Graham DI, Adams JH, Doyle D: Ischemic brain damage in fatal non-missile head injuries. J Neurol Sci 39:213-234, 1978
24. Gronwall D, Wrightson P: Delayed recovery of intellectual function after minor head injury. Lancet 2:605-609, 1974
25. Harrison MS: Notes on the clinical features and pathology of postconcussional vertigo, with especial reference to positional nystagmus. Brain 79:474-482, 1956
26. Heilman KM, Safran A, Geschwind N: Closed head trauma and aphasia. J Neurol Neurosurg Psychiatry 34:265-269, 1971
27. Heiskanen O, Sipponen P: Prognosis of severe brain injury. Acta Neurol Scand 46:343-348, 1970
28. Heiskanen O, Kaste M: Late prognosis of severe brain injury in children. Dev Med Child Neurol 6:11-14, 1974
29. Jennett B: Early traumatic epilepsy. Lancet 1:1023-1025, 1969
30. Jennett B: Predictors of recovery in evaluation of patients in coma. Adv Neurol 22:129-135, 1979
31. Jennett B, Teasdale G: Management of Head Injuries. Philadelphia, Davis, 1981, Ch 1
32. Kalsbeck WD, McLaurin RL, Harris BSH, Miller JD: The National Head and Spinal Cord Injury Survey: Major Findings. J Neurosurg 53:519-531, 1980
33. Keane JR: Blindness following tentorial herniation. Ann Neurol 2:186-191, 1980
34. Levin HS, Grossman RG: Behavioral sequalae of closed head injury. Arch Neurol 35:720-727, 1978
35. Levin HS, Grossman RG, Kelly PJ: Aphasic disorder in patients with closed head injury. J Neurol Neurosurg Psychiatry 39:1062-1070, 1976
36. Levin HS, Grossman RG, Rose JE, Teasdale G: Long-term neuropsychological outcome of closed head injury. J Neurosurg 50:412-422, 1979
37. Lewin W: Changing attitudes to the management of severe head injuries. Br Med J 2:1234-1239, 1976
38. Lezak MD: Living with the characterologically altered brain injured patient. J Clin Psychiatry 39:592-598, 1978
39. Lezak MD: Recovery of memory and learning functions following traumatic brain injury. Cortex 12:63-72, 1976

40. Mandleberg IA: Cognitive recovery after severe head injury, 2. J Neurol Neurosurg Psychiatry 38:1127-1132, 1975
41. Mandleberg IA: Cognitive recovery after severe head injury. J Neurol Neurosurg Psychiatry 29:1001-1007, 1976
42. Mandleberg IA, Brooks DN: Cognitive recovery after severe head injury, 1. J Neurol Neurosurg Psychiatry 38:1121-1126, 1975
43. Merskey H, Woodforde JM: Psychiatric sequelae of minor head injury. Brain 95:521-528, 1972
44. Miller E: Simple and choice reaction time following severe head injury. Cortex 6:121-127, 1970
45. Miller H: Accident neurosis. Br Med J 1:919-925, 1961
46. Nauta WJH: The problem of the frontal lobe: A reinterpretation. J Psychiatr Res 8:167-187, 1971
47. Oddy M, Humphrey M: Social recovery during the year following severe head injury. J Neurol Neurosurg Psychiatry 43:798-802, 1980
48. Ommaya AK, Gennarelli TA: Cerebral concussion and traumatic unconsciousness. Brain 97:633-654, 1974
49. Oppenheimer DR: Microscopic lesions in the brain following head injury. J Neurol Neurosurg Psychiatry 31:299-306, 1968
50. Plum F, Posner JB: The Diagnosis of Stupor and Coma, ed 2. Philadelphia, Davis, 1972, Ch 1
51. Richardson F: Some effects of severe head injury. Dev Med Child Neurol 5:471-482, 1963
52. Rowe MJ, Carlson C: Brainstem auditory evoked potentials in postconcussion dizziness. Arch Neurol 37:679-683, 1980
53. Seltzer B, Sherwin I: "Organic brain syndromes:" An empirical study and critical review. Am J Psychiatry 135:13-21, 1978
54. Shaffer D, Chadwick O, Rutter M: Psychiatric outcome of localized head injury in children, in Porter R, Fitzsimons DW (eds): Outcome of Severe Damage to the Central Nervous System (Ciba Foundation Symposium 34). Amsterdam, Elsevier, 1975, pp 191-213
55. Shapiro BE, Alexander MP, Gardner H, Mercer B: Mechanisms of confabulation. Neurology 31(9):1070-1076, 1981
56. Steadman JH, Graham JG: Head injuries: An analysis and follow-up study. Proc R Soc Med 63:23-28, 1970
57. Strich SJ: The pathology of severe head injury. J Neurol Neurosurg Psychiatry 19:163-185, 1956
58. Stuss DT, Alexander MP, Lieberman A, Levine H: An extraordinary form of confabulation. Neurology 28:1166-1172, 1978
59. Symonds C: Concussion and its sequelae. Lancet 1:1-5, 1962
60. Taylor AR: Post-concussional sequelae. Br Med J 3:67-71, 1967
61. Van Zomeren A, Deelman BG: Long-term recovery of visual reaction time after closed head injury. J Neurol Neurosurg Psychiatry 41:452-457, 1978
62. Victor M, Adams RD, Collins GH: The Wernicke-Korsakoff Syndrome. Philadelphia, Davis, 1971
63. Walshe KW: Neuropsychology. Edinburgh, Churchill Livingstone, 1978

64. Weinstein EA, Kahn RL: Denial of Illness. Symbolic and Physiological aspects. Springfield, Ill., Charles C. Thomas, 1955.
65. Whitty CWM, Zangwill OL: Traumatic amnesia, in Whitty CWM, Zangwill OL (eds): Amnesia, ed 2. London, Butterworths, 1977, pp 118-135

Commentary

Chapter 11 presented a clinically based outline of the neurobehavioral residua of brain trauma. The approach was almost entirely phenomenologic and carefully avoided attempts to quantitate the degree of the various mental disabilities. The literature of the past few years contains a number of quantitative studies of brain injury; almost without exception, however, the demand for finite, enumerable items has produced limited, distorted, and in some instances even dishonest results. The complex mixture of neurologic, mental, and psychiatric factors that make up the true picture of traumatic brain injury have been sacrificed to meet the limitations of the computer/statistician. Data of interest to an actuarial statistician are available, but the entire picture must be considered if the brain injured patient is to be helped. Initial understanding of the multifactorial problem must be based on a phenomenologic structure of the type presented by Dr. Alexander. From this chapter it is evident that not only are many facets of TBI treatable but, that for success, each facet must be treated in the context of the entire problem, not as the sole disturbance. The residua of brain injury are not easy to manage, but the information in this chapter has provided an excellent structure to aid the clinician.

One of the most common consequences of head trauma is the impairment of memory function called amnesia. The specific constellation of memory disturbances called amnesia can also be seen in many other clinical states, however. Memory disturbances have been studied for well over a century,[2] and great strides have been made in the study of memory in the past several decades. Much memory research has been limited to formal, academic studies that led to and/or support a variety of information and learning theories. Unfortunately, these studies offer comparatively little of practical importance for the physician charged with management of a patient with amnesia. Even in recent years, when there has been a surge of psychologic studies investigating amnesic patients, most of the emphasis has centered on theories of memory. During this time, however, clinicians and neuropathologists have been reporting their own findings on patients with memory dysfunction and have developed a solidly based theory of the neural function underlying memory.[1] In addition, the phenomenology of the type of amnesia associated with brain abnormality is sharply different from psychogenic amnesia. The next chapter will review current thoughts about the neurologic basis of memory impairment and from this base ideas regarding therapy can be developed.

REFERENCES

1. Brierly JB: The neuropathology of amnesic states, in Whitty CWM, Zangwill OL (eds): Amnesia. New York, Appleton-Century-Crofts, 1966, pp 150–180
2. Ebbinghaus H: Memory—A Contribution to Experimental Psychology. New York, Dover, 1964

D. Frank Benson, M.D.
Dietrich Blumer, M.D.

12
Amnesia: A Clinical Approach to Memory

Disturbances of memory produce a serious clinical problem. As a pure disturbance, memory disorders are neither common nor rare and are seen regularly by all practitioners caring for individuals with neurologic and psychiatric problems. Most often, the memory disturbance is part of a complex mixture of organic and/or psychogenic problems and is often difficult to isolate from the other components. To recognize the presence and seriousness of the memory disturbance, the clinician must have a clear picture of memory function and the signs of its disturbance in the comparatively pure state. Memory disturbance in this state is called amnesia.

DEFINITIONS

Amnesia can be defined rather simply as "a loss of the ability to form memories despite an alert state of mind."[1] Another definition merely says that amnesia is "a loss or impairment of memory functions secondary to cerebral malfunction."[7] Amnesia is a clinical condition and, as such, rather rigid operational qualities can be assigned. All definitions, however, depend ultimately on the meaning of the word memory, a complicated term, and before presenting a clinical definition of amnesia, some discussion of memory is indicated.

Memory is a frequently used word, having many different contexts and through the years a number of quite different meanings have developed. Most commonly, memory refers to reminiscences, particularly the events of earlier life that are recalled. "Memories" describe important lifetime events that are remembered. In a more selected usage, many think of memory with a Freudian implication. Alterations of memory function such as suppression, sublimation, and repression are major building blocks of the psychoanalytic theories. This work has so thoroughly infiltrated 20th Century thinking that most educated persons have some realization of memory distortion based on the Freudian theories.

In a more scientific manner, memory has been described as a function that could be altered by neurosurgical stimulation or ablation.[50] Based on clinical-physiologic studies, a memory was considered an engram, an individual bit of information stored in the brain, and these neurosurgical studies even suggested a specific storage area for memories in the temporal lobe.[51] From a totally different scientific approach, discussion of memory arose from the behavior of lower animal forms (planaria and mice were most popular) whose behavior was altered through ingestion or injection of a "knowledge enriched" media. Thus, a planarian that ingested material from another planaria already trained in the running of a maze appeared superior at learning the maze and the possibility that stored "memories" were transferred in this manner was suggested and explored in a number of animals.[40,41]

There is also a vast psychologic literature on memory, much of it focused on mountains of data that detail supraspan learning, the effects of primacy, interference, and other conditions that affect the learning of new material. Unfortunately, while of considerable theoretical interest, the psychologic approaches to memory, with a few notable exceptions, have not proved particularly helpful to the physician studying an individual with amnesia.

Physicians have developed some fairly sharp demarcations of memory functions over the years. These divisions are test-dependent to a considerable extent although they seem to fit both clinical and psychologic parameters and, as will be demonstrated, can be loosely correlated with the neuroanatomy, the neuropathology, and, quite probably, the neurophysiology of memory. For clinical purposes, memory can be divided into three distinct aspects. These have been given many different names over the years but for the purposes of this chapter will be called (1) immediate recall; (2) the ability to learn new material; and (3) the ability to retrieve previously learned information.

Immediate recall refers to the ability to reproduce, with total accuracy, information that has just been received. This has been called by a number of different names including primary memory,[60] short-term memory,[18,64] and immediate memory, etc. One distinct feature of this function is that the demand for extreme accuracy in recall limits the quantity of material that can be handled. It is better to refer to this function as immediate recall, not immediate memory or short-term

Amnesia

memory, as the information is not put into permanent storage (memorized) in this step. In fact, most of the information handled in this stage never enters storage to become a memory. Nonetheless, the ability to maintain a reasonable amount of information very accurately, even if only for a short period of time, is an essential initial step in the process of memory.

The ability to learn new material is the active step of learning; this is the act of memorizing, of putting something into memory store. This function also has been given many other names including recent memory and short-term memory. Some psychologists refer to this process as the selection and registration of information and also call this step consolidation of information. It appears probable that only a small portion of the information continuously entering the nervous system, and temporarily held in the immediate recall stage, actually enters the storage system to be held in memory. This process is complex and can be subdivided into a number of separate steps,[33] but for clinical purposes the entire process can be considered a single activity accurately defined as the ability to learn new material.

The retrieval of old, learned information has also been given many different names such as remote memory, long-term memory, and fund of information, etc. This function refers to the individual's ability to recollect information learned in the past. There is an obvious point of overlap between the ability to learn new material and the ability to retrieve this information, an overlap that can cause confusion in the evaluation of a memory defect. It seems certain, however, that these are different functions as demonstrated clinically by patients who have one function seriously impaired while the other remains normal or near normal.

While admittedly simplified, the division of memory into these three distinctly different functions greatly aids in understanding amnesia and allows development of an operational definition. The following four specific features should be present in each case that is to be called *amnesia.*

1. Immediate recall. The status of the immediate recall function must be normal or at very near normal levels. Any distinct abnormality of immediate recall renders it almost impossible to make a diagnosis of amnesia as the patient will be in a confusional state and the examiner cannot be certain that information is being held long enough to be learned.
2. Learning ability. In amnesia there is a serious impairment of learning. This is the prime clinical feature and must be present for a diagnosis of amnesia. Difficulty in learning alone, however, is not a sufficient criterion and two additional features must be considered.

3. Retrieval. The ability to retrieve old, overlearned information must be normal or at near normal levels for a diagnosis of amnesia. There is one important exception, however. Information learned in the recent past (usually a period of several years) will not be retrieved as well as material learned many years before the onset of amnesia, a condition called *retrograde amnesia*.

4. Cognitive function and personality. These two important behavioral functions should be normal or near normal for a diagnosis of amnesia. Significant abnormality in either suggests a more widespread disturbance (dementia).

It can be seen that amnesia is a specific clinical syndrome featuring good immediate recall, severe disturbance in the ability to learn, comparatively normal ability to retrieve old information, plus relatively normal cognitive and personality functions. A different use of the term amnesia is common, however, and deserves recognition. Many individuals, both professional and lay, use amnesia to designate the period of time during which new memories were not laid down, a blank in the patient's bank of ongoing memories. Thus, amnesia can refer to either the active disturbance of the learning process (the four criteria above) or the period in the past in which this disturbance occurred. While amnesia may refer to either the ongoing abnormality or the residua of this disturbance, the key process, the inability to learn, is always the same one. In addition to these specific findings, several other clinical conditions are frequently related to amnesia and deserve mention.

Anterograde Amnesia

This term designates the ongoing problem in learning following injury. This concept is used most often in cases of head trauma where amnesia is a major complication and it designates the period following the head injury during which the patient cannot lay down memories. A more commonly used term for this feature is posttraumatic amnesia (PTA). Correctly, anterograde amnesia can be used to designate any ongoing amnesia whereas PTA should refer only to the posttraumatic variety, a nicety that is often ignored.

Retrograde Amnesia

This term refers to a period of retrieval disturbance that precedes the onset of anterograde amnesia. It has long been recognized that individuals with amnesia have a period before the onset of the amnesia for which their ability to retrieve information is severely compromised. In recent years two distinct varieties of retrograde amnesia, a long retrograde amnesia and a short retrograde amnesia, have been described.[7,10,54]

Short retrograde amnesia is frequently noted as a permanent residual following significant head injury and is most often measured in seconds, a few minutes or possibly several hours. Most individuals who recover from a posttraumatic amnesia that has persisted for days will not remember the accident itself; their last preinjury memory may be minutes or even hours before the accident.

Some individuals, however, show a comparatively long retrograde amnesia, measured in years. The cutoff point between retrieval and inability to retrieve is not exact in these cases so that while there is severe inability to retrieve information learned for several years before the onset of amnesia, there are also lesser degrees of retrieval abnormality for some years preceding that. One study reported a period of retrograde amnesia extending 15 years before the onset of amnesia with retrieval for information learned previously being relatively normal.[56] One aspect of a long retrograde amnesia deserves emphasis; long retrograde amnesia is *always* associated with an ongoing anterograde amnesia. Thus, the presence of a long retrograde amnesia is a good indication of ongoing difficulty in learning new information, an important clinical determination.

Individuals who recover from amnesia may show a shrinkage from long retrograde amnesia to short retrograde amnesia.[10,54] At times, shrinkage is heralded by the return of memory lacunes, retained bits of information from previous memories. At other times, a progressive decrease in the duration of the retrograde amnesia is noted, first a return of the earlier learned memories with continuation until the retrograde amnesia has shrunk to encompass only minutes or hours before the onset of the amnesia. For the clinician, the crucial point is that the presence of long retrograde amnesia indicates ongoing learning difficulties.

Confabulation

Another condition of considerable importance often associated with amnesia is confabulation. For many years, confabulation was fully equated with amnesia ("the amnestic-confabulatory state" was a synonym for Korsakoff's psychosis). Actually, confabulation is usually a short-lived symptom, occurring only in the early period following onset of amnesia. Confabulation is characterized by responses to questions that are not only false but may appear bizarre or fantastic. The patient may express grossly inaccurate and apparently imaginary occurrences that appear psychotic, a state called fantastic confabulation.[58] More often, however, the confabulatory response is merely an incorrect answer readily provided for a general information question. Psychogenic motivation has been suggested for the incorrect answers but most psychologists and neurologists now believe that confabulation reflects an organic mental process.[5]

There is no easy explanation for confabulation; thus, Berlyne concluded that "the cause of confabulation remains obscure and no explanation is entirely adequate."[13] Barbizet suggested that confabulatory responses were produced by an individual who "cannot remember that he cannot remember."[4] In other words, when given questions for which they formerly knew the answer (e.g., what day is it today?, What is the name of this building?), the patient, not realizing the presence of a memory disturbance, offers the best available answer. The confabulatory response can almost always be traced to the patient's past knowledge and appears bizarre primarily because it is so far from the current context. Psychologic investigation has sought correlation of confabulation with suggestability, disorientation, degree of memory disorder, and other factors.[42] Correlation was not demonstrated with any of these factors. Rather, an inability to monitor their own responses and to be self-corrective was the single trait that correlated with confabulation. A recent series of clinical reports have described individuals who confabulated spontaneously; each patient had suffered severe, bilateral frontal lobe damage.[3,9,58] From this it has been suggested that confabulation appears when amnesia is complicated by bifrontal dysfunction, a postulation that has yet to be proved.

Forgetting

Almost everyone experiences instances when they cannot immediately retrieve perfectly well-known and eventually remembered information (such as the name of an acquaintance). This disturbance is different from amnesia as defined, but the disturbances can be quite difficult to separate. Forgetfulness occurs to everyone but can be sufficiently severe to be pathologic and is easily misinterpreted as amnesia. Forgetful individuals can learn new information but this may be difficult to prove because they "forget" (fail to retrieve) the information on request. Careful testing, particularly the use of structured questioning, can demonstrate the difference[20]; forgetting appears to be a disturbance in activating the retrieval process, not an inability to learn. Although forgetting is frequently seen clinically, there is almost no pathologic correlation data available. Frontal lobe malfunction is usually suggested as the major problem but this has never been well substantiated. Forgetting is a real phenomenon, experienced by all, but pathologic in certain disease states.

Forgetting must be differentiated from amnesia because the clinical-pathologic correlation data, so abundantly available for amnesia, does not hold for forgetting.

TESTS OF MEMORY FUNCTION

The testing of memory functions has long been popular with psychologists[26] and in recent years has become a true science. Many research centers throughout the world currently investigate memory and many detailed tests of memory function have been devised and perfected. Unfortunately, there are almost as many different memory tests as there are research centers; almost every center has developed its own battery including unique tests for both normal and brain damaged subjects. Inasmuch as the etiology of the amnestic disorders available to the various research centers varies considerably and the test batteries may be quite different, the results of current research are difficult to correlate. While excellent psychologic approaches to memory are available, there is presently considerable disagreement on the interpretation of the findings. Most clinical psychologists utilize standardized tests of memory and supplement them with research tests. Unfortunately, few of these tests are capable of dissecting out the different aspects of memory. In the hands of a skilled interpreter, some of these tests can be of help to the clinician but for diagnostic purposes, most are inadequate.

Because of this, the clinician must depend upon his own testing capabilities to diagnose amnesia. At present, informal clinical tests of memory function are the equal of the formal clinical and research tests and, for clinical purposes, are more pertinent. The informal clinical tests to be described will be divided into the three categories used in the definition—immediate recall, learning, and retrieval—although some overlap is unavoidable.

Tests of Immediate Recall

The classic test for determining immediate recall is the Digit Span. The examiner slowly recites numbers (one or two numbers per second) and the patient is instructed to repeat the numbers in the exact order presented. With success, an increased number of digits is offered until a span is reached that the patient cannot correctly reproduce. Normal is usually considered "the magic number seven, plus or minus two."[44] Variations may indicate IQ (higher IQ individuals perform somewhat better), anxiety (which decreases digit span), or pathologic attention abnormalities.

Normal individuals recall at least five digits and any lower total must be considered suspicious, most often of some form of confusional state. Metabolic or pharmacologic toxicity is the most common cause of organic confusion although brain trauma, increased intracranial pressure, inflammation, and a number of other central nervous system abnormalities can decrease attention (See Chapter 1 for additional details). Amnesia cannot be diagnosed with certainty in the presence of a confusional state. Some individuals in a severe confusional state (e.g., delirium tremens) can learn new information.

Other tests can be used to supplement the Digit Span. One is a variation of the "A" Test. Letters of the alphabet are recited at approximately two per second and the patient is instructed to raise his hand (or tap the table) each time the letter "A" is pronounced. Over a period of 45-60 seconds, normal individuals make no more than a single error; individuals with immediate recall problems may lose the entire purpose of the project or make false-positive and/or omission errors. A written variation of this task asks the patient to circle all the "A"'s in a paragraph.

Tests of the Ability to Learn

There are many clinical tests designed to test learning ability (recent memory); most are readily performed. Giving the patient a group of unrelated words, possibly including your own name, repeating them several times with a warning of a request to recall them after a period of some minutes is the classic bedside memory test. Most patients can remember three or four or even more unrelated words for 10-15 minutes without difficulty. Unfortunately, low intelligence, anxiety, and other factors can interfere. Individuals with a severe amnesia may fail totally at recall and often they will deny ever being told the words. There are many variations of this test. For instance, in England, a commonly used version offers a man's name and address plus the name of a flower and instructs the patient to recall this information after a period of 5-10 minutes. The Babcock sentence ("The one thing a nation needs in order to be rich and great is a large supply of wood") and supraspan word lists (10 or more unrelated words) are useful variations. The patient is asked to immediately recall as much as possible and the process is repeated until the patient has learned the information. Most normal subjects recall all of the words in a few trials; some may succeed in two trials, but four or five trials may be necessary. An amnesic patient will plateau (usually at about five to seven words of a supraspan list) and, while the recalled words may differ from one trial to the next, they never accomplish the entire test. These tests are all verbal. Related tests of a nonverbal nature request that the patient copy drawings and several minutes later redraw them without a model. Obviously, these memory tests can be contaminated by aphasia and constructional disturbances but, used intelligently, they can provide a good indication of the ability to learn.

One part of all standard mental status evaluations, orientation for time and place, specifically probes the ability to learn. Orientation questions are routinely asked but rarely analyzed. The individual with a memory problem often cannot state the exact day, date, month, or year and often confabulates, giving dates before the correct one. Similarly, orientation for place, unless in a familiar environment, must be learned and proves difficult for the amnesic patient. Thus, in a hospital or clinic, the amnesic patient often responds with a completely wrong place or a vague, nonspecific generalization. Orientation for person (at best a dubious mental status test item) is different and cannot be interpreted as a memory test. While orientation for time and for place are important tests of amnesia, they are among the earliest memory functions recovered, and memory testing limited to orientation questions is inadequate.

Tests of Retrieval Ability

This is the most difficult memory function to test accurately, not that the tests are difficult to perform but because the examiner cannot be certain what information the patient has in his store of knowledge. One frequent test requests the name of the president and then the names of preceding presidents. The current president is often named correctly, even by severely amnesic patients. In contrast, the preceding president recalled may be someone who served many years earlier. When the response is very poor, a cue, e.g., the first name of the president, can be given. Some amnesic patients easily provide the last name of presidents that served 20 or more years earlier while failing to recognize the more recent presidents, demonstrating both retrieval ability and a long retrograde amnesia. Other simple tests of retrieval probe the fund of knowledge (e.g., the capitals of various countries, the dates of major world events). If the patient has served in the Armed Forces, data concerning the time and place of enlistment and discharge, the primary duty assignments, etc. can be asked. Similarly, personal information such as wedding date, the year of graduation and name of school, the names of children, etc. can be asked. Unfortunately, the examiner does not usually know the correct answers and must base judgment on the confidence and speed of the patient's responses. With careful and intuitive testing, good estimates of the patient's ability to retrieve old information can be made.

Formal Psychologic Tests of Memory

A great variety of formal memory tests are performed routinely by psychologists. Most test a mixture of memory functions; none clearly provides the differentiating information that can be obtained from the bedside tests. Nonetheless, a number of these tests provide replicable quantitative estimates of memory function and are widely used.

Wechsler Adult Intelligence Scale[65]

A number of subtests of the WAIS actually test memory function. These include the Digit Span and Vocabulary Subtests; some of the more complex arithmetic and comprehension questions also demand memory function. Memory loss can only be interpreted, not demonstrated, from the results of these tests.

Wechsler Memory Scale[66]

This test was designed to provide quantitative information about memory functions that can be correlated with WAIS scores. Among the subtests are Digit Span and Visual Reproduction, which probe immediate recall, and Logical Memory and Paired Associate Learning, which quantify the ability to learn new material and can be correlated with the clinical tests of learning ability.

Learning Tests

Consonant Trigrams[52] is a verbal learning task that, when correlated with an interference task such as counting backwards, usefully gauges learning capability. The Rey Auditory-Verbal Learning Test[53] is a verbal supraspan test coupled with a complex interference task that provides a good indication of learning problems. Both tests can be contaminated by a number of non-memory malfunctions but, when coupled with other mental status information, offer good estimates of learning ability.

The Benton Visual Retention Test[12]

This is a widely used visual memory test which, in its original form, probed only immediate recall of nonverbal material. A recent alteration provides a nonverbal learning task but uses recognition rather than recall for response, a markedly different process.

Rey-Osterreith Figure[48]

While this test was originally designed to evaluate visual-spatial competency, a variation in which the patient is asked to redraw the figure some 15–20 minutes later, has become popular and provides a demanding test of nonverbal learning ability. Inasmuch as constructional competency has already been evaluated by the original copying task, nonverbal learning competency can be interpreted from the repeat drawing.

Many more standardized and semistandardized neuropsychologic tests of memory exist, and most clinical psychologists have their own battery of memory tests. With appropriate interpretation, information from formal memory testing provides valuable data for the evaluation of amnesia and is even more useful in quantitating memory function longitudinally.

CLINICAL VARIETIES OF AMNESIA

Using the strict operational criteria for amnesia outlined earlier, a number of clinical syndromes that feature amnesia can be described.

Korsakoff's Psychosis

This is one of the most specific and probably the most widely known of all amnesic conditions. The disorder has been recognized for almost a century and has been excellently reviewed by Victor, Adams, and Collins.[61] Only a cursory summary of important data need be presented. Korsakoff originally reported a syndrome featuring mental disorder and peripheral neuropathy.[62] While most often seen in alcoholics, it is now accepted that a nutritional deficiency (Vitamin B_1 [thiamine] deficiency) is the real problem. While Korsakoff emphasized the combination of memory impairment and peripheral neuropathy, the two do not always coexist and amnesia is the finding now related with the name Korsakoff. Many patients, however, do have additional neurologic problems, peripheral neuropathy being the most common. Confabulation is so common in the early stages of this disorder that for many years the term amnesic-confabulatory state was used as a synonym.

Korsakoff's psychosis most often occurs in an individual who has been drinking seriously for many months, usually obtaining almost all caloric intake from alcohol. The disease may start while drinking continues, or after some alteration (such as hemorrhagic gastritis) demands cessation of drinking. A confusional state with ataxia and ophthalmoplegia (Wernicke's polioencephalopathy) often occurs; this responds to thiamine therapy but a residual amnesia may be noted after recovery from the withdrawal confusion. The amnesia is characterized by good immediate recall (normal to supranormal), severe learning disability, comparatively good retrieval of old information except for a long retrograde amnesia,[56] plus comparatively well retained cognitive and personality features. The patient often appears somewhat passive but the change in basic personality is limited. The amnesia tends to improve over time. First the confabulation, often striking in the early period, will wane. Along with this, the patient can often state that "I appear to have something wrong with my memory." Victor and colleagues followed a sizeable number of individuals with Korsakoff's psychosis and demonstrated a considerable but incomplete improvement; approximately 25 percent improved sufficiently to return to their previous employment, another 25 percent returned to work at a lower level, another 25 percent were unable to work but managed well at home, and only about 25 percent needed custodial care because of ongoing amnesia.[61] Peripheral neuropathy, eye movement problems, convulsions, or other primary neurologic disorders of the initial stages routinely improve. With occasional exceptions, amnesia is the only long-lasting disability.

Posttraumatic Amnesia

Head trauma is the most common cause of amnesia but posttraumatic amnesia (PTA) frequently goes unrecognized, hidden by the many complex behavioral alterations that can follow brain injury. The patient is first stuporous or comatose and, with recovery, a confusional state is usually present. Recovery from these problems is accepted happily and the more stringent testing necessary to demonstrate amnesia is often omitted. Only by appropriate testing can it be demonstrated that the recovering head injury patient cannot learn new material. While PTA is extremely common (almost invariable) following serious brain injury, the duration is variable. PTA may persist only minutes or hours following injury but may last for days, weeks, or even months. Only rarely, however, does a permanent PTA persist. While PTA is ongoing, there is a long retrograde amnesia; with recovery of learning ability, this will shrink until only a short retrograde amnesia, usually involving minutes or seconds preceding the head trauma, remains. Lacunes, new memories formed during the period of PTA, are not uncommon. Strong emotional trauma associated with an incident is often suggested as the major factor in the formation and retention of a memory in the face of ongoing PTA.

Amnesic Stroke

A number of careful studies have outlined a clear-cut amnesia following cerebral vascular accident (CVA). The original reports of amnesic stroke described bilateral posterior cerebral artery occlusion and the amnesia was associated with cortical blindness[63]; subsequent reports, however, describe amnesia following left posterior cerebral infarction only.[11,30,47] Postmortem examinations of individuals with amnesia following CVA demonstrate involvement of the medial temporal regions and/or the posterior thalamus. In most cases that have come to autopsy, the pathology has been bilateral but in at least two autopsied cases the pathology was entirely unilateral (left).[30,47] Amnesia may follow bilateral middle cerebral stroke but the memory problem is then part of a severe dementia and the criteria for amnesia cannot be applied. There is one well-studied case of a true amnesia following anterior cerebral occlusion[14] in which the anterior columns of the fornix were destroyed. Amnesic stroke does exist and usually indicates posterior cerebral disease, either bilateral or left unilateral.

Postsurgical Amnesia

With the advent of unilateral temporal lobe resection as therapy for intractible temporal lobe seizures, a number of cases of amnesia following removal of one temporal lobe were reported. Milner carefully reviewed the originally reported cases and found evidence suggesting that the opposite (unoperated) temporal lobe was abnormal.[46] In addition, in a series of bilateral temporal lobe resections performed as treatment for serious mental disease, each patient developed a severe amnesia.[55] These studies suggest that one temporal lobe can be removed without producing memory disturbance but that bilateral temporal pathology leads to amnesia. In actuality, however, careful psychologic testing of patients following unilateral temporal lobectomy consistently demonstrates some decrease in the ability to learn new material.[46] There is decreased competency in the ability to learn verbal material following left temporal lobectomy; after right temporal lobectomy, the problem involves the learning of nonverbal material. Most physicians will see few patients with a postoperative amnesia but it is a recognized cause of relatively pure amnesia and surgical cases have been heavily used for psychologic investigations of memory function.

Postinfectious Amnesia

While a number of infections can produce sufficient brain damage to disturb memory function, one infectious disorder is particularly common as a source of amnesia. This is the encephalitis of herpes simplex, a virus with a predilection for limbic structures. Clinically, the onset is abrupt with fever, confusional state, aphasia, convulsions, and increased intracranial pressure, leading to stupor and coma. The disease is often fatal.

The patient often presents with indications of a space-occupying lesion and, in the past, surgical decompression was performed, often with poor outcome. Medical therapy (both anti-inflammatory and antiviral medications) is now available and has improved the recovery rate. In those patients who do recover, a long period of convalescence is common with mental abnormalities dominating the picture. The most prominent residual problem is amnesia, but in the early stages this is usually obscured by aphasia, seizures, dementia, and serious personality alterations. The latter findings usually improve or disappear and a severe amnesia is often the only residual.[24]

Anoxic Amnesia

The widespread use of cardiac resuscitation in the past decade has rescued many individuals from death due to acute cardiac and pulmonary arrest. A prolonged period of both cardiac and pulmonary arrest, however, causes severe cerebral anoxia, (not hypoxia) and the victim often suffers residual behavioral problems including amnesia. The initial recovery state from cerebral anoxia is almost always a deep coma that slowly lightens until the patient enters a period of agitated confusion. Many neurobehavioral complications such as aphasia, dementia, hallucinations, and seizures, etc. may be present but with appropriate management the patient improves, leaving a state of amnesia. In our experience anoxic amnesia is initially severe and only gradually improves. Improvement is slow (months or years) and often incomplete. The clinical features of anoxic and postencephalitic amnesia are strikingly similar, except for the dramatically different onset and the obviously different etiologies.

Postconvulsive Amnesia

It has long been recognized that a period of confusion (postictal state) follows many epileptic convulsions. As the postictal confusion clears, the patient may enter a postictal, nonlearning period but it is often difficult to identify this period of pure amnesia. Individuals who suffer multiple seizures may develop a prolonged and/or progressive learning disability; this may show the characteristics of amnesia but often other neurobehavioral abnormalities such as aphasia, agnosia, apraxia, cognitive defect, and constructional disturbance, etc. coexist. While amnesia—a period of nonlearning—is a hallmark of an epileptic seizure,[14] prolonged amnesia is not a common seizure residual.

The period of amnesia following a seizure can include purposive movements, a state called automatism. The acts performed during this period are often rather simple and repetitive but may be increasingly complex; they are consistently routine and well-practiced actions, not novel activities. The most frequently quoted complex automatism is that of the physician Z, reported by Hughlings Jackson[32]; Z is reported to have competently treated a patient with pneumonia while in a postictal amnesic state. On occasion the actual seizure may be short, almost unnoticeable, but lead to a postictal amnesia state. This is exceptional and in most instances the amnesia follows a distinct seizure.

Only rarely is postictal amnesia prolonged. Two such situations deserve mention. Poriomania is a state of wandering that may last for minutes, hours, or, in a few reported cases, several days.[36] Whether poriomania is truly postictal or part of an ongoing seizure has never been settled and differentiating it from a dissociative fugue state (see later) remains difficult if not dubious. A second condition, somewhat better defined, is temporal lobe status in which a series of complex-partial seizures with interictal confusion and/or amnesia can lead to a prolonged period of nonlearning.[27] While actually a product of ongoing seizures, the amnesic state may be among the most prominent clinical features of temporal lobe status.

Artificially induced seizures, such as electroconvulsive therapy (ECT) may cause memory disturbance. Again, an acute confusional state characterizes the initial postseizure status but clears, leaving a true amnesia. The duration of post-ECT amnesia varies considerably, usually only minutes or hours after a few "shocks"; with more treatments, however, the period of amnesia becomes longer. Whether a permanent amnesia can result from ECT remains an open question. Well-controlled before-and-after studies of depressed patients treated with ECT consistently demonstrate an improvement in memory,[57] but the presence of serious depression affecting the pre-ECT memory status must be recognized. Some individuals do develop an increased memory problem after receiving ECT. Most often an associated dementing disorder can be demonstrated in these individuals, suggesting that the ECT has been used to treat a dementia that was misdiagnosed as depression. Isolated case reports suggest that a permanent amnesia condition may be produced by excessive ECT. Each report remains anecdotal, however; there is no solid evidence of permanent residual amnesia caused by ECT. The judicious use of ECT does not seem to produce a memory disturbance.

Transient Global Amnesia

Bender[6] and Fisher and Adams[29] reported a small series of individuals with episodes characterized by an acute, short period of amnesia, a disturbance now called transient global amnesia (TGA). The amnesic episode usually lasts from 12 to 36 hours after which ongoing memory function returns, leaving the patient unable to recall events during the period of TGA. Most individuals have only a single episode of TGA, most are middle-aged or older, and most show no significant behavioral abnormalities once the episode is completed. One striking clinical feature of TGA is a tendency for repetitive questioning by the patient. The response is accepted but soon the same question is asked. The apparent inability to remember the answer usually alerts family members and medical attention is sought. Examination during active TGA reveals no evidence of visual abnormality, no paresis or other significant neurologic disturbance. Amnesia is usually the only behavioral abnormality demonstrated.[19] The condition spontaneously disappears and, except for the absence of memory for the period of the episode, there is no residual.

The etiology of TGA has remained obscure. One early suggestion was that TGA was caused by a medial temporal lobe seizure discharge. Considerable investigation has failed to confirm this. Among the other postulated causes, the most popular concerns a transient vascular insufficiency, primarily involving the posterior cerebral circulation and thereby affecting the medial aspect of the temporal lobe. The absence of visual field defect remains difficult to explain. TGA has been reported with diverse conditions including the aura of classic migraine headache, overdose of medications, deep temporal lobe tumors, and following alterations in peripheral body temperature. It would appear that there is no single cause of transient global amnesia.

Psychogenic Amnesia

One of the most common uses of the term amnesia concerns a psychogenic disturbance in which the patient claims inability to remember. Psychodynamic theory suggests that amnesia can occur when the patient attempts to hide from an overwhelming psychic trauma by totally dissociating the self from the environment. The clinical features of psychogenic amnesia differ considerably from the description of amnesia mentioned earlier and the clinician should have little difficulty differentiating psychogenic from organic amnesia. Most specifically, the pertinent memory loss in psychogenic amnesia concerns personal information. This often includes the individual's own name (the most highly overlearned of all information) plus inability to retrieve information concerning family, job, or home address, etc. Patients with psychogenic amnesia have good vocabulary, retain normal social graces, and can often discuss both current and past information better than personal information. Depression is frequently present and problems such as abandonment of family, threat of arrest, overwhelming business reversals, or other major personal problems should be sought. Psychogenic amnesia is a remarkably inefficient defense mechanism and indicates a severe underlying psychologic problem. While distinctly different from the other types of amnesia, psychogenic amnesia deserves attention in differential considerations as it indicates a serious problem that deserves recognition; treatment is considerably different from that used for the other varieties.

Fugue States, Dissociative Reactions, and Multiple Personalities

Finally, a comparatively rare group of disorders in which memory alteration is an important feature but in which the features of amnesia are unclear deserves discussion. In this group, the patient can carry out extensive, complex, and often quite natural acts, lasting many hours or days, for which they claim no memory. As noted in the section on psychogenic amnesia, a rational psychodynamic theory of these actions, the dissociative state, is available. This has not proved universally satisfactory, however, and there is now scattered evidence indicating that organic pathology underlies some of these situations. The most dramatic problems of this type are the patients with multiple personalities; they may switch from hypermoral to amoral activities with little or no apparent knowledge of the alternate personality. Multiple personality is far more common in women. Usually considered a serious psychodynamic problem, a recent report suggests that at least some are associated with temporal lobe seizure abnormality.[43]

In a similar manner, fugue states are usually thought to represent a psychic defense mechanism; far more frequently than could be anticipated, however, they occur in individuals with evidence of some type of organic brain abnormality. While seizure disorder, particularly complex-partial seizure, is commonly associated with fugue states,[28] this is not a constant association.

At present, it is unclear whether the above disorders represent an unusual manifestation of psychogenic disease, are primarily due to some organic brain abnormality, or are a combination—a specific psychic reaction possible only in the face of abnormal brain control. Each case deserves separate and careful investigation with efforts to locate both psychogenic and organic problems. It is only the presence of amnesia for a variable period that suggests association with the organic amnesic disorders discussed above but this is sufficient to warrant close scrutiny.

CLINICAL PSYCHOLOGIC INVESTIGATIONS

As noted, psychologists have been studying memory and learning for almost a century. Much investigation has used normal subjects, utilizing a vast variety of techniques to prove or disprove theories of learning and information handling, etc. While this material offers a valuable corpus of normative data against which amnesia and other memory disturbances can be compared, most of the postulations have remained just that and surrounding these mountains of data is a cloud of confusion. The theories of learning will not be reviewed here.

Many psychologists and related investigators, on the other hand, now use amnesia patients as research subjects and have created a variety of ingenious memory tests. Only a few can be discussed but some are pertinent to current discussions of amnesia and deserve mention.

One of the first contemporary investigators to use clinical psychologic testing to investigate amnesia was George Talland who with his co-investigators studied individuals with chronic Korsakoff's psychosis. Many standardized tests and some original tests were administered.[60] From this work three well-defined memory disorders called primary, secondary, and tertiary were postulated. Descriptively, these are identical to the three memory disturbances mentioned earlier.

Brenda Milner is another early contributor whose laboratory remains active. Patients who have undergone unilateral temporal lobectomy have been studied by careful pre- and postoperative memory testing. Dr. Milner and her colleagues have demonstrated significant differences in memory disturbances following left or right temporal surgery, specifically a verbal memory defect following left lobectomy and nonverbal learning disturbances after right.[46] Many innovative techniques have been devised to demonstrate the specialized memory loss in these patients.

Another innovative team is Elizabeth Warrington and the psychology research group at the National Hospital, Queen Square, London. Dr. Warrington has investigated many facets of memory; possibly most pertinent are the studies of retrograde amnesia and "short term memory."[64] Again, innovative techniques for memory testing have been produced and findings of consequence have been demonstrated in a variety of amnesic conditions.

Another productive laboratory is the Psychology Research Section of the Boston Veterans Administration Hospital where Drs. Nelson Butters and Laird Cermak have performed extensive testing on a sizeable group of amnesic patients, most with Korsakoff's psychosis. Their major tool has been the Peterson-Peterson (consonant trigram) technique but many other memory tests, both standardized and innovative have been used and their work covers other clinical causes of memory disorder.[18,22]

Several more recent contributions deserve mention. Dr. Larry Squire and his associates in San Diego have used a combination of standardized and original tests in quantifying the long-term outcome of memory following electroshock therapy for depression[57] as well as other varieties of amnesia. Memory testing at the National Institutes of Mental Health, particularly in the laboratory of Herbert Weingartner and associates, has focused on the memory disturbances in Huntington's disease and on pharmacologic therapy for amnesia.[67]

Although this short review omits many laboratories currently performing significant work, it emphasizes that much effort is being expended in the study of amnesia. Several major problems have surfaced that add to the current confusion but appear to be correctable. The first concerns the tremendous variety of psychologic test procedures in use. Every laboratory doing research on memory has devised its own battery of memory tests. While some are standardized, many are either variations of standard tests or totally unique. Thus, comparison of results from one laboratory to another is limited. A second source of current confusion concerns the variety of disease processes evaluated. Some laboratories test brain tumor or brain trauma cases, others postalcoholic Korsakoff amnesia, while others evaluate electroshock therapy and herpes encephalitis, etc. The combination of different test procedures administered to different types of amnesia has produced divergent results that have proved difficult to reconcile. Much of the work done in the psychologic research is valid, but better correlation between laboratories is needed. The future should see more standardization of the test procedures and further advances in psychologic testing techniques for memory research.

NEUROANATOMIC BASIS OF MEMORY

The clinical studies of amnesia have developed a neuropathology of memory. This material has been reviewed a number of times[1,15,31] but as additional information has been obtained, alterations have been made in the proposed anatomic basis of memory. We will outline current thoughts on the neuroanatomic basis of learning, of immediate recall, of retrieval of old, overlearned information and, finally, the hemispheric lateralization of memory function.

First, the anatomic basis of learning presents an area of considerable discussion and considerable agreement. The mamillary bodies, the posterior portion of the hypothalamus, have long been known to be sclerosed (gliotic) in Korsakoff's amnesia. On the basis of straight clinical/pathologic correlation it is usually assumed that the mamillary bodies are of importance for the task of learning. While there is some disagreement,[31,61] most investigators concur that the mamillary bodies are significant for the act of learning.

A second area consistently suggested is the hippocampus and/or the surrounding perihippocampal structures of the medial temporal lobe. Stroke and surgical ablation are the most clear-cut clinical examples of medial temporal pathology causing amnesia, although both herpes encephalitis and brain trauma also involve this region primarily. The medial temporal structures, particularly the hippocampus and perihippocampal structures, appear important for learning new material.

Inasmuch as both the hippocampus and the mamillary bodies are parts of the limbic system,[49] the fornix, the white matter pathway that connects these nuclear areas, would appear important for memory function. This is not a recognized situation, however. Early investigators suggested that the fornix could be sacrificed bilaterally without difficulty.[21,23] In later years, it was suggested that this is not true and there are several well-documented cases of amnesia following bilateral fornix section[45,59] or infarction.[16] While still controversial, it appears that the inner core of the limbic system—the hippocampus, fornix, and mamillary bodies—are all significant for learning new material.

Recent work on the anatomic basis of Korsakoff's amnesia by Victor, Adams and Collins implies that another crucial area for learning, at least in the Korsakoff type of amnesia, is the dorsal medial nucleus of the thalamus.[61] In their postmortem series all cases with severe amnesia had considerable cell loss in this thalamic area whereas a few did not show serious mamillary body sclerosis. This finding has never been fully replicated (or accepted) but the quality of their investigation demands recognition of this finding. Subsequent clinical studies imply that diencephalic pathology exclusive of the fornix and mamillary bodies may produce amnesia.[37]

Finally, in a recent clinical/anatomic correlation study, Horel suggested that none of these areas were truly crucial and that the most important anatomic site underlying the production of amnesia was the temporal stem (isthmus) of the left posterior temporal region.[31] Horel's theory was based on good anatomic studies but has not found widespread agreement or duplication.

In summary, a number of anatomically separate areas are said to be involved in the neuroanatomic basis of learning. While this has been the source of disagreement, it is important to recognize that many more areas of the brain are not implicated. Thus, no cortical structure, none of the basal ganglia or other extrapyramidal structures and no brain stem structures appear to be essential for learning. Only the structures in and around the inner limbic system and selected portions of the thalamus have been suggested as crucial for competency in learning.

Information concerning the anatomic basis of the function called immediate recall is considerably less definite. Logic, plus some rather circumstantial clinical evidence, suggests that immediate recall is the product of a cortical-cortical reverberating circuit. Interference with this circuitry through pathologic destruction, metabolic malfunction, or psychologic interference inhibits immediate recall. Thus, seriously decreased immediate recall (digit span) follows acute cortical pathology, particularly if it involves the left hemisphere, many metabolic and toxic disturbances such as drug intoxication, uremia, etc., and even the simple interference of demanding that some other mental function be performed before the return of the information.[17] It would appear that immediate recall, the first step in putting information into memory, demands an active and intact network of neural connections that can reverberate material between cortical areas over a relatively short period of time.

The third major memory function (the retrieval of old information) is even more difficult to place in a specific anatomic focus. On the basis of intuitive guessing, the retrieval of previously learned information appears to depend on a complex network of cortical and subcortical circuits. Support stems from those few clinical situations in which retrieval of old information alone is disturbed. One example is the word selection of pure anomic aphasia in which much concerning a given item can be remembered except the specific name.[8] In this syndrome, pathology is almost constantly present in the posterior inferior temporal cortex (Brodmann area 37). While possibly not a "storage area" in the computer sense, this cortical area appears essential for the function of specific name selection.

On the other hand, the shrinking of a long retrograde amnesia to a short retrograde amnesia suggests an additional functional area for the retrieval of old, learned material. Information that could not be retrieved during the period of long retrograde amnesia becomes available again with recovery from PTA. This information is not relearned; it has remained in "storage" but cannot be retrieved while there is an ongoing amnesia. Thus, some retrieval activity is linked to the ability to learn and, based on the earlier discussion, this function apparently involves the inner limbic structures. Full retrieval ability appears dependent upon both subcortical and cortical circuitry. That much well-learned information can be retrieved without the limbic circuitry, however, is obvious because, even during periods of ongoing amnesia, material that was learned many years previously is still available.[56]

Finally, mention should be made of the hemispheric lateralization of memory functions. As noted earlier, Milner demonstrated a difference in the type of memory disturance depending upon which temporal lobe was removed. The left temporal lobe is more active in verbal memory whereas the right temporal lobe is more active in nonverbal functions. While either area can be surgically removed without seriously jeopardizing memory function, demanding tests of verbal and nonverbal function successfully demonstrate this temporal lobe specialization. Other suggested hemispheric lateralizations of memory functions such as the site of long-term storage can be conjectured but not proved by present data.

In summary, there is a considerable body of knowledge concerning the neuroanatomic basis of memory but much remains unclear. There are many excellent psychologic studies of memory and there are also excellent anatomical studies of amnesia but, unfortunately, the two do not coincide. Not only are there problems in definition but most cases that are well-studied pathologically have not had an intense clinical workup while those with in-depth psychologic studies have not come to postmortem. Future research should correct the definition problem, and much of the clinical information should be correlated with pathologic findings. Until then, controversy will remain.

TREATMENT OF AMNESIA

At the present time, there is no single medication or treatment that acts as a remedy for amnesia. Most amnesics do show some degree of improvement with time but there is no proof that any of the improvement is based on specific therapy.

Thiamine is routinely given to individuals with the Wernicke-Korsakoff syndrome and has a remarkable effect on most of the abnormalities; the ataxia, ophthalmoplegia, and confusional state are rather rapidly ameliorated, often improvement in the ataxia and eye findings can be seen within hours. There is no evidence to suggest that the thiamine therapy alters the amnesia component. Attempts to treat chronic Korsakoff's psychosis with massive doses of a thiamine analogue, tetrahydrofurfuryl disulfide (TTFD), have produced only a slight suggestion of improvement.[35] Other drugs have been tried in amnesia and show some results. For instance, physostigmine, a central cholinergic agonist, has been said to help some varieties of memory disturbance,[25] but trials with this and related medications in many centers using patients with memory disturbances produced only questionable results.[2,34] More recently, a series of studies of the therapy for amnesia has been based on a theory that one source of amnesia might be interference with diencephalic neurotransmitter systems.[39] A number of drugs proved ineffective but one, clonidine, produced suggestive results.[38] This study questioned, however, whether the drug effected the learning aspect of amnesia or produced a general activation. Thus, research on the pharmacologic influence on learning has failed to provide a drug treatment for amnesia or produce a strong pharmacologic-clinical theory of memory function.

A number of behavioral treatments have been used to manage amnesia. Mnemonic devices, rote drill, and even setting information to music or other conditioning paradigms have all been tried and all have demonstrated some ability to instill information to severely amnesic patients. Retrieval of the information, however, depends on the specific behavioral cue. Most information learned by behavioral conditioning is retrieved only if the behavioral cue is given; information requested without the specific cue will not be retrieved. Thus, individuals taught a melodic response for place orientation can respond correctly only if cued with the melody; if asked where they are without the melodic cue, they can provide no information. Psychotherapy in a variety of forms has been tried without success in amnesia. The only exception is psychogenic amnesia; while this condition is usually self-limited, there is often a need for psychiatric management of the underlying condition.

At best, therapy for amnesia is extremely limited and most often is of no benefit. Although research continues, there is presently no true therapy for acquired learning deficits.

PROGNOSIS AND OUTCOME

Despite the severe limitations of therapy, the outlook is not entirely unfavorable. Posttraumatic amnesia is usually self-limited; it is only the exceptional, severely brain damaged individual who does not eventually show a considerable return of the ability to learn new material. The status on recovery may not be at the premorbid level but it is almost impossible to obtain firm data on this point. By definition, and in actual practice, transient global amnesia is self-limited. Most cases of anoxic amnesia improve but only partially and this occurs over a prolonged period. Individuals with postherpetic amnesia usually show improvement, some having nearly total improvement and many more enjoying a partial resolution of the amnesia. Korsakoff's psychosis has a variable prognosis but there is also a definite tendency for improvement in this disorder. Confabulation disappears fairly early and the follow-up study of Victor et al. demonstrated that many Korsakoff patients improved significantly.[61] Finally, while the long-term outlook for psychogenic amnesia depends upon the underlying disease process, the memory problem can usually be corrected fairly easily; it is the underlying psychiatric problem that prompts guarding of the long-term prognosis.

In summary, amnesia is a specific clinical entity, the result of a finite number of specific disease processes. While there is no specific treatment for amnesia, some degree of improvement usually occurs. It is important that amnesia be separated from other alterations in mental function, particularly from aphasia, agnosia, dementia, and, most difficult, forgetfulness. Completely different treatments and different prognoses are present in these disorders. Amnesia should be considered a specific neurobehavioral abnormality with a specific anatomic substrate. Hopefully, in the future there will be a specific treatment or treatments.

REFERENCES

1. Adams RD, Victor M: Delerium and other confusional states, in Wintrobe MM, Thorn GW, Adams RD, et al (eds): Harrison's Principles of Internal Medicine, vol. 1, ed 6. New York, McGraw-Hill, 1970, pp 185-193
2. Albert ML, Feldman RG, Willis AL: The "subcortical dementia" of progressive supranuclear palsy. J Neurol Neurosurg Psychiatry 37:121-130, 1974
3. Alexander MP, Stuss DT, Benson DF: Capgras syndrome: A reduplicative phenomenon. Neurology 29:334-339, 1979
4. Barbizet J: Defect of memorizing of hippocampal-mamillary origin: A review. J Neurol Neurosurg Psychiatry 26:127-135, 1963
5. Barbizet J: Human Memory and Its Pathology. San Francisco, Freeman, 1970
6. Bender MB: Syndrome of isolated episode of confusion with amnesia. J Hillside Hosp 5:212-215, 1956
7. Benson DF: Amnesia. South Med J 71:1221-1227, 1978
8. Benson DF: Aphasia, Alexia, and Agraphia. New York, Churchill-Livingstone, 1979
9. Benson DF, Gardner H, Meadows JC: Reduplicative paramnesia. Neurology 26:147-151, 1976
10. Benson DF, Geschwind N: Shrinking retrograde amnesia. J Neurol Neurosurg Psychiatry 30:457-461, 1967
11. Benson DF, Marsden CD, Meadows JC: The amnesic syndrome of posterior cerebral artery occlusion. Acta Neurol Scand 50:133-145, 1974
12. Benton AL: A multiple choice type of visual retention test. Arch Neurol Psychiatry 64:699-707, 1950

13. Berlyne N: Confabulation. Br J Psychiatry 120:31-39, 1972
14. Blumer D: Temporal lobe epilepsy and its psychiatric significance, in Benson DF, Blumer D (eds): Psychiatric Aspects of Neurologic Disease. New York, Grune & Stratton, 1975, pp 171-198
15. Brierly JB: The neuropathology of amnesic states, in Whitty CWM, Zangwill OL (eds): Amnesia. New York, Appleton-Century-Crofts, 1977, pp 150-180
16. Brion S, Pragier C, Guerin R, Teitgen MMC: Korsakoff syndrome due to bilateral softening of fornix. Rev Neurol (Paris) 120:255-262, 1969
17. Brown JR: Short-term memory. Br Med Bull 20:8-11, 1964
18. Butters N, Grady M: The role of temporal processing factors in the short-term memory performance of patients with Korsakoff's and Huntington's disease. Neuropsychologia 15:701-706, 1977
19. Byer JA, Crowley WJ Jr: Musical performance during transient global amnesia. Neurology 30:80-82, 1980
20. Caine ED, Ebert MH, Weingartner H: An outline for the analysis of dementia: The memory disorder of Huntington's disease. Neurology 27:1087-1092, 1977
21. Cairns H, Mosberg WH Jr: Colloid cyst of the third ventricle. Surg Gynecol Obstet 92:545-570, 1951
22. Cermak LS, Butters N: The role of interference and encoding in the short-term memory of Korsakoff patients. Neuropsychologia 10:89-95, 1972
23. Dott NM: Hypothalamus—Surgical aspects, in Clark WEL, Beattie J, Riddoch G, Dott NM (eds): The Hypothalamus. London, Oliver & Boyd, 1938, pp 131-164
24. Drachman DA, Arbit J: Memory and the hippocampal complex. Arch Neurol 15:52-61, 1966
25. Drachman DA, Leavitt J: Human memory and the cholinergic system. Arch Neurol 30:113-121, 1974
26. Ebbinghaus H: Memory—A Contribution to Experimental Psychology. New York, Dover, 1964
27. Engel J Jr, Ludwig BI, Fetell M: Prolonged partial complex status epilepticus: EEG and behavioral observations. Neurology 28:863-869, 1978
28. Escueta AV, Boxley J, Stubbs N: Prolonged twilight state and automatisms: A case report. Neurology 24:331-339, 1974
29. Fisher CM, Adams RD: Transient global amnesia. Acta Neurol Scand 40(suppl 9):7-83, 1964
30. Geschwind N, Fusillo M: Color naming defects in association with alexia. Arch Neurol 15:137-146, 1966
31. Horel JA: The neuroanatomy of amnesia: A critique of the hippocampal memory hypothesis. Brain 101:403-445, 1978
32. Jackson JH: Selected Writings. Taylor H (ed). London, Hodder & Stoughton, 1932
33. Kinsbourne M, Wood F: Short-term memory processes and the amnesic syndrome, in Deutsch D, Deutsch JA (eds): Short-Term Memory. New York, Academic Press, 1975
34. Legros JJ, G'lot P, Seron X, et al.: Influence of vasopressin on learning and memory. Lancet 1:41-42, 1978

35. Leigh D: Personal communication, 1977
36. Mayeux R, Benson DF, Alexander M, et al.: Poriomania. Neurology 29:1616–1619, 1979
37. McEntee WJ, Biber MP, Perl DP, Benson DF: Diencephalic amnesia: A reappraisal. J Neurol Neurosurg Psychiatry 39:436–441, 1976.
38. McEntee WJ, Mair RG: Memory enhancement in Korsakoff's psychosis by clonidine: Further evidence for a norodrenergic deficit. Ann Neurol 7:466–470, 1980
39. McEntee WJ, Mair RG: Memory impairment in Korsakoff's psychosis: A correlation with brain norodrenergic activity. Science 202(4370):905–907, 1978
40. McConnell JV, Jacobsen R, Humphries BM: The effects of ingestion of conditioned planaria on the response level of naive planarias: A pilot study (or "you are what you eat"). Worm Runners Digest 3:41–47, 1961
41. McGaugh JL, Madsen MC: Amnesic and punishing effects of electroconvulsive therapy. Science 144:182–185, 1964
42. Mercer B, Wepner W, Gardner H, Benson DF: A study of confabulation. Arch Neurol 34:429–433, 1977
43. Mesulam MM: Dissociative states with abnormal temporal lobe EEG. Arch Neurol 38:176–181, 1981
44. Miller GA: The magical number seven, plus or minus two: Some limits on our capacity for processing information. Psychol Review 63:81–97, 1966
45. Milner B: Discussion of "Loss of Recent Memory Following Section of the Fornix." Trans Am Neurol Assoc 84:78–79, 1959
46. Milner B: Amnesia following operation on the temporal lobes, in Whitty CWM, Zangwill OL (eds): Amnesia. London, Butterworths, 1966, pp 109–133
47. Mohr JP, Leicester J, Stoddard LT, Sidman M: Right hemianopsia with memory and color deficits in circumscribed left posterior cerebral artery infarction. Neurology 21:1104–1113, 1971
48. Osterrieth PA: Le test de copie d'une figure complexe. Arch Psychologie 30:206–356, 1944
49. Papez JW: A proposed mechanism of emotion. Arch Neurol Psychiatry 38:725–743, 1937
50. Penfield W, Mathieson G: Memory. Arch Neurol 31:145–154, 1974
51. Penfield W, Perot P: The brain record of auditory and visual experience: A final summary and discussion. Brain 86:595–696, 1963
52. Peterson LR, Peterson MJ: Short-term retention of individual verbal items. J Exp Psychol 58:193–198, 1959
53. Rey A: L'examen psychologigue dans les cas d'encephalopathie traumatique. Arch Psychologie 28:286–340, 1941
54. Russell WR, Nathan PW: Traumatic amnesia. Brain 69:280–300, 1946
55. Scoville WB, Milner B: Loss of recent memory after bilateral hippocampal lesions. J Neurol Neurosurg Psychiatry 20:11–21, 1957
56. Seltzer B, Benson DF: The temporal patterns of retrograde amnesia in Korsakoff's disease. Neurology 24:527–530, 1974

57. Squire LR, Miller PL: Diminution of anterograde amnesia following electroconvulsive therapy. Br J Psychiatry 125:490-495, 1974
58. Stuss DT, Alexander MP, Lieberman A, Levine H: An extraordinary form of confabulation. Neurology 28:1166-1172, 1978
59. Sweet WH, Tallande GA, Ervin FR: Loss of recent memory following section of the fornix. 84:76-82, 1959
60. Talland GA: Deranged Memory—A Psychonomic Study of the Amnesic Syndrome. New York, Academic Press, 1965
61. Victor M, Adams RD, Collins GH: The Wernicke-Korsakoff Syndrome. Philadelphia, Davis, 1971
62. Victor M, Yakovlev P: S.S. Korsakoff's psychic disorder in conjunction with peripheral neuritis. Neurology 5:394-406, 1955
63. Victor M, Angevine J, Mancall E, Fisher CM: Memory loss with lesions of hippocampal formation. Arch Neurol 5:244-263, 1961
64. Warrington EK, Shallice T: The selective impairment of auditory verbal short-term memory. Brain 92:885-896, 1969
65. Wechsler D: The Measurement and Appraisal of Adult Intelligence. Baltimore, Williams & Williams, 1958
66. Wechsler D: A Standardized memory scale for clinical use. J Psychol 19:87-95, 1945
67. Weingartner H, Gold P, Ballenger JC, et al.: Effects of vasopressin on human memory functions. Science 211:601-603, 1981

Commentary

Several features of Chapter 12 deserve emphasis. First, the division of memory function into several totally different activities (immediate recall, learning, and retrieval of old learned material), while widely accepted, is routinely lost in everyday discussion. Any attempt to discuss "memory" without separation of such basically different functions is bound to produce confusion and, unfortunately, much contemporary work in this field fails at this level. Recognition of the three almost totally distinct divisions leads to improved clinical delineation, almost obvious separation of psychogenic and organic memory disturbances, and a rational clinical/anatomic basis for the different memory functions. A second point deserves emphasis and reinforces the first. Not all of the brain is involved in all portions of the complex activity called memory. Recognition of the separate functions underlying memory allows considerable understanding of the influence of various neuroanatomically localized activities on the behavior of a patient and at least a teasing insight into the complex integrative brain actions underlying mental operations. Yet another important point, however, is the demonstration that all memory problems cannot be readily explained by this neuroanatomic model. For instance, the abnormal memory functions underlying fugue state, possession, multiple personality, and psychogenic amnesia need clarification. Future investigations starting from the base of current knowledge should help resolve these questions.

The next two chapters will also deal with disorders that involve the borderland between neurology and psychiatry, problems that can be considered neurobehavioral problems. Neither disorder is usually considered in this light, however. One, multiple sclerosis, is usually looked upon as a classic neurologic disorder; it has many psychiatric complications, however, most of which revolve around the combination of organic mental alterations and the individual's reaction to a chronic disease. In a nearly opposite manner, stuttering has long been considered a psychiatric problem, closely related to emotional tension; only recently has there been a renewed interest in the part that an underlying neurologic dysfunction may play in stuttering. First, Drs. Trimble and Grant will provide an overview of the many psychiatric problems that can be encountered in the clinical management of individuals with multiple sclerosis.

Michael R. Trimble, M.R.C.P., F.R.C. Psych.
Igor Grant, M.D., F.R.C.P.(C)

13
Psychiatric Aspects of Multiple Sclerosis

Multiple sclerosis (MS) is a chronic recurring disorder of the nervous system, which in many cases leads to the development of demyelinating plaques in the cortex and subcortical structures. Consequent neuronal dysfunction often leads to a variety of disturbances of behavior which can be devastating for the individual and his family. In addition, the knowledge of living with such a disorder, with the sudden and unpredictable catastrophic loss of activity that occurs, in itself often leads to emotional disturbances in patients; this is often not adequately dealt with in treatment.

Following an initial historic overview, discussion of the neuropsychiatric research on MS which has emerged since 1950 will be divided into two separate categories: the investigations into psychiatric disturbances, particularly personality change, depression, and psychosis, and studies of neuropsychologic deficits, usually detected in early stages only by standardized neuropsychologic tests. The latter may present either as isolated cognitive disorders or as general progressive dementia. Although both aspects are interrelated, as the literature will show, it is helpful in the initial analysis to view them separately.

HISTORIC INTRODUCTION — EARLY LITERATURE

Although early descriptions of MS are found in the work of Cruveilhier and Carswell from the 1830s, it was Charcot and Vulpian from the Salpêtrière who clearly delineated it as a clinical entity and provided accounts of its pathology and symptomatology. Charcot's original description of the psychopathology is provided in full:

> Most of the patients affected by multilocular sclerosis whom I have had occasion to observe, have presented at a certain stage of the disease a truly peculiar facies. The look is vague and uncertain, the lips are hanging and half open; the features have a stolid expression, sometimes even an appearance of stupor. This dominant expression of the physiognomy is almost always accompanied by a corresponding mental state, which deserves notice. There is marked enfeeblement of the memory; conceptions are formed slowly; the intellectual and emotional faculties are blunted in their totality. The dominant feeling in the patients appears to be a sort of almost stupid indifference in reference to all things. It is not rare to see them give way to foolish laughter for no cause, and sometimes, on the contrary, melt into tears without reason. Nor is it rare, amid this state of mental depression, to find psychic disorders to arise which assume one or other of the classic forms of mental alienation.[14]

He went on to describe a female patient who was frequently seized with causeless fits of uncontrolled laughter, and another who was usually subject to "melancholia" but from time to time was seized with "ambitious mania." A third patient had delusions of grandeur, and a fourth had auditory and visual hallucinations and persecutory delusions.[14]

In England, Gowers suggested that although mental changes were common in the disease, they were usually slight; he observed that: "There may be failure of memory, but especially frequent is an undue complacency and contentment, which, under the increasing disability, is distinctly unnatural."[22] Several other authors around this time noted the presence of this unusual "euphoric" state, including Wilkes,[67] Oppenheim,[45] and Seiffer.[57] The latter two authors, as well as Raecke[52] and Duge,[18] all observed intellectual changes, including enfeeblement, impaired memory, and defective association of ideas, in some patients.

One of the first more comprehensive accounts of the mental changes in MS was given by Brown and Davis.[10] They noted mental alterations in 90 percent of cases and suggested that because the alterations were often overshadowed by physical symptoms they were frequently disregarded. In their experience, a slight elevation of mood was common; thus patients suffering from a serious disease would fail to see the seriousness of their condition and lack any deep concern about it. There was a marked inconsistency between the patient's mood and his physical disability. Depression, they reported, was rare and unaccompanied by mental slowing or retardation, but it could be severe and lead to suicide attempts. They noted the tendency of symptoms to change and that emotional disturbances were sometimes very brief and unexplainable. As the disorder progressed, however, the euphoria increased, and they suggested grandiose elaboration as a possible late development. Brown and Davis were equivocal regarding intellectual decline. They believed that although mental deterioration may or may not occur, it was probably present in the majority of cases. Some patients, they noted, had only mild memory disturbances and were entirely aware of the disturbances.

Cottrell and Wilson provided the first systematic study on this subject.[15] They examined 100 patients using a semistructured interview which specifically inquired about emotional disorders. Fifteen patients had the disease less than a year, although the majority were affected for 3 years or longer. Euphoria was present in 63 percent of their sample, while only 10 percent were depressed or dysphoric. Eutonia, a sense of physical as opposed to mental well-being, occurred in 84 percent, and the authors believed this symptom was fundamentally significant. Only two of their patients had intellectual deterioration, although quantification and detailed studies were not carried out. Noting the frequent pathologic changes in the periventricular region, they argued that some mental change was universal, and that it occurred with greater frequency than any other neurologic symptom in this disease.

Sugar and Nadell examined 28 patients and generally agreed with Cottrell and Wilson. Their study reported euphoria in 54 percent, eutonia in 50 percent, and depression ("increase in pessimism") in 36 percent of patients. No patient was reported as mentally deteriorated.[60]

In contrast to these opinions, Ombrédane confirmed the opinion expressed earlier by Runge that intellectual deficits were common. In a study of 50 patients, he found intellectual deficits present in 36. He believed that euphoria occurred concomitantly with decreased intellectual capacity. Depression was noted to occur earlier in the disease, and this gave way to euphoria as the disorder progressed with advancing intellectual deterioration.[44]

In complete antithesis to the above opinions, however, a few authors failed to document mental changes as a common symptom of multiple sclerosis. For example, Sachs and Friedman, recognizing the problems of diagnostic confusion with central nervous system (CNS) syphilis, found emotional instability in only 17 percent of 141 cases of MS.[56]

Following these early studies, with the exception of some explorations into the personalities of sufferers (see below), few authors investigated these aspects of MS until the 1950s. Since then, several systematic investigations have been carried out. These will now be discussed and differing aspects of psychopathology will be examined.

PSYCHIATRIC DISORDERS—LITERATURE SINCE 1950

Disorders of Affect and Euphoria

Braceland and Giffin examined 75 patients between the ages of 18 and 58 with MS of varying severity, noting in particular the psychiatric symptomatology.[7] Ten percent of the 75 patients were characterized as euphoric, and in 20 percent the predominant mood was that of depression. Approximately 18 percent of their sample had lability, and 12 percent had an unusual degree of irritability. All of the patients who exhibited euphoria showed evidence of widespread cerebral disease, although not all showed quantitative intellectual deficits.

In the first controlled study of this subject, Pratt investigated the psychiatric morbidity in 100 patients with the disease compared with 100 others with alternative organic disease of the CNS, and paid particular attention to psychiatric and emotional changes that followed the onset of the illness.[50] The mood of the patients with MS was found to be significantly more cheerful since the onset of illness was noted, as was a tendency to laugh and cry more easily. Six patients stated that after the onset of their disease they had an increase in bodily well-being. In this study, Pratt also examined the intellectual changes that occurred (see below), and was able to confirm that an increase in euphoria was associated with intellectual deterioration and with neurologic disability.

Surridge elaborated on Pratt's investigations.[61] The incidence of psychiatric disturbance, as noted at a psychiatric interview, in a sample of 108 patients who had had MS for more than 2 years was compared to that of a control sample of 39 patients suffering from muscular dystrophy. Depression was noted in 18 percent of the MS patients, and was severe in 4 percent. The incidence of depression was 13 percent in the control group and was not rated as severe in any. Overall, however, these differences were not significant. Euphoria was seen in 26 percent of the MS patients and in none of the controls—a highly significant difference. In terms of the quality of depression, the author claimed that most states of depression, if not all, had a psychogenic and reactive origin. Of particular importance was his observation that many patients who appeared euphoric at first glance also showed signs and symptoms of depression during a more in-depth interview. Surridge confirmed Pratt's correlation between increasing euphoria and increasing deterioration. In addition, the euphoric group showed more disability and incontinence than the depressed or control groups, and exaggerated emotional expression showed a significant association with intellectual deterioration and the degree of physical disability.

Whitlock and Siskind recently undertook a specific study of depression in MS.[66] In their study, 30 patients without signs of dementia underwent psychiatric interview, and depression was assessed using the Beck Scale. A control group was selected from patients with other chronic or progressive neurologic syndromes and was matched for age and sex. Disorders in the control group included Friedreich's ataxia, muscular dystrophy, motor neurone disease, dystrophia myotonica, and polyneuritis. Both groups were well matched for general disability, but the MS patients had significantly higher depression scores, although a correlation between the degree of the depression and the disability existed in both groups.

In this study, more MS patients experienced episodes of depression before the onset of the neurologic disabilities versus the control group—an observation recorded by several other authors. For example, Young et al. described five patients with mental changes as an early and prominent symptom of MS—the latter diagnosis being supported by follow-up and cerebrospinal fluid (CSF) findings.[70] Two of his patients were profoundly depressed, one required electroconvulsive therapy (ECT) and admission to a psychiatric unit for retardation, depression, and feelings of guilt and worthlessness. Similar observations were recorded by Mur et al.[42] and Goodstein and Ferrell[20] and lead to the conclusion that depression may be one of the first signs of MS. In the case of Bignami et al., depression occurred before the onset of other neurologic symptoms in a patient who had rapidly progressive MS, and who at autopsy was noted to have areas of demyelination in the diencephalon.[6]

In contrast to Surridge, Whitlock and Siskind suggested that the symptomatology of depression in this illness was endogenous, with the characteristic symptoms of guilt, suicidal thoughts, and diurnal mood changes.[66] They cited two patients, including one of their own, who developed a manic-depressive illness associated with MS; in one patient plaques were noted in the temporal lobes, thalamus, and periventricular grey matter.

If, as the above results suggest, depressive illness is significantly associated with MS, the possibility of suicide is a risk that must be considered. Little accurate epidemiologic evidence is available on this point, although 8 of 295 patients studied by Kahana et al. killed themselves during follow-up.[32] The suicide rate in this study was 14 times higher than that of the general population of Israel, where the sample was taken.[36]

Psychosis

The relationship between schizophrenia-like psychosis and MS was reviewed by Davison and Bagley.[16] Noting that Gowers referred to rare cases of insanity in the disorder, they were able to trace 39 acceptable reports from 26 authors. In 14 patients, the neurologic and psychiatric signs and symptoms appeared at about the same time as the onset of MS; coincident onset of the psychotic illness occurred within 2 years of the development of the neurologic abnormalities in 24 patients (61.5 percent). Several authors had recorded episodes of psychosis before the neurologic symptomatology, and the close resemblance of the clinical picture to process schizophrenia was noted. There was little evidence that patients had a genetic predisposition to the schizophrenia, although few authors had actually studied this. They concluded that the frequency of a schizophrenia-like psychosis in MS was not greater than chance expectation. The clustering of the psychosis onset around the time the neurologic abnormalities appeared, however, and the rarity of schizophrenic family history suggested that the demyelinating disease and the psychosis were not wholly independent.

Since that review, Surridge reported 1 case in 108 of schizophreniform psychosis, a prevalence similar to the control group. In our experience, the occurrence of psychosis in the setting of clear consciousness is rare; i.e., in marked contrast to its prevalence in partial epilepsy (see Chapter 2). In the absence of further studies, the conclusions of Davison and Bagley must remain.

Personality Changes and Hysteria

Although it is unlikely that a disease such as MS, in which demyelination of various areas of the CNS occurs, would fail to lead to clearly demarcated changes of personality, this issue has been confused by the inadequate methods used to assess personality change, the practical impossibility of assessing personality before the onset of neurologic disease, and the question of personality bias. Personality bias, a concept which states that certain patients tend to develop certain diseases due to their premorbid personality, is a theme that flowered in the 1940s with the era of psychosomatic medicine. The latter idea was particularly discussed by Langworthy, who suggested that poor emotional adjustment was a premorbid problem in many patients with MS.[35] He thought that these patients showed immaturity in interpersonal relationships and sexual adjustment, and he supported these ideas with anecdotal case histories. This theory was investigated by Pratt who tried to make a retrospective assessment of premorbid personality by allotting patients to appropriate classes following the schemes of Jung (extraversion-introversion) and Sheldon (viscerotonia, cerebrotonia).[50] No differences emerged between the MS and control patients. In addition, there were no differences noted for hysterical manifestations, obsessional traits, psychopathy, childhood environment, or early separation from parents.

In the study by Surridge, MS and muscular dystrophy patients both showed personality changes, although the type of change was different.[61] The MS group showed a significant tendency to irritability and apathy, whereas the controls showed increased patience and tolerance. The fact that intellectual deterioration tended to coexist with apathy and irritability suggested to him that the latter were the result of CNS damage.

Several authors have attempted to assess personality in MS by using standardized and validated rating scales. The majority have used the Minnesota Multiphasic Personality Inventory (MMPI). Several have noted elevations of the so-called neurotic triad—hypochondriasis, depression, and hysteria.[3] Ross and Reitan, however, showed that elevation of these subscales was not specific for MS, and are seen following other CNS disorders.[55] More recently, Peyser et al. assessed 55 patients with MS on several rating scales including the MMPI.[48] They used cluster analysis to define subgroups of patients, and concluded that there may be as many as six different patterns of psychiatric symptomatology linked with various demographic, neurologic, and neuropsychologic variables.

The association between hysteria and MS was well ingrained in the earlier literature, and was particularly highlighted by Brain,[8] who said of Cottrell and Wilson's study: "Their valuable analysis omits, however, one symptom of importance—the predisposition of hysteria which clinical experience has long associated with the disease." Brain's comment contrasts with Wilson's, which suggested that hysterical phenomena were rare, and that their development in MS was a mere coincidence.[68] The problem was examined in more detail by Pratt, who concluded that anxiety and hysteria were not major manifestations of patients with disseminated sclerosis.

At least two problems have contributed to this confusion. First, "hysteria" is an imprecise term used by some to describe symptoms (e.g., of conversion or dissociation) and by others to describe a personality style (a certain constellation of features including dramatism, verbal imprecision, lability, shallowness of affect, seductiveness, and a tendency to be dependent and demanding in interpersonal relationships). Hysterical symptoms are seen in association with a broad range of psychiatric and medical disorders, and do not presuppose an underlying hysterical personality.[23] Indeed, hysterical symptoms are often the harbingers of disease as yet undiagnosed, and several authors have reported a high association of this diagnosis with organic disorders.[40,58,65] The hysterical personality is not known to be associated with any particular illness, although such personalities may present with atypical symptoms such that diagnosis of any underlying medical illness is delayed or missed.[63]

The second cause of confusion is related to the fact that conversion symptoms and MS both tend to occur in young people, especially women, and that the initial symptoms of MS may be nonspecific, evanescent, and unaccompanied by clearly detectable neurologic signs. It is only with the passage of time that the diagnosis becomes clear and earlier misclassification becomes apparent.

NEUROPSYCHOLOGIC DEFICITS— LITERATURE SINCE 1950

We use the term neuropsychologic to describe abilities whose disruption is generally indicative of cerebral dysfunction. Neuropsychologic testing embraces sensation and motor skills, as well as attention, perception, thinking, and memory.[24]

As noted in the introduction, despite 75 years of clinical observation of patients with MS, the neuropsychologic correlates of the disorder still remained unclear in the 1950s. Most observers agreed that cognitive decline occurred in some cases, but there was little agreement over the prevalence, qualitative features, or natural history of the MS-associated cognitive deficit. This was due, in part, to the disparate populations sampled by different investigators—i.e., reports based on patients from psychiatric institutions, or on a mixture of both psychiatric and neurologic patients which tended to note more organic mental change,[9,44] in contrast to those studies from neurologic hospitals where only negligible changes are recorded.[15,60] In addition, standardized and validated methods for assessing cognitive function were not generally available until the late 1940s and early 1950s, when the pioneering work of Wechsler[64] and Halstead[26] permitted reliable testing of patients for the first time.

Burgmeister and Tallman used the newly developed Wechsler-Bellevue scale on 40 patients with MS and found a scatter of subtest scores that suggested "a lowering of the present level of functioning" and a difficulty in assimilating new material quickly.[11]

Using the Rorschach test, they also found that their patients had "difficulties in organizing abilities and in handling abstract ideas such as are found among patients with organic disturbances." Diers and Brown noted that while 24 patients with MS had a normal distribution of their full-scale

IQ, they performed poorly on digit span, block design, object assembly, and digit symbol subtests of the WAIS.[17] Although the latter three are timed tests which require motor speed and dexterity, and do not necessarily reflect cerebral pathology, the authors could not explain the poor digit span result and suggested that it might be due to either anxiety or cerebral dysfunction.

One of the major problems of interpretation of these results is that decline of cognitive ability is usually inferred either by comparing patients with controls, or by seeking discrepancies among various abilities that may represent selective impairments.[53] An important contribution in this area was that of Canter who was able to directly assess deficit in a group of 23 World War II veterans with MS who had several years earlier—before the onset of their illness—performed the Army General Classification Test (AGCT) on entry into the service.[13] He noted a significant fall in the AGCT scores for the group as a whole; the greatest drop occurred in patients classified as "severe" from the neurologic standpoint. In the second part of this study, Canter administered the Wechsler-Bellevue test to 47 MS patients and 38 controls on two occasions separated by a 6-month interval. As would be expected from a practice effect, the controls improved on retest, whereas the patient scores actually declined. The MS patients performed more poorly than controls on 8 out of 11 of the Wechsler scale subtests, the most marked difference being in block design.

The first neuropsychologic study of MS to meet modern standards of experimental design and methodology was that of Ross and Reitan.[55] They had three groups of 13 subjects matched for age, educational level, and IQ as determined on the Wechsler-Bellevue scale. Subjects included MS patients, patients with intracranial masses or trauma, and nonbrain-damaged control subjects. The control group contained some patients with psychiatric illness and others with noncerebral neurologic problems. The tests administered included the Halstead battery, the MMPI, and the Rorschach test. The MS patients performed worse than the nonbrain-damaged controls on 6 of 10 Halstead tests, and on a global impairment index. The MS patients' test results resembled the intracranial lesion group on most subtests, and their most obvious difficulties were in simple motor skills and more complex perceptual-motor problem-solving tasks. Although the group mean on a sensitive test of abstracting ability (category test) was in the impaired range for the MS patients, the comparison with controls did not reach statistical significance. In this study, the presence of the third group with psychiatric and other medical disorders suggested that the neuropsychologic deficits in the MS patients were not artifacts related to depression, anxiety, preoccupation with their illness, or to problems with cooperation during testing.

Several other investigations reported in the 1950s should be mentioned. Pratt estimated intellectual changes by noting subjective complaints of poor memory and clinical impressions of intellectual deterioration at interview.[50] He also measured conceptual quotient scores using the Shipley-Hartford test in 50 patients, and gave 64 patients the Raven's Progressive Matrices. Impairments were noted in 15-28 percent of patients, depending on the method of assessment. On the Progressive Matrices, a progression of neuropsychologic impairment was suggested by the finding that patients in the most severe group neurologically had the worst performance on this task of nonverbal reasoning. Two later studies have supported these observations. Knehr found no impairment in Progressive Matrices among 11 ambulatory MS patients,[33] while Staples and Lincoln reported that more severely disabled patients with the disease manifested considerable impairments on this task.[59]

Baldwin examined 34 women with MS against a similar number of controls matched for age, education, and Stanford-Binet vocabulary attainment.[3] The majority of the patients were markedly handicapped. Small differences were noted on the Shipley-Hartford Conceptual Quotient, and no association was found between the disability level and the test results. Unfortunately, several authors have criticized the reliability of the tests used as indicators of cerebral dysfunction.[13,39]

Parsons et al. confirmed Diers and Brown's observation that patients with MS maintained their verbal IQ scores while showing a deficit on performance tests.[46] In studies comparing patients to a matched control medical-surgical group, these investigators also noted differences on the Grassi Block Substitution Test, a visual-perceptual-motor task with four levels of difficulty, the lowest level requiring simple concrete responses while the highest level required abstract and flexible responses. The inferior performance of the MS group was reported to be the result of inaccuracy rather than just slower motor speed, and they were much worse on the more abstract tasks than on the simple ones.

Over the years, several studies have used the Wechsler-Bellevue or WAIS (or portions of them) in evaluating MS patients. Because these studies were uncontrolled, a brief summary of their findings is sufficient; it is stressed, however, that few conclusions can justifiably be drawn from such investigations. Harrower and Kraus reported that the verbal IQ declined with increased neurologic impairment;[27] Fink and Houser concurred.[19] Hirschenfang and Benton noted lowering of the arithmetic, similarities, and digit-span scores in their patients (only verbal subtests of the WAIS were given);[28] Marsh concluded that her patients performed better on verbal than performance subtests of the WAIS, but that scores on both were in the average range.[37]

Other studies at this time included that of Surridge, discussed above, who noted that almost two thirds of the MS patients had some intellectual deficit;[61] this was most often an impairment in memory for recent events and a decline in conceptual thinking.[31] In that study there was also an association between the extent of the intellectual impairment and the degree of the physical disability. In a study of 295 patients from Israel with MS, Kahana et al. concluded at follow-up (mean, 17.3 years after the onset of the disease) that 25 percent of patients had "organic mental syndrome." This figure is consistent with that of Muller who reported a rate of 28 percent for an organic mental syndrome on follow-up (mean, 20 years after onset of the disease).[41] Finally, several case reports have documented the presence of dementia as a prominent feature in selected patients with MS—in some it was the presenting feature of the illness.[5,34,70]

The early work of Ross and Reitan led to a number of more recent investigations employing the Halstead-Reitan Neuropsychologic Test Battery (HRB) or subelements of it.[55] Several studies have yielded comparable results, showing that patients with MS demonstrate neuropsychologic deficits suggestive of brain damage, but that the pattern of this deficit differs from that encountered among other patients with diffuse brain disease such as dementia.[21,38,54] Multiple sclerosis patients exhibit greatest difficulty with time-based, simple motor tasks (e.g., tapping speed, peg insertion) and perceptual problem-solving tasks involving a motor element (e.g., tactual performance test, certain performance elements of the WAIS). Multiple sclerosis patients often performed worse on these tests than other brain damaged patients.

Abstracting ability (category test), on the other hand, although impaired in comparison to "normal" controls, seems better preserved among the MS patients than among those with other forms of brain damage. Over-learned language skills (e.g., vocabulary, information) are best preserved, which tends to be true also of brain damaged control patients, except when lesions affect areas of the brain that determine language ability.[21,38,54]

Recent studies have examined the relationship of neuropsychologic variables to illness duration and types of neurologic presentation and emotional response, as well as the neuropsychologic deficits found in relatively early MS. Ivnik confirmed that neuropsychologic performance deteriorates with increasing length of illness and demonstrated the progression of deficits in examinations a year apart.[29,30] Beatty and Gange demonstrated impaired verbal memory in patients who were otherwise relatively intact.[4] Peyser et al. found that about half of their patients, who were thought to have clinically intact cognitive abilities, showed deficit in abstracting ability.[49] There was also evidence that neuropsychologic deficit was related to the type of neurologic presentation. Thus twice as many patients with visual system symptoms had impaired abstracting abilities when compared with those who did not.

A companion report from the same group presented a promising attempt to unite converging neuropsychologic, psychiatric, and neurologic information.[48] Using cluster analysis, they were able to separate their patients into six descriptive groups on the basis of combinations of reported length of disease, age of diagnosis, Kurtzke Disability Scale scores, category test scores, Purdue Pegboard assembly scores, MMPI data, age, and sex. Although the authors can be criticized for using too many variables for the limited number of subjects (55) in this cluster analysis, their attempt is interesting and their findings are intriguing. One group, for example, consisted of young patients with short duration of the disease who were cognitively intact and had little neurologic disability. Their psychologic adjustment was based on denial. A group of older patients had the disease a long time, were disabled, had cognitive deficit, and considerable psychopathology as measured on the MMPI. Another group of older patients with moderate physical impairment had onset at a later age; they were cognitively intact and showed MMPI evidence of depression and preoccupation with symptoms typical of chronically medically ill subjects. Another smaller group had little objective disability (either physical or neuropsychologic), but had evidence of conversion hysteria on the MMPI rating scale. It is hoped that further investigations of this sort will lead to a more comprehensive classification of the subtypes of presentation of the disorder.

PSYCHIATRIC DISORDERS RESEMBLING MULTIPLE SCLEROSIS

In any series of patients diagnosed as having MS, there will be several in whom subsequent follow-up suggests that the diagnosis was incorrectly given. Of particular concern are those patients who present with psychopathology which for one reason or another, leads to a diagnosis of MS in the absence of clearly-defined neurologic illness. The most important point regarding the problem of hysteria, briefly discussed above, is that the presentation of symptomatology in medicine can be markedly influenced by personality factors; failure to assess these factors adequately can lead to diagnostic confusion.

There is one group of patients who initially present with histories of fleeting neurologic symptoms and then develop, for example, a progressive paraplegia which leads to eventual confinement in a wheelchair.

Somewhere in the course of their medical consultations, a doctor discusses the possibility of MS and this is taken by the patient as a definitive diagnosis. Gradually, as consultations progress, the possible diagnosis of MS becomes definite, and the patient's environment and activities become organized to these ends. Assessment of such patients is often extremely difficult, although ultimately it is clear that the initial diagnosis was probably amiss, since after a long history of neurologic disability, neurologic signs remain distinctly difficult to actually document. The typical hysterical personality is not necessarily seen in this sort of patient, and only very close dissection of the patient's history, coping style, and current interpersonal relationships may give a clue as to the origin of such behavior. Some of these patients cling to the diagnosis of MS and, while accepting further investigations and consultations, become acutely distressed should anyone raise the possibility that a revision of their diagnosis is warranted.

Another group of patients who must be recognized are those suffering from Briquet's syndrome,[69] also termed somatization disorder.[1] The essential features of this syndrome have been clearly defined by Guze and colleagues:[69] Patients are all young women, polysymptomatic, and characteristically have a history containing an excessive number of surgical operations and hospitalizations associated with numerous vague complaints.[51] In one early series, blurred vision occurred in 62 percent of patients, transient blindness in 20 percent, double vision in 10 percent, urinary retention in 43 percent, paralyses in 33 percent, and paresthesias in 80 percent.[51] These symptoms typically intermingled with others, were recurrent, and led to multiple hospitalizations for investigations, often with surgical exploration. Such patients can occasionally be misdiagnosed as having MS. The importance of recognizing this disorder is that it is intractable, and patients with Briquet's syndrome present severe management problems; they are also vulnerable to having iatrogenic morbidity added to their symptom complex as a result of unnecessary investigations and explorations.

Anxiety states, both acute and chronic, can present with somatic complaints and a diagnosis of MS. Thus symptoms may include somatic complaints that resemble the punctuated history of MS, particularly anesthesias and tingling, tremor, frequency of micturition, and sometimes weakness and giddiness and gait disturbances with a tendency to fall. Higher cognitive disturbances, such as memory loss, confusion, and amnesia may also take an intermittent course and lead to diagnostic difficulty.

In contrast, depressive illness or more clearly defined psychotic states such as schizophrenia, are rarely confused with MS. The exception is a case of masked depression with somatization which, taking a recurrent unipolar course, leads to episodic bouts of neurologic symptoms, again in the absence of clearly-defined neurologic signs. Fatigue, particularly associated with fleeting aches and paresthesia, may lead to diagnostic difficulty, and the actual diagnosis may only become clear with time.

Recognition of these problems clearly requires a familiarity with psychiatric diagnosis on the part of the examining physician, and emphasizes the need for psychiatric referral in cases where the clinical progress seems out of keeping with the diagnosis of MS.

PSYCHIATRIC DISORDERS FOLLOWING TREATMENT FOR MULTIPLE SCLEROSIS

Of the several treatments available for managing MS, adrenocorticotropic hormone (ACTH) or prednisolone are often given in the acute phase of the illness, usually begun in high doses and gradually reduced. Such treatment may alter the affective state of the patient or be associated with the onset of psychosis. Steroid administration is generally associated with euphoria, although a florid psychosis has been reported in up to 10 percent of patients. The latter effect manifests within 3 weeks of starting treatment and usually occurs in the first 7 days. It is more likely to occur with higher doses of steroids, takes no specific form, and may be associated with electroencephalographic changes, especially slowing of background rhythms.[25] There is some suggestion that ACTH is more likely to induce such changes than corticosteroids;[62] this is in keeping with the now recognized psychoactive properties of ACTH fragments. Although disturbance of consciousness occurs in up to one third of patients with the psychosis, the differential diagnosis can often be difficult to make in these situations since the psychosis may occur in the setting of clear consciousness, and its cause may not be clear, i.e., an exacerbation of the MS or a side effect of steroid treatment. In view of the relative infrequency of psychosis in untreated MS, however, it is likely that most of these cases represent steroid-induced phenomena. Where possible, the dose of steroids should be reduced and the psychosis treated symptomatically with antipsychotic medication.

Other medications used in the management of MS are occasionally implicated in producing psychiatric disturbance. In a recent case report, for example, the sudden cessation of baclofen produced a psychotic manic state which responded to haloperidol.[2]

TREATMENT OF PSYCHIATRIC DISORDERS IN MULTIPLE SCLEROSIS

It is clear that psychopathology is common in MS, and that the problems patients face involve a number of therapeutic specialists, including neurologists, psychiatrists, physiotherapists, social workers, occupational therapists, and rehabilitation officers. As with all chronic conditions, patients should have someone they can turn to; this person does not have to be medically qualified, but should be familiar with all aspects of the disease in order to discuss problems and worries as they arise in the patient's life. Counseling and psychotherapy may be particularly useful here, especially where marital problems exist. Paulley suggested that many MS patients demonstrate emotional dependence, passivity, and problems in separation from key figures, and that more formal psychotherapy is useful in managing these problems.[47] Indeed, he suggested that psychotherapy today, especially couple therapy, may offer more promise than other forms of treatment, and that anyone with a sufficient understanding of psychodynamics should be able to provide valuable aid. Many marriages deteriorate because of the disease, and if the basic relationship is inadequate, the MS may become a scapegoat for all ensuing difficulties. Patients often fear rejection; they might worry, especially if they develop sexual disabilities, that their spouse will seek extramarital relationships for satisfaction. Strain may also arise in situations where euphoria and denial are great, in which patients fail to acknowledge their limitations and put quite impossible strains upon other members in the family.[12]

The use of psychotropic drugs in MS has not been studied extensively. Such agents should be considered when frank psychopathology becomes evident. If antidepressants are called for, those which cause minimal side effects should be used. These considerations tend to limit the usefulness of the tricyclic compounds. In particular, their ability to cause micturition difficulties, postural hypotension, and sweating may be distressing to the patient with MS, and newer compounds may be preferred. If hypnotic action is required, a more sedating antidepressant such as mianserin may be useful; in patients for whom a more alerting response is required, nomifensine or flupenthixol in the day time are reasonable alternatives. For psychotic symptoms, antipsychotic medications will be required. The phenothiazines and butyrophenones are the most common compounds, and choice will depend to some extent on the amount of sedation required. The butyrophenones, i.e., haloperidol, are less hypnotic, but are associated with the ready production of extrapyramidal complications such as dystonias, Parkinsonism, and, after prolonged use, tardive dyskinesia. Whatever psychotropic drug is chosen, it appears that MS patients require smaller doses than would otherwise be used. The complications of long-term antipsychotic drug therapy include severe extrapyramidal problems which can be misinterpreted as progression of MS. Electroconvulsive therapy is not contraindicated in MS, and may be used where the clinical situation demands it. In cases of severe depression and suicidal ideation, where the possibility of suicide is very high, ECT should be considered as the first choice of treatment.

CONCLUSIONS

Although many studies have investigated the mental state of patients with MS, much work still has to be done, particularly with newer techniques of neuropsychiatric investigation. Most studies emphasize that some change in mentation occurs at some stage of the disease in the majority of patients, although there are obvious exceptions to this, particularly the early studies from neurologic clinics. The use of more refined techniques and a more widespread population of patients will allow more deficits to be detected.

Although depression is a particularly common psychiatric problem, further studies on its phenomenology are needed. The exact interrelationship between the disease process and the presentation of depression is unclear at this stage, although evidence implies that the tendency for a more euphoric picture to emerge increases as CNS damage increases. Presentation of euphoria certainly suggests that cognitive deficits will also be found, although it should be remembered that under the veneer of euphoria many patients are in fact depressed.

The unusual eutonia repeatedly described by clinical observers may be a mental state that is relatively specific to MS; it is qualitatively different both from the fatuous euphoria of patients with clearly defined frontal lobe damage, and the affectively consistent feelings of well-being described in manic-depressive illness. Psychosis is rare in MS and, if anything, is seen more commonly as a result of treatment.

The more sophisticated neuropsychologic studies have indicated that the majority of patients with MS show some evidence of disturbed ability suggesting cerebral involvement, but that in the early stages the deficit may well be isolated and subtle. As the disorder progresses, the deficits worsen. In the middle phase of the disease, a relatively characteristic pattern of disorder may exist in which perceptual motor deficits are impaired while abstracting and memory deficits are not detected. Aphasia in this condition is relatively rare. In the late stages, frank dementia is often seen, although this rarely may be a presenting sign of the disorder.

There is no evidence of a predisposing MS personality. Although the disorder clearly leads to personality changes, the results may depend on the characteristic coping styles of individual patients. Diagnostic difficulties often arise in the early stages of this disease, not only vis-a-vis other neurologic disorders, but also with respect to psychiatric disorders. In cases of diagnostic doubt, comprehensive neuropsychiatric investigations are helpful; in difficult cases, follow-up by physicians acquainted with the progression of both neurologic and psychiatric disease is recommended.

REFERENCES

1. American Psychiatric Association: Diagnostic and Statistical Manual of Mental Disorders, ed 3: Washington DC, APA, 1980
2. Arnold ES, Rudd SM, Kirschner H: Manic psychosis following rapid withdrawal from baclofen. Am J Psychiatry 137:1466–1467, 1980
3. Baldwin MV: A clinico-experimental investigation into the psychologic aspects of multiple sclerosis. J Nerv Ment Dis 115:299–342, 1952
4. Beatty PA, Gange JJ: Neuropsychological aspects of multiple sclerosis. J Nerv Ment Dis 164:42–50, 1977
5. Bergin JD: Rapidly progressing dementia in disseminated sclerosis. J Neurol Neurosurg Psychiatry 20:285–292, 1957
6. Bignami A, Gherardi D, Gallo G: Sclerosi a placche acuta a localizzazione i potalamica con sintomolyogia a psychica do tipo malinconico. Riv Neurol 31:240–268, 1961
7. Braceland FJ, Giffin ME: The mental changes associated with multiple sclerosis. Res Publ Assoc Res Nerv Ment Dis 28:450–455, 1950
8. Brain WR: Critical review: Disseminated sclerosis. Q J Med 23:343–391, 1930
9. Brown S, Davis TK: The mental symptoms of multiple sclerosis. Assoc Res Nerv Ment Dis 2:76–82, 1922
10. Brown S, Davis TK: The mental symptoms of multiple sclerosis. Arch Neurol Psychiatry 7:629–634, 1922
11. Burgmeister BB, Tallman G: Rorschach patterns in multiple sclerosis. Rorschach Research Exchange 9:111–122, 1945
12. Burnfield A, Burnfield P: Common psychological problems in multiple sclerosis. Br Med J II:1193–1194, 1978
13. Canter AH: Direct and indirect measures of psychological deficit in multiple sclerosis. J Gen Psychol 44:3–50, 1951
14. Charcot JM: Lectures on the Diseases of the Nervous System Delivered at La Salpetriere. London, New Syndenham Society, 1877, pp 194–195

15. Cottrell SS, Wilson SAK: The affective symptomatology of disseminated sclerosis. A study of 100 cases. J Neurol Psychopathol 7:1–30, 1926
16. Davison K, Bagley CR: Schizophrenia-like psychoses associated with organic disorders of the central nervous system: Review of the literature, in Herrington RN (ed): Current Problems in Neuropsychiatry. Kent, England, Headley Brothers, 1969
17. Diers WC, Brown CC: Psychometric patterns in multiple sclerosis 1. Wechsler-Bellevue patterns. Arch Neurol Psychiatry 63:760–765, 1950
18. Duge, Ein Beitrag zur Kenntnis der Psychosen bei der Multiplen Sklerose des Gehirns und Rükenmarks. Deutsche Zeitschrift. Nervenheilkunde, 51, 459–512, 1914. Cited by Ross AT, Reitan RM: Intellectual and affective functions in multiple sclerosis. Arch Neurol Psych 73:663–677, 1955
19. Fink SL, Houser AB: An investigation of physical and intellectual changes in multiple sclerosis. Arch Phys Med Rehabil 47:56–61, 1966
20. Goodstein RK, Farrell RB: Multiple sclerosis presenting as a depressive illness. Dis Nerv Sys 38:127–131, 1977
21. Goldstein G, Shelly CH: Neuropsychological diagnosis of multiple sclerosis in a neuropsychiatric setting. J Nerv Ment Dis 158:280–290, 1974
22. Gowers WR: A Manual of Diseases of the Nervous System, 2nd Ed. London, Churchill, 1893
23. Grant I: Behavioral Disorders. New York, Spectrum, 1979
24. Grant I, Reed R: Neuropsychological testing, in Wiederholt WC (ed): Neurology for Non-neurologists. New York, Academic, 1982
25. Hall RCW, Popkin MK, Stickney SK, Gardner ER: Presentation of the steroid psychoses. J Nerv Ment Dis 167:229–236, 1979
26. Halstead WC: Brain and Intelligence: A Quantitative Study of the Frontal Lobes. Chicago, University of Chicago Press, 1947
27. Harrower MR, Kraus J: Psychological studies on patients with multiple sclerosis. Arch Neurol 66:44–51, 1951
28. Hirschenfang S, Benton JG: Note on intellectual changes in multiple sclerosis. Percept Mot Skills 22:786, 1966
29. Ivnik RJ: Neuropsychological stability in multiple sclerosis. J Consult Clin Psychol 46:913–923, 1978
30. Ivnik RJ: Neuropsychological test performance as a function of duration of multiple sclerosis-related symptomatology. J Clin Psychol 39:304–307, 311–331, 1978
31. Jambor KL: Cognitive functioning in multiple sclerosis. Br J Psychiatry, 115:765–775, 1969
32. Kahana E, Leibowitz U, Alter M: Cerebral multiple sclerosis. Neurology 21:1170–1176, 1971
33. Knehr CA: Differential impairment in multiple sclerosis. J Psychol 54:443–451, 1962
34. Koenig H: Dementia associated with multiple sclerosis. Trans Am Neurol Assoc 93:227–228, 1968
35. Langworthy OR: Relation of Personality problems to onset and progress of multiple sclerosis. Arch Neurol Psychiatry 59:13–28, 1948

36. Leibowitz U, Kahana E, Jacobson SG, Alter M: Cause of death in multiple sclerosis. Progress in multiple sclerosis, research and treatment, in Leibowitz U (ed): Proccedings of an International Symposium, May 1970. New York, Academic Press, 1970
37. Marsh G: Disability and intellectual function in multiple sclerosis. J Nerv Ment Dis 168:758-762, 1980
38. Matthews CG, Cleeland CS, Hopper CL: Neuropsychological patterns in multiple sclerosis. Dis Nerv Sys 31:161-170, 1970
39. Meehl PE, Jeffery ME: The Hunt-Minnesota Test for organic brain damage in cases of functional depression. J Appl Psychol 30:276, 1946
40. Merskey H, Buhrich NA: Hysteria and organic brain disease. Br J Med Psychol 48:359-366, 1975
41. Muller R: Studies on disseminated sclerosis with special reference to symptomatology, course, and prognosis. Acta Med Scand 133 (Suppl 222):1, 1949
42. Mur J, Kumpel G, Dostal S: An anergic phase of disseminated sclerosis with psychiatric course. Confin Neurol 28:37-49, 1966
43. O'Malley PO: Severe mental symptoms in disseminated sclerosis. J Irish Med Assoc 55:115-127, 1966
44. Ombredrane A: Sur les Troubles Mentaux de la Sclerose en Plaques. These de Paris, 1929. Quoted by Surridge D in: An investigation into some psychiatric aspects of multiple sclerosis. Br J Psychiatry 155:749-764, 1969
45. Oppenheim (1896). Quoted by O'Malley PO in: Severe mental symptoms in disseminated sclerosis. J Irish Med Assoc 55:115-127, 1966
46. Parsons OA, Stewart BA, Arenberg D: Impairment of abstracting ability in multiple sclerosis. J Nerv Ment Dis 125:221-225, 1957
47. Paulley JW: The psychological management of multiple sclerosis. Practitioner 218:100-105, 1977
48. Peyser JM, Edwards KR, Poser CM: Psychological profiles in patients with multiple sclerosis. A preliminary investigation. Arch Neurol 37:437-440, 1980
49. Peyser JM, Edwards KR, Poser CM, Filskov SB: Cognitive function in patients with multiple sclerosis. Arch Neurol 37:577-579, 1980
50. Pratt RTC: An investigation of the psychiatric aspects of disseminated sclerosis. J Neurol Neurosurg Psychiatry 14:326-335, 1951
51. Purtell JJ, Robins E, Cohen ME: Observations on the clinical aspects of hysteria. JAMA 146:902-909, 1951
52. Raecke J: Psychische Storungen bei der Multiplen Sklerose. Arch Psychiatrie (Berlin) 41:482-518, 1906
53. Reitan RM, Davison L: Clinical Neuropsychology: Current Status and Applications. Washington DC, VH Winston, 1974
54. Reitan RM, Reed JC, Dyken M: Cognitive, psychomotor, and motor correlates of multiple sclerosis. J Nerv Ment Dis 153:218-224, 1971
55. Ross AT, Reitan RM: Intellectual and affective functions in multiple sclerosis. Arch Neurol Psychiatry 73:663-677, 1955
56. Sachs B, Friedman ED: General symptomatology and differential diagnosis of disseminated sclerosis. Arch Neurol Psychiatry 7:551-560, 1922

57. Seiffer H: Ueber psychiche in besondere Intelligenzstorungen bei multipler sklerose. Arch Psychiatrie 40:253–283, 1905
58. Slater E: Diagnosis of "hysteria." Br Med J I:1395–1399, 1965
59. Staples D, Lincoln NB: Impairment in multiple sclerosis and its relation to functional abilities. Rheumatol Rehabil 18:153–160, 1979
60. Sugar C, Nadell R: Mental symptoms in multiple sclerosis: A study of 28 cases with review of the literature. J Nerv Ment Dis 98:267–280, 1943
61. Surridge D: An investigation into some psychiatric aspects of multiple sclerosis. Br J Psychiatry 155:749–764, 1969
62. Truelove SC, Witts LJ: Cortisone and corticotrophin in ulcerative colitis. Br Med J I:387–393, 1959
63. Trimble MR: Neuropsychiatry. New York, Wiley, 1981
64. Wechsler D: The Measurement of Adult Intelligence. Baltimore, Williams & Wilkins, 1944
65. Whitlock FA: The aetiology of hysteria. Acta Psychiatri Scand 43:144–162, 1967
66. Whitlock FA, Siskind MM: Depression as a major symptom of multiple sclerosis. J Neurol Neurosurg Psychiatry 43:861–865, 1980
67. Wilkes S: Lectures on Diseases of the Nervous System. London, Churchill, 1878
68. Wilson SAK: Neurology. London, Arnold, 1940
69. Woodruff RA, Goodwin DW, Guze SB: Psychiatric Diagnosis. New York, Oxford University Press, 1974
70. Young AC, Saunders J, Ponsford JR: Mental change as an early feature of multiple sclerosis. J Neurol Neurosurg Psychiatry 39:1008–1013, 1976

Commentary

It has long been recognized that behavioral abnormalities involving both psychiatric and neurologic causation are present in MS and that these are complicated and multiple has also been recognized. Actually, the problem has been sufficiently complex that, although many have tried, clinicians have rarely been successful in fully describing and discussing the multiple factors. Drs. Trimble and Grant have not only succinctly reviewed the massive collection of material on the behavioral abnormalities of MS but have organized it into a cohesive and reasonable format which permits recognition of individual traits of a patient within the total context of the neuropsychiatric complications of MS. In addition, based on this structure, the authors provide a rational format for investigation of the behavioral difficulties and, based on the findings of such research, offer a rational plan for therapy. For certain, not all of the behavioral problems of MS have been solved but the authors have developed a usable structure incorporating the information necessary to begin understanding these problems. Chapter 13 truly reflects a full neurobehavioral approach, and notes both neurologically and psychiatrically derived behavioral problems occurring in combination.

Finally, this volume concludes with a review and update of an easily recognized but bewilderingly enigmatic disorder—stuttering. While common and long studied, the phenomenon of stuttering has avoided any fully acceptable explanation. Mechanical explanations (based on early concepts of lateralized cortical function) were popular at the turn of the century but gave way to comprehensive psychogenic theories of causation. In turn, despite considerable creativity, these theories have proved inadequate and led to renewed search for the causes of stuttering. Dr. Rosenfield reviews this background and complements the review with a comprehensive update of reported research and current research directions in the attempt to understand stuttering. While offering no easy answers for the victim, improved recognition of the multiple factors not only provides some comfort for the stutterer but also considerable hope for improved management.

David B. Rosenfield, M.D.

14
Neuropsychiatric Aspects of Stuttering

The purpose of this chapter is to present current thinking about stuttering. It is not intended to be a detailed review of mechanisms of voice production but rather a review of current ideas that hopefully will be of importance for the practicing psychiatrist and neurologist.

DEFINITION

Stuttering is a pan-global, pan-cultural phenomenon that is noted in all languages.[53] It is characterized by words which are improperly patterned in time and by repetitive dysfluencies.[53] One to two percent of all populations are afflicted with this disturbance.[1,36] One can gain insight into mechanisms of speech and language by examining the phenomenon of stuttering.

Some query whether there is a difference between stuttering and stammering. This is an old European distinction, with stuttering refering to clonic repetitions of sound (b-b-b-book) and stammering refering to a tonic abnormality (b-------book). Stutterers can learn to modify aspects of their sound output such that clonic disturbances are produced as tonic disturbances. Thus, the distinction between stammering and stuttering has little meaning. The secondary characteristics of stuttering, i.e., grimacing and bizarre facial contortions, are usually "learned" responses that are

---

This work was supported by the Ariel Foundation and the Perkins Foundation.

associated with the struggle of speech production and are readily controlled by speech therapy.

HISTORY

Many individuals have attempted to explain stuttering. Hippocrates commented about *trauloi* (stuttering as well as other speech disturbances), but it was not until Aristotle that we note any particular focus upon this speech disturbance. Aristotle thought that *ischnophonia* resulted from improper body humor interaction. This thesis was promulgated for nearly 1600 years under the aegis of Galen. In 1583, Mercurialis wrote the first detailed review on stuttering. His *Treatise on the Diseases of Children* agreed with Galen and Aristotle that stuttering resulted from abnormal humoral interactions in the body.[41]

Bacon's *Sylva Sylvarum*, published in 1627, marked the advent of scientific reason. It was no longer sufficient to quote Aristotle or Galen as a source of knowledge; theories had to be based upon observable data. In this setting, Morgagni (1682–1771) sought to ascertain whether stutterers had physical abnormalities which accounted for their abnormal speech. He believed that abnormalities of the hyoid bone (then thought to be a major organ of speech) accounted for stuttering. Later, Erasmus Darwin, a Locke "associationist," contended that stuttering resulted from bonafide physiologic interactions. The 19th Century witnessed Warren and Dieffenbach addressing physical abnormalities of stutterers, the latter resecting portions of their tongue.[41]

The 20th century has witnessed theories pertaining to interhemisphere competition (Orton,[34] Travis,[50] Jones[23]) as well as disturbances of self-concept (Johnson,[21,22] Sheehan[47]). The historic continuum of stuttering has witnessed its leaving philosophic permutations and entering neurologic realms, demanding attention to cerebral laterality, laryngeal-auditory-cerebral feedback circuits, and neurolaryngeal physiology.

THEORIES AND MECHANISMS

Any theory of stuttering must explain several phenomenon. First, there is a genetic factor. Nelson has demonstrated a 90 percent concordance rate in monozygotic twins versus a 20 percent concordance rate in dizygotic twins.[33] Further, Kidd and his colleagues have elegantly demonstrated that the incidence of stuttering follows particular mathematical genetic models. His studies have also helped explain the strong male sexual bias of stuttering.[24]

There are other phenomena of stuttering which must be addressed by any theory. A stutterer's fluency is markedly enhanced during singing; indeed, stutterers do not stutter when they sing. White noise, whispering, and speaking during inhalation promote fluency. Also, one notes that stutterers frequently stutter on transitions from voiced (i.e., "z") to voiceless (i.e., "s") sounds and at particular loci in the sentence (i.e., at the beginning of phrases and sentences).[53]

One of the more popular theories of stuttering pertains to "abnormal" cerebral dominance. This theory, initially promulgated by Stier and Sachs in Germany, was popularized in the United States by Orton[34] and Travis.[50] The Orton-Travis theory of "incomplete" cerebral dominance contends that stuttering results from incomplete lateralization of language. This results in the two hemispheres competing with each other and somehow producing stuttered speech. Children learning to talk have repetitive dysfluencies because they lack fully developed cerebral dominance for language.[4] As this dominance is established, the child speaks more fluently.

Since handedness reflects lateralization of speech (99 percent of right-handed people have language in their left hemisphere as opposed to only 60 percent of left-handed individuals),[4] investigators focused attention upon the relationship between handedness and stuttering, contending that stutterers should have an increased prevalence of non-right-handedness. A wide disparity of results soon emerged. Estimates of left-handedness among groups of stutterers ranged from 2 to 21 percent; ambidexterity ranged from zero to 61 percent. The reasons for these discrepancies were due to various definitions of stuttering, ambidexterity, and handedness. In addition, their methods of ascertaining which individuals were stutterers was faulty—one cannot ascertain the prevalence of stuttering in a classroom by simply asking the teacher. There are many "closet stutterers," stutterers who alter their word choice and frequently appear to be fluent. These individuals use words/sentences which they can fluently produce instead of using words upon which they would stutter. School teachers often times do not know that they are stutterers.[7,8,10,11,30,31,49] (In my medical school class of 200, I was informed by a committee analyzing those with handicaps that we had one stutterer in our class of 200. I was involved in research projects and had already tested four bonafide stutterers.)

The relationship between stuttering and shift of handedness has long been a moot point.[8,21] Ballard believed that altering a child's hand preference might well cause stuttering.[3] He contended that 17 percent of left-handed children who had been forced to write with their right hand became stutterers. Wallin reported that over 9 percent of stutterers in a school population had been shifted from left- to right-handed writing, while only 2 percent of all pupils had been shifted. However, 80 percent of the shifted stutterers had been stutterers before learning how to write.[55] McAllister cites a study by Inman in which left-handed training was given to mentally retarded children; 5 months later, several of the children stuttered.[30] Parson evaluated atempts at trying to eliminate left-handedness in the school system and did not note the onset of any stuttering.[35] The issue of a forced shift in handedness altering speech output has never been substantiated.

As a result of these discrepancies pertaining to handedness and stuttering, the thesis of altered cerebral laterality in stutterers became less popular. The later advent of electroencephalography refocused attention toward an organic component but, again, many investigators reached conclusions that differed from their colleagues and the issue was unsettled.[15,38,51,52]

The thesis of altered cerebral laterality in stutterers then lay dormant until Jones, a neurosurgeon, reported that he had had occasion to operate upon four stutterers who had developed, subsequent to their stuttering, cerebral disease necessitating surgical intervention.[23] He was aware that language could reside in both hemispheres of stutterers and was concerned that his contemplated surgery might render the stutterers aphasic (i.e., would the stutterer undergoing left brain surgery become aphasic if classic areas of speech were surgically resected? Could the same happen to the right?). He obtained this information by performing a Wada test.[54]

The Wada test involves injecting sodium amobarbital, a short-acting barbituate, into the carotid artery. Each carotid artery supplies the ipsilateral cerebral hemisphere (although sometimes there is a crossover of blood flow) and the barbituate transiently anesthetizes the ipsilateral hemisphere. Patients are temporarily rendered hemiplegic on the side contralateral to the injection and become aphasic if the language-dominant hemisphere was exposed to the barbituate.

Jones noted that all four stutterers became aphasic following barbituate injection in either their right or their left carotid artery, thus indicating that both hemispheres significantly contributed to language. Each patient required unilateral intracranial surgery for treatment of the underlying cerebral disease. All four were aphasic following surgery but recovered language function completely and all four ceased stuttering. A repeat Wada test elicited aphasia only after injection on the nonoperated side. They no longer had bilateral speech representation and they no longer stuttered.

Jones' paper is intriguing but several criticisms should be noted. All but one of his four patients were left-handed, implicating bilateral language representation. All but one had a strong family history of left-handedness, further implicating bilateral language representation.[59] He did not state how the presence or absence of stuttering was ascertained. It would be interesting to know whether they had still "lost" the stutter several years following surgery and not just over the short period described in his paper. The strongest obstacle to accepting his findings is the fact that there are patients who have bilaterally positive Wada tests but who do not stutter.[32] In addition, why should bilateral speech/language representation produce a stutter rather than make one mute, aphasic, schizophrenic, or, perhaps, more fluent than others?

Subsequent investigators have pursued Wada testing in stutterers.[2,29] In total, 11 stutterers have had bilateral Wada studies; 5 had bilateral speech representation. One of these was an individual who had developed stuttering-like behavior along with aphasia following head trauma.[2] This discrepancy in data may reflect the fact that stuttering is not a homogeneous disturbance.

Jones' report sparked new interest in the possibility of cerebral dominance aberrations causing stuttering. Investigators soon employed techniques for analyzing cerebral dominance which were not as invasive as the angiography required for the Wada test. One of these techniques is the dichotic listening paradigm.

The hallmark of dichotic listening studies is the systematic manipulation of acoustic parameters of auditory stimuli. In this paradigm, different auditory stimuli are simultaneously presented to each ear. Although the cochlea of each ear is neurally attached to both hemispheres, a group of listeners consistently report hearing the stimulus in only one ear when different speech sounds are simultaneously presented to both ears. Kimura has demonstrated that verbal signals (words, digits) are more accurately reported from the right ear (i.e., left hemisphere), than from the left (i.e., right hemisphere) in a simultaneous dichotic presentation.[25,26] The reverse is true for melody.[28]

Curry and Gregory investigated stutterers' performance in a dichotic listening paradigm.[9] They tested 20 adult stutterers (19 men, 1 woman) and 20 appropriate controls. All were allegedly right-handed. They employed several dichotic tasks, one of which was the dichotic word test. This involved the recognition of pairs of consonant-vowel-consonant words of high familiarity, presented in groups of six pairs with 0.50 seconds separating each pair. After each group of six words had been presented, the subjects attempted to recall the 12 different words in any order without concern for which words had been presented to any particular ear. There were 12 groups of 6 pairs in the test. The anticipated right ear superiority was significantly less for stutterers than for nonstutterers. Seventy-five percent of the nonstutterers had right-ear scores that were higher than left; this was true for only 45 percent of the stutterers. Kimura contends that such reversals of ear superiority occur in cases of known reversals of hemispheric dominance as confirmed by Wada tests.[25]

The nonstutterers' mean, absolute between-ears difference score was more than twice that of the stutterers. The exact meaning of this finding is unknown, but it may well be that it reflects the degree of dominance; i.e., if the magnitude of hemispheric language asymmetry is determined by the functional difference between the ipsilateral and contralateral ear responses, perhaps the degree of dominance which stutterers have is less than normal.

Quinn also investigated dichotic listening in stutterers with a method similar to that mentioned above.[37] He examined 60 right-handed stutterers (53 men, 7 women) with matched controls. He noted no difference between the two groups, but did observe that 12 individual stutterers had left-ear scores that were higher than right-ear scores; only two nonstutterers had this "reversal." He subsequently realized that 5 of these 12 stutterers were left-handed golfers. The remaining seven were strongly right-handed. Thus, though the initial report suggested that the population was entirely right-handed, some were more right-handed than others.

Brady and Berson compared 35 right-handed adult (men and women) stutterers' dichotic performance to that of a nonstuttering population.[6] Similar to Quinn, they were unable to confirm Curry and Gregory's group differences; however, they did note that six stutterers and no normals had a left ear advantage.

Dorman and Porter evaluated 16 right-handed adult stutterers (12 men, 4 women) and compared them to 20 controls (10 men, 10 women).[14] Subjects had to write responses to nonhuman speech, consonant-vowel dichotic stimuli. There was no difference between stutterers and nonstutterers.

Studies of child stutterers also fail to demonstrate dichotic listening differences between stutterers and control groups. Slorech and Noehr examined 15 stutterers, age 6.25–9.0 years.[48] The stutterers did not differ from the controls in the recognition of digit pairs. Gruber and Powell dichotically examined 28 right-handed children stutterers and controls, using digit pairs.[19] They failed to find significant dichotic differences for either group. (One should note that since 4 percent of children stutter compared to only 1 percent of adults,[50] the mechanisms and types of stuttering referred to may be different from that in adults. Also, Kimura failed to find significant differences between ear performances and dichotic tasks presented to 7- to 9-year-old normal girls.[27])

Neuropsychiatric Aspects of Stuttering

Rosenfield and Goodglass contended that perhaps the above studies lacked agreement because investigators looked at stuttering as a homogeneous syndrome. Perhaps stuttering was like pneumonia (some types being due to a fungus, some due to a bacteria, some due to a virus, etc.). Since handedness was an issue in stuttering, perhaps only individuals of homogeneous handedness, as determined by a stringent handedness questionnnaire, constituted a valuable experimental group. Also, since the prognosis and prevalence for stuttering among men and women is different, perhaps only individuals of one sex should be evaluated. Since children have a much better prognosis for losing their stutter than do adults,[5] perhaps adults should not be mixed with children. Consequently, these authors investigated an allegedly homogenous group of stutterers, those who were strongly right-handed adult men, and compared them to controls. After running the experiment once, they waited a week and then repeated it. They found that a significantly greater number of stutterers than controls consistently failed to show the expected ear laterality for consonant-vowel sounds (i.e., pa, ka) or melodies.

If stutterers have abnormalities in cerebral dominance, why should that make them stutter? Why not make them talk faster, be mute, or be schizophrenic? Why do they not stutter on all words or on all sounds? How do we know that the dichotic listening paradigm, a paradigm which ascertains language laterality viś-a-viś sound *input*, is an index of cerebral dominance at the moment of stuttering, a moment of sound *output*. If stutterers have "abnormal" dominance, how do we know that it does not only occur at the moment of stuttering, and is not a constant abnormality that would be detected during an experiment involving a listening task. These are all major issues and are currently being investigated.

Perhaps we can gain more insight into the vagaries of cerebral dominance in stuttering if we have a better understanding of the physiologic mechanics of sound production. Speaking involves moving the vocal cords (vocal folds). The vocal cords are composed of skeletal muscle. There are intrinsic brain stem reflexes involving laryngeal receptor systems that make the cords abduct upon inspiration and adduct during expiration.[57,58] In order to produce speech, one must exercise cerebral control over these intrinsic laryngeal mechanisms. Speech necessitates that the vocal cords move in and move out. This can only be accomplished by exercising supra-brain stem control over the above mentioned intrinsic laryngeal/brain stem reflexes. Were it just left to the larynx, so to speak, the cords would always be adducted as we exhale; they would not go through the abducted/adducted movements that are so typical of speech. How is this accomplished?

When we utter a voiced sound (i.e., "b," "g," "d,") we excite the adductors of the vocal cords and inhibit the abductors. Opposite cord movement occurs when we utter sounds that are voiceless (i.e., "p," "k," "f"). This cord action occurs 0.05-0.55 seconds before actual output of sound, and 0.05-0.10 seconds before any changes in air pressure transpire under the vocal cords. The vocal cords contract before any air pressure changes occur under the glottis (the opening between the vocal cords). This "prephonatory tuning" is thought to be under voluntary/learned control and to relate to corticobulbar fibers.Prephonatory tuning is followed by phonation, involving modulation and stabilization of laryngeal reflexes as they relate to subglottic mucosal receptors, stretch-sensitive myotatic mechanoreceptors, and articular (i.e., located in the joints of the larynx) mechanoreceptors. Lastly, there is acoustic-auto-monitoring of speech that involves voluntary and involuntary pathways.[57,58] It is this automonitoring that becomes compromised when normal individuals become totally deaf, resulting in changes in their articulatory patterns.

The laryngeal system of stutterers does not work appropriately. The normal abductor/adductor reciprocity of laryngeal muscles is absent in stutterers.[16] In many stutterers, when they enter a stuttering block, the adductors and abductors contract at the same time. When they attempt to fake a stuttering block, they are unable to produce this cocontraction and when a nonstutterer fakes a block, he is unable to produce this cocontraction.

A precise temporal relationship normally exists between the voluntary prephonatory setting of vocal musculature and the continuous reflex readjustment of the laryngeal muscle movment. All of this must somehow be influenced by the hemisphere that is dominant for language. If stutterers are genetically predisposed toward abnormalities in cerebral dominance, it may be difficult for them to learn to overcome the intrinsic laryngeal reflexes which must be overcome to produce speech. In the same way that a child learns bladder control, often by trial and error, the average child learns (through trial and error, i.e., stumbling dysfluencies) to speak fluently. Blocks are frequently located at the beginning of sentences and phrases because that is where the majority of inspirations occur, an act which results in abduction of the vocal cords and a resetting/reinitiation of intrinsic laryngeal mechanisms. Singing results in fluency, perhaps due to the fact that subglottic pressures are much higher for singing (10-20 cm of water at 70 d B) than for normal speech (3-7 cm of water), thus placing more stress on the cords and necessitating their tensing in order not to bow out.[46,58] This change in muscle tone alters laryngeal muscle tone and perhaps alters larnygeal reflex mechanisms.[58] Stutterers do not stutter when they inhale while speaking, [53]possibly because this results in decreased subglottic pressure with a consequent alteration of major reflex stimuli. More men stutter than women possibly because of the difference (especially at an early age) in the language laterality, women having a "stronger" left hemisphere than their male counterparts, thus being more able to control the fine motor system of the larynx.

If individuals stutter because they have difficulty in controlling intrinsic laryngeal reflexes, a difficulty that is overcome by the above mentioned maneuvers, then perhaps one should find nonstutterers who, subsequent to brain damage, become stutterers as a result of having lost appropriate motor control over the larynx. Indeed, this is the case. In 1972, Rosenfield reported the first case of an individual who, subsequent to brain damage, became a stutterer in the absence of aphasia.[40] Language mechanisms were intact; motor control of speech was not. This has subsequently been substantiated by others.[20,39,45] Brain lesions in either the left or the right hemisphere can cause a nonstutterer to become a stutterer, but the deficit is transient unless both hemispheres are involved. This probably reflects the fact that motor control mechanisms of speech are bilaterally represented. One should note that the "acquired stutterers" differ from "developmental stutterers" in that the former, unlike the latter, frequently stutter throughout sentences and phrases and oftentimes while singing.

If stuttering is due to the inability of the individual to exercise appropriate motor control over laryngeal mechanisms, one might expect stutterers to have altered speech production following institution of a new sound source—i.e., stutterers might not stutter following laryngectomy, a procedure subsequently associated with esophageal speech. An advertisement in a journal for laryngectomee patients queried whether there were any stutterers who had had a laryngectomy performed. Four stutterers had stopped stuttering following laryngectomy and use of esophageal speech or electronic sound sources.[42,43] Another finding was also reported. There were some individuals who had never previously stuttered who transiently became stutterers following their laryngectomy.[17] This may well be a result of difficulties in dealing with a new sound source. It does not seem unreasonable to discover nonstuttering individuals who, when given a new sound source (i.e. esophageal speech, electronic voicing), become stutterers.

There are many psychiatric theories pertaining to the genesis of stuttering.[5,53] Psychotherapy has been nonproductive as a cure, although it certainly may help stutterers in their adjustment and self-concept. Johnson contended that individuals became stutterers due to their parents having excessively focused upon the child's speech.[21] Once the child "learned" that he was a stutterer, the appellation stuck and the individual became a stutterer. This theory does not explain the sexual bias, fluency during singing, and the other phenomenon noted above. In general, psychogenic explanations of the phenomenon of stuttering have proved inadequate.

TREATMENT

There are many forms of speech therapy, excellently reviewed elsewhere.[5,16] Psychiatric therapy is a useful adjunct in many instances. Most forms of speech therapy relate to altering laryngeal mechanisms so that the sounds are produced more easily. Thus, gentle-onset speech, air-flow therapy, and behavioral modification of speech all have a role.[18,56]

The Edinburgh Masker is an electronic device that helps many stutterers.[12] It takes advantage of the fact that stutterers often do not stutter if they cannot hear themselves talk.[53] A small apparatus is attached over the larynx and a stethoscope is inserted into the ears. When the stutterer initiates phonation, a loud sound is produced and he literally cannot hear himself speak. Although slightly cumbersome, this device is usually effective and can be used as an adjunct to speech therapy.

There have been many recent advances in the realm of the voice sciences. It can be anticipated that the next several years will witness major advances in our understanding of many speech disturbances including stuttering and that improved means of therapy will become available from this improved understanding.

REFERENCES

1. American Speech and Hearing Association; White House Conference Report: Speech disorders and speech correction. J. Speech Hear Disord 17:129-37, 1957
2. Andrews G. Quinn PT, Sorby WA: Stuttering: An investigation into cerebral dominance for speech. J Neurol Neurosurg Psychiatry 35: 414-418, 1972
3. Ballard PB: Sinistrality and speech. J Exper Ped 1:298-310, 1912
4. Benson DF, Geschwind N: The aphasias and related disturbances, in Baker AB, Baker LH (eds): Clinical Neurology. Hagerstown, Maryland, Harper and Row, 1977
5. Bloodstein O: A Handbook on Stuttering. Chicago, National Easterseal Society, 1975
6. Brady JP, Berson J: Stuttering, dichotic listening and cerebral dominance. Arch Gen Psychiatry 32:1449-1453, 1975
7. Bryngelson B: Sidedness as an etiological factor in stuttering. J Gen Psychol 47:204-217, 1935
8. Bryngelson B, Rutherford B: A comparative study of laterality of stutterers

and non-stutterers. J Speech Hear Disord 2:15-16, 1937
9. Curry FK, Gregory H: The performance of stutterers on dichotic listening tasks thought to reflect cerebral dominance. J Speech Hear Res 12:73-82, 1965
10. Daniels EM: An analysis of the relation between handedness and stuttering with special reference to the Orton-Travis theory of cerebral dominance. J Speech Dis 5:309-326, 1940
11. Despert JL: Psychosomatic study of fifty stuttering children: I. Social, physical and psychiatric findings. Am J Orthopsychiatry 16:100-113, 1946
12. Dewar A, Dewar AD, Austin WTS, Brash HM: The long-term use of an automatically triggered auditory feedback masking device in the treatment of stammering. Br J Disord Commum 14:219-229, 1979
13. Dimond SJ: Neuropsychology: A Textbook of Systems and Psychological Functions of the Human Brain. London, Butterworth, 1980
14. Dorman MF, Porter RJ: Hemispheric lateralization for speech perceptors in stutterers. Cortex 11:181-185, 1975
15. Douglass LC: A study of bilaterally recorded electroencephalograms of adult stutterers. J Exp Psych 32:247-265, 1943
16. Freeman FJ, Ushijima T: Laryngeal muscle activity during stuttering. J Speech Hear Res 21:538-562, 1978
17. Freeman F, Rosenfield D: A note on source in stuttering. J Fluency Dis, (in press)
18. Gregory HH: Controversies About Stuttering Therapy. Baltimore, University Park Press, 1979
19. Gruber L, Powell RL: Responses of stuttering and non-stuttering children to a dichotic listening task. Percept Mot Skills 38:263-264, 1974
20. Helm NA, Butler RB, Benson DF: Acquired stuttering. Neurology 28:1159-1165, 1978
21. Johnson W: A study of the onset and development of stuttering. J Speech Disord 7:251-257, 1942
22. Johnson W. Stuttering, in Johnson W, Moeller D (eds): Speech Handicapped School Children. New York, Wiley, 1967
23. Jones RK: Observations on stammering after localized cerebral injury. J Neurol Neurosurg Psychiatry 29:192-195, 1966
24. Kidd KK, Heimbuch RC, Records MA: Vertical transmission of susceptibility to stuttering with sex-modified expression. Proc Natl Acad Sci USA 78:606-610, 1981
25. Kimura D: Cerebral dominance and the perception of verbal stimuli. Can J Psychol 3:166-171, 1961
26. Kimura D: Some effects of temporal lobe damage on auditory perception. Can J Psychol 15:156-165, 1961
27. Kimura D: Speech lateralization in young children as determined by an auditory test. J Comp Physiol Psychol 56:899-902, 1963
28. Kimura D: Left-right differences in the perception of melodies. J Exp Psychol 16:355-358, 1964
29. Lussenhop AJ, Boggs JS, La Borwit LJ, Walle EL: Cerebral dominance in

stutterers determined by Wada testing. Neurology 23:1190-1192, 1973
30. McAllister AH: Clinical Studies in Speech Therapy. London, University London Press, 1937
31. Mileson R, Johnson W: A comparative study of stutterers, former stutterers and normal speakers whose handedness has been changed. Arch Speech 1:61-86, 1936
32. Milner B, Branch C, Rasmussen T: Evidence for bilateral speech representation in some non-right-handers. Trans Am Neuro Assoc 91:306-308, 1966
33. Nelson SE, Hunter N, Walter M: Stuttering in twin types. J Speech Hear Disord 10:335, 1945
34. Orton ST: A physiological theory of reading disability and stuttering in children. N Eng J Med 199:1045-1052, 1928
35. Parson BS: Left-handedness. New York, Macmillan, 1924
36. Porfert AR, Rosenfield DB: Prevalence of stuttering. J Neurol Neurosurg Psychiatry 41:954-956, 1978
37. Quinn PT: Stuttering—cerebral dominance and dichotic word test. Med J Aust 2:639-642, 1972
38. Rheinberger MB, Karlin IW, Beuman AB: Electro-encephalographic and laterality studies of stuttering and non-stuttering children. Nerv Child, 2:117-133, 1943
39. Rosbenbek TC, Messert B, Collins M, Wertz R: Stuttering following brain damage. Brain Lang 6:82-96, 1978
40. Rosenfield DB: Stuttering and cerebral ischemia. N Eng J Med 287:991, 1972
41. Rosenfield DB: The history of stuttering. Presented at the 33rd Annual Meeting of the American Academy of Neurology, Toronto, Canada, April 27-May 2 1981
42. Rosenfield DB: Theories of stuttering. Invited presentation at the Vocal Fold Physiology Conference, Madison, Wisconsin, May 31-June 4 1981
43. Rosenfield DB, Freeman F: Stuttering and laryngectomy. Presented at the 34th Annual Meeting of the American Academy of Neurology, Washington D.C., April 1982
44. Rosenfield DB, Goodglass M: Dichotic testing of cerebral dominance in stutterers. Brain Lang 11:170-180, 1980
45. Rosenfield DB, Miller S, Feltovitch M: Brain damage causing stuttering. Presented at the 105th Annual Meeting of the American Neurological Association, Boston, September 7-10, 1980
46. Rubin HJ, LeCover M, Vernard W: Vocal intensity, subglottic pressure and airflow in relationship to singers. Laryngoscope 73:973-1015, 1963
47. Sheehan JG: Stuttering: Research and Therapy. New York, Harper and Row, 1970
48. Slorach N, Noehr B: Dichotic listening in stuttering and dyslalic children. Cortex 9: 295-300, 1973
49. Spadino EJ: Writing and Laterality Characteristics of Stuttering Children. New York, Columbia University Teachers College, 1941
50. Travis LE: Speech Pathology. New York, Appleton-Century, 1931
51. Travis LE, Knot JR: Brain potentials from normal speakers and stutterers. J Psychol 2:137-150, 1936

52. Travis LE, Knott JR: Bilaterally recorded brain potentials from normal speakers and stutterers. J Speech Disord 2:239-241, 1937
53. Van Riper C: The Nature of Stuttering. Englewood Cliffs, New Jersey, Prentice-Hall, 1971
54. Wada J, Rasmussen T: Intracarotid injection of sodium amytal for the lateralization of cerebral speech dominance: Experimental and clinical observation. J Neurosurg 17:266-282, 1960
55. Wallin JE: A census of speech defectives among 89,057 public-school pupils—a preliminary report. Sch Soc 3:213-216, 1916
56. Webster RL: Evolution of a target-based behavorial therapy for stuttering. J Fluency Dis 5:303-320, 1980
57. Wyke B: The neurology of stammering. J Psychosom Res 15:423-432, 1971
58. Wyke B, Kichner JA: Neurology of the larynx, in Hinchcliffe R, Harrison D (eds): Scientific Foundation of Otolaryngology. London, William Heinemann, 1976
59. Zuriff EB, Bryden MP: Familial handedness and left-right differences in auditory and visual perception. Neuropsychologia 7:179-187, 1969

Index

Accident neurosis, traumatic brain injury and, 227–228
ACTH (adrenocorticotropic hormone), for multiple sclerosis, 292
Acute confusional state. *See* Confusional state, acute
Adams, R. D., 96, 261, 265, 270
Adler, G., 61
Affective changes. *See* Emotional changes
Agnosias:
  in Alzheimer's disease, 96, 110
  in Pick's disease, 104, 110
Aggression (aggressive behavior), 59. *See also* Episodic dyscontrol; Explosive behavior; Violent behavior
Akathisia, 206
Alcoholic dementia, 149–164
  alcoholic neuropsychiatric disorders related to, 157–162
    chronic and nutritional disorders, 161–162
    functional psychiatric disorders, 160–161
    intoxication phenomena, 159
    withdrawal phenomena, 159–160
  cause of, 154–156
  clinical descriptions of, 150
  natural history and outcome of, 156–157
  pathologic findings in, 153
  prevalence of, 154
  psychologic impairment in, 150–154
Alcoholic hallucinosis, 160

Alcoholism, pain-prone disorder and, 185, 186
Aluminum intoxication, Alzheimer's disease and, 101
Alzheimer's disease, 90, 93–103, 124, 145–146
  clinical course of, 94–97
  histopathologic alterations in, 98–101
  laboratory findings in, 97–98
  management of, 102–103
  neurochemical studies of, 101
  pathogenesis of, 101–102
  Pick's disease differentiated from, 109–111, 120
Ammonshorn sclerosis in epilepsy, 27
Amnesia, 251–278
  in Alzheimer's disease, 95
  anoxic, 264
  anterograde. *See* Posttraumatic amnesia (PTA)
  after a cerebral vascular accident, 262–263
  clinical psychologic investigations of, 268–269
  clinical syndromes that feature, 261–267
  in complex-partial seizures, 32–35
  definition of, 251, 253–254
  in Korsakoff's psychosis, 261
  postconvulsive, 264–265
  postinfectious, 263–264
  postsurgical, 263
  prognosis and outcome of, 273–274

315

psychogenic, 266-267
retrograde, 254-255
transient global (TGA), 265-266
after traumatic brain injury, 229-230, 234-235, 237-239, 244, 254, 255, 262
treatment of, 272-273
Amytal test, intravenous, in acute confusional state, 12-13
Anger in epilepsy, 40
Anterograde amnesia. *See* Posttraumatic amnesia (PTA)
Antianxiety agents for episodic dyscontrol, 64
Anticholinergics for tardive dyskinesia, 208-210
Anticholinergic syndrome, acute confusional behavior and, 11
tranquilizers for, 16, 17
Anticonvulsants
for epilepsy, 40, 41, 43
for episodic dyscontrol, 63-64
Antidepressants
for episodic dyscontrol, 64-65
in multiple sclerosis, 293
Antitestosterone agents for episodic dyscontrol, 65-66
Anxiety states, multiple sclerosis and, 291
Aphasia
acute confusional state differentiated from, 6-7
in Alzheimer's disease, 95-96, 110, 127
in epilepsy, 32
in Pick's disease, 104, 110, 127
in subcortical dementia, 127
traumatic brain injury and, 232, 241
Apraxia
in Alzheimer's disease, 96
traumatic brain injury and, 232
Aristotle, 302
Arousal in acute confusional state, 3, 22
Asunti, T., 79
Attention
in acute confusional state, 3, 22
traumatic brain injury and
minor injury, 227
severe injury, 233-234, 236
Attention deficit syndrome, episodic dyscontrol and, 62
Aura, epileptic, 30-32
continuous, 34
Automatisms (automatic actions), 264-265
in epilepsy, 32-34

Bach-Y-Rita, G., 56
Bacon, Francis, 302
Bagley, C. R., 77, 284
Baldwin, M. V., 288
Ballard, P. B., 303-304
Barbizet, J., 256
Bear, D. M., 27
Beard, A. W., 76, 78, 79
Beatty, P. A., 289
Behavioral change
in organic brain disorders, 172-174
after traumatic brain injury, 239-241, 244
Bender, M. B., 265
Benson, D. F., 241
Benton, J. G., 288
Benton Visual Retention Test, 260
Benzodiazepines for acute confusional state, 16
Beresford, H. R., 67
Berglund, M., 152
Bergman, H., 154, 155
Berlyne, N., 256
Berson, J., 306
Bignami, A., 283
Blessed, G., 100, 124
Blumer, D., 65
Bond, A., 64
Bowman, K. M., 150
Braceland, F. J., 282
Brady, J. P., 306
Brain, W. R., 285
Brain
atrophy of. *See also* Cerebral atrophy Cortical atrophy
in Alzheimer's disease, 98, 110
in Pick's disease, 105-106, 110
structural lesions of, acute confusional state and, 10
Brain injury. *See* Traumatic brain injury
Bricolo, A., 232
Briquet's syndrome, 291
Brown, C. C., 286-288
Brown, J. H., 104
Brown, S., 280, 281
Bruens, J. H., 76, 80, 81, 83, 85
Bucco-lingual masticating syndrome, 198
Burgmeister, B. B., 286
Butters, N., 268

Canter, A. H., 287
Carlen, P. L., 153, 154, 157, 162
Carlson, C., 226-227

Index

Cerebral atrophy in alcoholic dementia, 153
Cerebral blood flow in Alzheimer's disease, 98
Cerebral vascular accident (CVA), amnesia following, 262-263
Cermak, L., 268
Chandler, B. C., 152
Charcot, J. M., 279-280
Chemical poisoning, dementia caused by, 135-136
Cholinergic agents, in tardive dyskinesia therapy, 208
Chorea, parkinsonism contrasted with, 197
Chouinard, G., 208
Christensen, E., 200
Circumstantiality/viscosity, in epilepsy, 27, 38-39
Clifton, G. L., 222
Closed head injury. See Traumatic brain injury
Clozapine, parkinsonism and tardive dyskinesia and, 210-211
Cognitive impairment
  in alcoholic dementia, 151-152
  in functional and organic disorders, 169-171
  in functional disorders, 170-171
  in organic brain disorders, 171-172
  after traumatic brain injury, 237-241, 243-244
Cohen, K. L., 204
Cohn, R., 108
Coid, J., 159
Collins, G. H., 261, 270
Coma, after traumatic brain injury, 229-232
Complex-partial seizures (CPS), 26-28. See also Epilepsy
  ictal phase of, 30-33
Computerized tomography (CT)
  in Alzheimer's disease, 97-98
  in dementia, 130-131
  in Pick's disease, 105, 110
Concussion. See Traumatic brain injury—minor
Confabulation, 255-256
  after traumatic brain injury, 234, 236-237
Confusional state, acute, 1-23
  clinical evaluation of, 12-14
  clinical manifestations of, 2-6
    clinical course, 5
    clouding of consciousness, 2-3

    emotional and personality changes, 4
    hallucinations, 3-4, 6-8
    illusions, 3
    incoherence of thought, 3
    psychomotor activity, alterations in, 5
    sleep disturbances, 5
  definition of, 1
  differential diagnosis of, 6-8
  etiology of, 8-12, 21-22
    medications and other drugs, 9, 18
    metabolic disturbances, 10
    neurologic diseases, 10-11
    structural lesions of the brain, 10
    surgery, 11, 18
  management of, 13, 15-17
    environmental manipulations, 13, 15
    extended recovery, 17
    sleep, 15-16
    tranquilization, 15-17
  prevention of, 17-18
  terminology for, 2
  after traumatic brain injury, 233-235
Confusional state, chronic, 128-129
Consonant Trigrams, 260
Constantinidis, J., 105, 108-109
Corsellis, J. A. N., 106
Cortical atrophy, in alcoholic dementia, 153
Cortical dementias. See Dementias—cortical
Cortical lesions. See Traumatic brain injury
Cottrell, S. S., 281, 285
Courville, C. B., 153, 221-222
CPS. See Complex-partial seizures
Crapper, D. R., 101, 102
Creutzfeldt-Jakob disease, 111
Criminal responsibility, episodic dyscontrol and, 67
Cummings, J. L., 104, 105, 107, 110
Curry, F. K., 305-306

Dalton, K., 60, 65
Davis, T. K., 280, 281
Davison, K., 77, 284
DeBoni, U. 102
Deja vu, in epilepsy, 31-32
Delirium tremens (DTs)
  alcoholic dementia and, 159-160
  tranquilizers for, 16, 17
Delusions
  in acute confusional state, 4
  in epilepsy, 82, 83

Dementia
  acute confusional state differentiated from, 6
  alcoholic. *See* Alcoholic dementia
  confusional state in, 17
  cortical, 93–121
    Alzheimer's disease. *See* Alzheimer's disease
    differential diagnosis, 125–131
    infectious processes that cause dementias, 111–112
    multi-infarct dementias, 111, 128
    Pick's disease. *See* Pick's disease
  definition of, 123, 125
  differential diagnosis of, 125–131
    computerized tomography (CT), 130–131
    EEG findings, 131
    laboratory tests, 129–131
    language and speech disturbances, 127
    memory disturbance, 127
    pseudodementia, 167–176
    psychologic tests, 129
    psychomotor retardation, 127–129
  epileptic, 42
  future considerations, 145–146
  incidence of, 123–124
  memory disturbance in, 127
  pseudo-. *See* Pseudodementia
  subcortical, 93. *See also* treatable or reversible *below*
    differential diagnosis, 125–131
  treatable or reversible, 124–125, 128–146
    chemical poisoning as cause of, 135–136
    chronic neurologic states as cause of, 139
    deficiency states as cause of, 137–138
    drug poisoning as cause of, 136–137
    endocrine diseases as cause of, 133
    infectious diseases as cause of, 134–135
    intracranial tumor as cause of, 138–139
    psychogenic states as cause of, 140–141
    systemic diseases as cause of, 132–133
    trauma as cause of, 141–142
    vascular diseases as cause of, 134
  treatment of, 142–144
  unitary approach to, 124
Denervation hypersensitivity, 202–204
Denial of illness, after traumatic brain injury, 234

Depression, 174
  acute confusional state differentiated from, 8
  amnesia and, 265–267
  cognitive changes in, 170
  dementia and, 140–141
  in epilepsy, 40
  multiple sclerosis and, 281–283, 291–292
  pain-prone disorder and, 181–182, 184–187
  pseudodementia and, 170, 174
  psychomotor retardation in, 127, 128
  traumatic brain injury and, 228–229, 242
Diers, W. C., 286–288
Dissociative reactions, 266, 267
Diuretics, for episodic dyscontrol, 65
Dongier, S., 77, 78
Dopamine
  epilepsy-psychosis relationship and, 78, 85–86
  tardive dyskinesia and, 208, 211
Dopamine receptors
  in parkinsonism, 201–203
  in tardive dyskinesia, 200–204, 207
Dorman, M. F., 306
Dostoevsky, F., 40
Down's syndrome, Alzheimer's disease and, 94
Dreaming, acute confusional state and, 4, 5
Dreamy state, in epilepsy, 31–32
Driver, M. V., 81
Drugs (other than medications). *See also* Medications
  acute confusional state and, 9–10, 18
  dementia caused by, 136–137
Duchen, L. W., 104, 105, 107, 110
Duge, 280
Dyscontrol. *See* Episodic dyscontrol
Dyskinesias, withdrawal and covert, 206
Dysphasia. *See* Aphasia

Echeverria, M. G., 75–76
Ehlers, C. L., 60
Electroconvulsive therapy (ECT)
  amnesia caused by, 265
  for tardive dyskinesia, 209
Electroencephalogram (EEG) abnormalities
  in acute confusional state, 12
  in Alzheimer's disease, 97–98
  in dementia, 131, 138, 139
  in epilepsy, 43

Index

epilepsy-psychosis relationship and, 77, 78
in episodic dyscontrol, 56-59
in Pick's disease, 105
Elliott, F. A., 49, 51, 56-58, 61, 62, 65
Elliott, W. A., 156
Emotional changes
  in acute confusional state, 4
  in multiple sclerosis, 280-283
  in organic brain syndromes, 174-175
  after traumatic brain injury, 240-243
Emotionality, in epilepsy, 27, 39-41
Encephalitis of herpes simplex, amnesia caused by, 263-264
Endocrine diseases, dementia caused by, 133
Engel, George, 181-182, 188
Environmental factors, in episodic dyscontrol, 61-63
Epilepsy (seizure disorders), 25-48. *See also* Complex-partial seizures
  amnesia and, 32-35, 264-265
  ictal manifestations of, 30-33
    amnesic state, 32-33
    automatisms, 32
    autonomic changes, 33
    dreamy state, 31-32
    hallucinations, illusions, and other misperceptions, 31
    motor alterations, 32
    primictal stage (aura), 30-32
    speech utterances, 32
  interictal behavior manifestations in, 36-41
    deepened emotionality, 39-41
    hypergraphia, 39
    hypometamorphosis (viscosity-circumstantiality), 38-39
    hyposexuality, 37-38
  medications for, 25-26
  postictal phase of, 33-36
    automatisms, 34
    continuous aura, 34
    poriomania, 35
    sexual arousal, 36
    temporal lobe status, 34
    violent, explosive behavior, 35
  prodromal manifestations of, 29-30
  psychologic response to, 43-44
  psychotic complications of, 41-43, 73-90
    affinity between epilepsy and psychosis, 78-80
    antagonism between psychosis and epilepsy, 77-78
    historical background, 75-77
    laterality of focus and, 80-81
    mechanisms of chronic interictal psychosis, 84-86
    phenomenology of psychosis, 82-83
    pseudoseizures (hysteroepilepsy), 42-43
    schizophrenia-like psychosis, 41-42, 83, 84, 89-90
    toxic psychosis or epileptic dementia, 42
    traumatic brain injury as cause of, 241-242
Episodic dyscontrol (explosive behavior), 49-74
  biologic factors in, 57-61
    EEG findings, 58-59
    genetic factors, 61
    limbic dysfunction, 59
    neuroendocrine relationships, 60
    neurotransmitter function, 60
    psychosurgical experience, 59-60
  case histories of, 52-55
  clinical findings associated with, 56
  definition, 50-52
  demographic data, 57
  EEG abnormalities in, 56-59
  in epilepsy, 35
  evaluation of, 62-63
  forensic and ethical issues, 67
  laboratory findings in, 56-57
  psychosocial factors in, 61-63
  treatment of, 63-66
    antianxiety agents, 64
    anticonvulsants, 63-64
    antidepressants, 64-65
    antitestosterone agents, 65-66
    diuretics, 65
    lithium, 65
    propranolol, 65
    psychotherapy, 66
    surgery, 59-60, 66
    temporal lobectomy, 66
    underlying conditions, treatment of, 66
Ergomania, pain-prone disorder and, 184-186
Erving, F. R., 50, 51, 61, 80
Esquirol, J. E. D., 75
Ethical issues, in episodic dyscontrol, 67

Euphoria
  in dementia, 175
  in multiple sclerosis, 280–283
Explosive behavior. *See* Episodic dyscontrol
Extrapyramidal syndrome, 195, 197
Extrapyramidal system, 196–197

Falret, J., 75
Faurbye, A., 198
Ferrell, R. B., 283
Fink, S. L., 288
Fisher, C. M., 265
Fleminger, J. J., 167
Flor-Henry, P., 76, 80–83, 84
Folstein, M. F., 170
Fordyce, W. E., 180
Forgetting, 256–257. *See also* Amnesia; Memory disturbances
Fornix, memory and, 270
Freud, S., 40
Friedman, E. D., 281
Fugue states, 267
Functional disorders
  cognitive changes in, 170–171
  distinction between organic and, 168–171

Gange, J. J., 289
Gastaut, H., 27, 35
Genetic factors, in episodic dyscontrol, 61
Gennarelli, T. A., 221, 222
Gianotti, G., 97
Gibbs, F. A., 80
Giffin, M. E., 282
Gilchrist, E., 243
Glaser, G. H., 80
Glaus, A., 76
Gloor, P., 59
Goddard, G. V., 60
Goodglass, M., 307
Goodstein, R. K., 283
Goodwin, D. W., 159
Goudsmit, J., 102
Gowers, W. R., 5, 280
Graham, D. I., 224
Granulovacuolar degeneration, 100
Gregoriadis, A., 81
Gregory, H., 305–306
Griesinger, W., 75
Gronwall, D., 227
Grossman, R. G., 240

Gruber, L., 306
Gruhle, H. W., 76
Gudmundsson, G., 79
Gustafson, L., 98
Guthrie, A., 156

Haase, G. R., 110
Halgren, E., 59
Hallucinations
  in acute confusional state, 3, 6–8
  in epilepsy, 31, 82, 83
Hallucinosis, alcoholic, 160
Haloperidol, for acute confusional state, 16
Halstead, W. C., 286
Handedness, stuttering and, 303–307
Harner, R. N., 97
Harrison, M. S., 226
Harrower, M. R., 288
Heath, R. G., 66
Heilman, K. M., 241
Hermann, B. P., 40
Herpes simplex, encephalitis of
  amnesia caused by, 263–264
Higher intellectual functions, in acute confusional state, 3
Hill, D., 76, 89
Hippocrates, 302
Hirschenfang, S., 288
Hollender, M. H., 175
Horel, J. A., 270
Horvath, T. B., 150
Houser, A. B., 288
Humphrey, M., 247
Huss, Magnus, 150
Hydrocephalus, traumatic brain injury
  and, 231–233, 238
Hyperactivity, in acute confusional state, 5
Hypergraphia, in epilepsy, 39
Hypometamorphosis, in epilepsy, 38
Hyposexuality, in epilepsy, 27, 37–38
Hysteria, multiple sclerosis and, 285–286
Hysterical epileptic seizures, 42–43

Illusions
  in acute confusional state, 3
  in epilepsy, 31
Immediate recall, 252–253
  anatomic basis of, 271
  tests of, 257–258
Impulse dyscontrol. *See* Episodic dyscontrol

Index

Inattention. *See* Attention
Infections
  acute confusional state and, 10
  amnesia caused by, 263-264
  dementia caused by, 134-135
Inman, 304
Intermittent explosive disorder. *See* Episodic dyscontrol
Intoxication, pathologic
  alcoholic dementia and, 159
Irritability, in epilepsy, 35
Ivnik, R. J., 289

Jackson, J. H., 31, 265
Jacob, H., 97
Janz, D., 33
Jellinek, E. M., 150
Jennett, B., 229, 242
Jensen, I., 76, 80, 81, 83
Jervis, G. A., 103, 108
Johnson, W., 302, 309
Jones, R. K., 302, 304-305
Jus, A., 199, 207

Kahana, E., 293, 289
Kidd, K. K., 302-303
Kidd, M., 102
Kimura, D., 305, 306
Kindling, of the mesolimbic dopamine system in epilepsy, 85-86
Klawans, H. L., 208
Klüver-Bucy syndrome
  in Alzheimer's disease, 96, 110
  partial inverse, 27, 28
  in Pick's disease, 104, 110, 111
Knehr, C. A., 288
Korsakoff, 261
Korsakoff's psychosis (Korsakoff's syndrome), 150, 161-162, 261-262, 268, 270, 272-274
Kraepelin, E., 40, 78, 94
Kraus, J., 288
Kristensen, O., 76, 81, 83, 84

Lader, M., 64
Landolt, H., 77, 78
Language disturbances. *See* Aphasia
Langworthy, O. R., 284
Larsen, J. K., 76, 80, 81, 83
Larson, T., 95
Learning. *See also* Memory
  neuroanatomic basis of, 269-272
Learning ability, 253
  after temporal lobe resection, 263
  tests of, 258-259
Learning tests, 260
Lee, T., 203
Legal issues, in episodic dyscontrol, 67
Le Roux, A., 104
Levin, H. S., 237, 240
Lewin, W., 232
Lewis, A., 150
Lewis, D. O., 56
Lezak, M. D., 237-238, 240
Limbic system, in episodic dyscontrol, 58-59
Lincoln, N. B., 288
Lindsay, J., 79, 81
Lingual-facial-buccal dyskinesias, 197-198, 207
Lion, J. R., 61
Lipowski, Z. J., 170
Lishman, W. A., 96, 104
Liston, E. H., Jr., 174
Lithium
  for episodic dyscontrol, 65
  for tardive dyskinesia, 209
Loeser, J. D., 180

McAllister, A. H., 304
McHugh, P. R., 170
Madden, D. J., 61
Malamud, N., 58
Maletzky, B. M., 51
Mamillary bodies, memory and, 269-270
Mandleberg, I. A., 234
Mania, acute confusional state differentiated from, 8
Mannerisms, in tardive dyskinesia, 205
Mark, V. H., 50, 51, 59, 61
Marsh, G., 288
Maudsley, H., 76
Mayer-Gross, W., 104
Medications. *See also* Drugs; *and specific types of medication*
  acute confusional state caused by, 9
  dementia caused by, 136-137
  for epilepsy, 25-26
Melzack, R., 180
Memory
  definition of, 251-252
  functions of, 252-253

hemispheric lateralization of, 272
neuroanatomic basis of, 269–272
tests of, 257–261
  formal tests, 260–261
  immediate recall, 257–258
  learning ability, 258–259
  retrieval ability, 259–260
Memory blackouts, in alcoholic dementia, 159
Memory disturbances. *See also* Amnesia
  in Alzheimer's disease, 94, 95
  in dementias, 127
  in Pick's disease, 105
Mercurialis, 302
Metabolic disturbances, acute confusional state and, 10
Migeon, C., 65
Miller, H., 228
Milner, B., 263, 268, 272
Misperceptions. *See* Perceptual disturbances
Monroe, R. R., 50–52, 56–58, 61
Montague, A., 62
Mood changes, in epilepsy, 31–32, 40–41
Morel, B. A., 75
Morgagni, G. B., 302
Muller, R., 289
Multi-infarct dementia, 111, 128
Multiple personality, 267
Multiple sclerosis (MS), 279–299
  early studies of, 279–281
  hysteria and, 285–286
  neuropsychologic deficits in, 286–290
  personality changes in, 284–285
  psychiatric disorders following treatment for, 292
  psychiatric disorders resembling, 290–292
  schizophrenia-like psychosis and, 284
  treatment of psychiatric disorders in, 293–294
Mur, J., 283

Nadell, R., 281
Narabayashi, H., 60
Nauta, 58
Nelson, S. E., 302
Neumann, M. A., 108
Neuroendocrine relationship, in episodic dyscontrol, 60
Neurofibrillary tangles, 98–102

Neuroleptics
  for episodic dyscontrol, 64
  tardive dyskinesia caused by, 197–206, 210–212, 217
  in tardive dyskinesia therapy, 207–208
Neurologic diseases, acute confusional state and, 10–11
Neurotransmitters
  in episodic dyscontrol, 60
  in tardive dyskinesia therapy, 208
Niedermeyer, E., 56
Noble, E. P., 154
Noehr, B., 306
Nott, P. N., 167
Nutritional deficiency, dementia caused by, 137–138

Oddy, M., 243
Ohye, C., 202
Ombrédane, A., 281
Ommaya, A. K., 221, 222
Onari, 103
Oppenheim, Hermann, 188–190, 193, 280
Oppenheimer, D. R., 224, 226
Organic disorders
  behavioral and affective changes in the diagnosis of, 171–175
  distinction between functional and, 168–171
Orton, S. T., 302, 303
Ounsted, C., 79, 81
Owen, F., 203

Pain, chronic, 178–194. *See also* Pain-prone disorders
  depression and, 181–182
  as a neurologic or psychologic phenomenon, 179–180
  treatment for, 181
Pain-prone disorder, 182–194
  clinical presentation of, 182–184
  demographic data, 182
  family history and, 184–185
  Oppenheim's treatise on traumatic neuroses, 188–190
  premorbid traits, 184
  psychodynamic factors in, 185–186
  treatment of, 186–188
Paranoia
  in Alzheimer's disease, 94, 95
  in epilepsy, 82

Paraphasias, 6-7
Paresis, general, 112
Parker, E. S., 154
Parkinson's disease (parkinsonism), 197
  drug-induced, 200-203, 210, 211
  tardive dyskinesia differentiated from, 204-205
Parson, B. S., 304
Parsons, O. A., 152, 288
Paulley, J. W., 293
Perceptual disturbances. *See also* Hallucinations; Illusions
  in acute confusional state, 3, 6-8
  complex-partial seizures and, 31
Perez, F. I., 97
Perez, M. M., 76, 81, 83, 84
Personality changes
  in acute confusional state, 4
  in alcoholic dementia, 151
  in Alzheimer's disease, 95
  in multiple sclerosis, 284-285
  after traumatic brain injury, 239-240, 243-244
Petit-mal status, epilepsy associated with, 42
Peyser, J. M., 295, 289
Physostigmine, for anticholinergic syndrome, 17
Pick, Arnold, 103
Pick bodies, 106-107
Pick cells, 107-108
Pick's disease, 103-112
  Alzheimer's disease differentiated from, 109-111, 120
  cellular alterations in, 106-108
  clinical course of, 103-105
  etiology and pathogenesis of, 108
  histopathologic alterations in, 105-106
  laboratory findings in, 105
  management of, 108-109
Pillutla, V. S., 79
Polatin, P., 96, 110
Pond, D. A., 76, 82
Poriomania, 265
  in epilepsy, 35
Porter, R. J., 306
Postconcussion syndrome (PCS), 226-229
Posttraumatic amnesia (PTA), 229-230, 234-235, 237-239, 244, 254, 255, 262
Powell, R. L., 306

Pratt, R. T. C., 282, 284-285, 288
Progressive multifocal leukoencephalopathy, 111-112
Propranolol, for episodic dyscontrol, 65
Pseudodementia, 164-165, 167-177
  diagnosis of, 167-176
  behavioral and affective changes in organic disorders, 171-175
  cognitive impairment, 169-171
  functional and organic disorders, distinction between, 168-169
Pseudoseizures (hysteroepilepsy), 42-43
Psychologic tests, for dementia, 129
Psychomotor retardation, in subcortical dementia, 127-129
Psychosis, epileptic. *See* Epilepsy—psychotic complications of
Psychotherapy
  for dementia, 143-144
  for episodic dyscontrol, 66
Pyramidal system, 196

Quinn, P. T., 306

Raecke, J., 280
Rapid eye movement (REM) sleep
  in acute confusional state, 5
  pain-prone disorder and, 186
Rehabilitation
  of chronic pain patients, 187-188
  of traumatic brain injury patients, 243-244
Reifler, B., 174
Reitan, R. M., 285, 287, 289
Repetitive behavior, in epilepsy, 32, 33
Reserpine, in tardive dyskinesia therapy, 207
Retrieval, 253
  anatomic basis of, 271-272
Retrieval ability, tests of, 259-260
Retrograde amnesia, 254-255
Rey Auditory-Verbal Learning Test, 260
Reynolds, E. H., 78
Rey-Osterreith Figure, 260-261
Riley, T., 56
Robertson, E. E., 104
Rochford, G., 96
Rodin, E., 26, 27, 43, 80
Ron, M. A., 153, 155, 167-168
Rosenfield, D. B., 307, 309

Ross, A. T., 285, 287, 289
Roth, M., 101, 124
Rowe, M. J., 226–227
Rubovits, R., 208

Sachs, B., 281
St. Hillaire, J. M., 59
Schizophrenia
  acute confusional state differentiated from, 7–8
  tardive dyskinesia and, 203, 204, 207, 210–211
Schizophrenia-like psychosis
  in epilepsy, 41–42, 83, 84, 89–90
  multiple sclerosis and, 284
Seiffer, H., 280
Seizure disorders. *See* Epilepsy
Senile plaques, in Alzheimer's disease, 99–102
Sexual arousal, in epilepsy, 36
Sexuality. *See* Hyposexuality
Sheehan, J. G., 302
Sherwin, I., 76, 81
Sim, M., 95
Sindrup, E. H., 76, 81, 83, 84
Siskind, M., M., 283
Sjogren, T., 96, 110
Slater, E., 76, 78–80, 82, 84
Sleep disturbances
  in acute confusional state, 5, 15, 18
  pain-prone disorders and, 184, 186, 187
Slorech, N., 306
Smith, H. M., 198–199
Smith, J. S., 59
Somatization disorder, 291
Spatz, 103
Speech disturbances. *See also* Aphasia
  in Alzheimer's disease, 96
Squire, Larry, 269
Stammering, 301. *See also* Stuttering
Staples, D., 288
Stevens, J. R., 40, 79, 84
Stimulants, for episodic dyscontrol, 65
Stroke, amnesic, 262–263
Stuttering, 301–310
  cerebral dominance and, 303–307
  definition of, 301–302
  dichotic listening studies of, 305–307
  early literature on, 302
  genetic factors in, 302–303
  physiologic mechanics of sound production and, 307–309
  psychiatric theories of, 309–310
  treatment of, 310
  Wada test for, 304–306
Sugar, C., 281
Suicide
  among epileptic patients, 43–44
  among multiple sclerosis patients, 283
Surgery
  confusional state after, 11–12, 18
  for episodic dyscontrol, 59–60, 66
Surridge, D., 282, 284
Sussman, I., 95
Symonds, C., 85

Talland, G., 268
Tallman, G., 286
Tardive dyskinesia (TD), 193–217
  akathisia differentiated from, 206
  clinical manifestations of, 197–198
  definition of, 198
  differential diagnosis of, 204–206
  epidemiology of, 198–199
  neuropathology of, 199–200
  pathogenesis and pathophysiology of, 200–204
    blockade of dopamine receptor sites, 200–201
    hypersensitivity of dopamine receptor sites, 201–204
    hypothalamic hypersensitivity, 204
  parkinsonism differentiated from, 204–205
  pharmacologic therapy for, 206–211
  prognosis for, 211
  recommendations for decreasing the incidence of, 210–211
  spontaneous lingual-facial-buccal dyskinesias differentiated from, 198
Tarter, R. E., 152
Taylor, A. R., 228
Taylor, D. C., 76, 81
Temkin, O., 25
Temporal hyperconnection syndrome, in epilepsy, 28, 36, 37, 44
Temporal lobectomy
  ability to learn after, 263
  for episodic dyscontrol, 66
Temporal lobe status, 265
  in epilepsy, 34
Tests of memory function, 257–261

formal tests, 260-261
immediate recall, 257-258
learning ability, 258-259
retrieval ability, 259-260
Tetrabenazine, in tardive dyskinesia therapy, 207
Thioridazine, parkinsonism and tardive dyskinesia and, 210-211
Tomlinson, B. E., 101, 124
Toone, B., 81, 84
Toxic psychosis, in epilepsy, 42
Tranquilization, in acute confusional state, 15-17
Transient global amnesia (TGA), 265-266
Trauma
　amnesia caused by, 262
　dementia caused by, 141-142
Traumatic brain injury (TBI), 218-248
　amnesia caused by, 229-230, 234-235, 237-239, 244, 254, 255, 262
　behavioral consequences of, 223, 225, 239-241, 244
　epidemiology of, 219-221
　minor, 225-229
　　accident neurosis, 227-228
　　depression, 228-229
　　postconcussion syndrome, 226-227
　pathophysiology of, 221-225
　severe, 229-244
　　aphasia caused by, 241
　　coma following, 229-232
　　confusional state following, 233-235
　　definition of, 230
　　depression caused by, 242
　　epilepsy caused by, 241-242
　　independent self care, 235-238
　　intake criteria, 229-230
　　intellectual independence, 239-241
　　long-term outcome, 242-244
　　mute responsiveness following, 232-233
　　outcome criteria, 230-242
　　unresponsive vigilance following, 231-232
Traumatic neuroses, Oppenheim's treatise on, 188-190
Travis, L. E., 302, 303
Trimble, M. R., 76, 81, 83, 84
Tumor, intracranial
　dementia caused by, 138-139
Turner, W. A., 76

Uhrbrand, L., 198
Uno, M., 60
Unresponsive vigilance, after traumatic brain injury, 231-232

Vascular diseases, dementia caused by, 134
Victor, M., 96, 261, 262, 270
Violent behavior. See also Episodic dyscontrol
　in epilepsy, 35, 40
Viscosity/circumstantiality, in epilepsy, 27, 38-39
Visuo-spatial skills
　in Alzheimer's disease, 95
　in Pick's disease, 105
Von Meduna, L., 77

Wada test, for stuttering, 304-306
Warrington, E., 268
Wechsler, D., 286
Wechsler Adult Intelligence Scale, 260
Wechsler Memory Scale, 260
Weingartner, H., 269
Wernicke-Korsakoff syndrome, 161, 162, 272
Wernicke's [polio]encephalopathy, 161, 162, 261
Whitlock, F. A., 283
Whitty, C. W. M., 236
Wilkes, S., 280
Wilkinson, D. A., 153, 154, 162
Wilkinson, M., 243
Williams, H. W., 108
Willis, T., 75
Wilson, S. A. K., 281, 285
Winokur, G., 185
Wisniewski, H. M., 108
Withdrawal phenomena, alcoholic dementia and, 159-160
Wrightson, P., 227

Yde, A., 78-79
Young, A. C., 283
Yudofsky, S., 65

Zangwill, O. L., 236

     a
2 b
3 c
4 d
5 e
6 f
7 g
8 h
9 i
8 0 j